OCCUPATIONAL STRESS IN THE CARE OF THE CRITICALLY ILL, THE DYING, AND THE BEREAVED

OCCUPATIONAL STRESS IN THE CARE OF THE CRITICALLY ILL, THE DYING, AND THE BEREAVED

MARY L. S. VACHON
Clarke Institute of Psychiatry
Toronto, Ontario, Canada

● HEMISPHERE PUBLISHING CORPORATION
A member of the Taylor & Francis Group

New York   Washington   Philadelphia   London

OCCUPATIONAL STRESS IN THE CARE OF THE CRITICALLY ILL, THE DYING, AND THE BEREAVED

    4 5 6 7 8 9 0   B C B C   8 9

This book was set in Press Roman by Hemisphere Publishing Corporation. The
editors were Christine Flint Lowry and Elizabeth Maggiora; the production
supervisor was Miriam Gonzalez; and the typesetter was Rita Shapiro.
BookCrafters, Inc. was printer and binder.

Library of Congress Cataloging-in-Publication Data

Vachon, Mary L. S.
    Occupational stress in the care of the critically ill,
the dying, and the bereaved.

    (Series in death education, aging, and health care)
    Bibliography: p.
    Includes index.
    1. Terminal care—Psychological aspects. 2. Medical
personnel—Job stress. 3. Adjustment (Psychology)
I. Title. II. Series. [DNLM: 1. Adaptation,
Psychological. 2. Critical Care—psychology. 3. Grief.
4. Occupational Diseases—etiology. 5. Stress—
etiology. 6. Terminal Care—psychology. WM 172 V119o]
R726.8.V33   1985   616'.029'019   85-8716
ISBN 0-89116-318-2
ISSN 0275-3510

This book is dedicated to my parents
Margaret Mary *and the late* ***Walter Suslak***
who gave me life and the courage to meet challenges,
and to
Bruce, Wolfgang Adeodatus, *and* ***Alexa Amadeus***
who have helped me to learn much of what I know
about stress, social support, and coping.

Contents

Foreword

Readers have much in store, much to ponder, and much to enjoy in the pages to come. Though difficult to grasp at times, theirs will be the pleasure and enjoyment that good copers find in accomplishment. This, in my opinion, is the theme of the book. I am confident that most other professionals who grapple with occupational stress will also appreciate its scope and understanding.

Let readers therefore get on with a most illuminating experience. Dr. Vachon has managed to be gentle, delightful, and scholarly. She is truly, compassionately concerned about the plight of colleagues who care for the critically ill, the dying, and the bereaved. She knows how often and unrecognized are their efforts to cope with sometimes uncopable problems.

Her main question sounds very simple: How do *you* keep functioning in your job? But the question is both deceptive and evocative; it could also mean to ask another, more existential question, which no one could answer: How do *you* manage to preserve your sanity and equilibrium in a job that constantly demands more than skill, knowledge, and dedication?

Dr. Vachon recognizes that stress and distress are almost inevitable in this field. This prompts still another question: Why do people choose such a field in the first place? The work is unending, and frustration is frequent. Where do the rewards and compensation come from? I assume that few health professionals who do this type of work are passively assigned. They elect the field, finding that danger, technology, and confrontation with death on almost daily terms can be rewarding, even exhilarating. I suspect that more professionals volunteer to do this risky work as a personal challenge, to see if they can at length maintain quiet accomplishment and significant endurance, despite emotional and social vulnerability.

One benefit from the demystification of medicine and the secularization of medical professionalism is that the public has now come not to expect miracles, but to watch out for mistakes. Medicine—and I refer to all health professionals—is vulnerable on all fronts, not just to litigation, but to accepting inevitable disappointment and frustration in critical-care work. This applies, in my opinion, to any health professional whose daily job confronts the likelihood of death and despair.

Altruism begins at home; taking careful care is a personal obligation toward oneself. Before putting oneself at the service of others, it is only prudent to care for one's own well being. This is particularly urgent among professionals who care for the critically ill, the dying, and the bereaved, since blatant commercialism is never the reason for undertaking such work. On the contrary, it is a field in which recognition is limited, self-esteem is bombarded, and exhaustion a common consequence. Nevertheless, such professionals have not adopted the lessons of consumerism for themselves, as if they are reluctant to concede vulnerability to a variety of difficulties and dangers.

The benchmark of excellence in psychosocial research is to elucidate and expound upon general principles that colleagues can then apply with positive practical results. Occupational stress is a more difficult problem to research. The more opportune result is that colleagues will recognize that psychosocial problems can cluster within themselves, and will not go away. There is no virtue in self-suffering, no redemption in insisting upon exhaustion and emotional poverty. Those who unwittingly follow such a course, believing that they are only being true to medical ideals, become their own adversaries. Vulnerability is a human quality, not a fatal disease. But burnout is the all too common end-stage when stress is not dealt with. In her research, Dr. Vachon has diplomatically not been specific about who fails to cope and what happens to them.

To cope well means to reflect, examine, instruct oneself, learn from others, tolerate shortcomings, preserve an optimistic viewpoint, and perform skillfully, though short of perfection. This lesson is difficult to teach, but capable of being learned.

Support is a common nostrum almost casually and complacently recommended for occupational stress. The trouble is that none of us can be sure what support means. Dr. Vachon noticed that few of her colleagues found much benefit from so-called support groups, and that there is much variety in what people report doing about difficulties at work. It should be recognized that most people who can share problems with others have already taken a strong step toward better coping. Support has a negative value when it implies that a person is admitting to a state of helplessness. To cope better, therefore, means that we must admit to ourselves that we are doing quite well with the demands put on us, but that we want to do better, and deserve respect for what we are doing and hope to do. Careful delineation of a problem, together with acknowledging distress, is a respectable way of helping oneself, and even healing oneself. Regardless of how much one enjoys the challenge and thrill of performing competently on the edge of danger, it is still prudent to recognize fatigue, boredom, resentment, and shortcomings, and to do something about them besides complain.

Coping is a valuable skill, often appreciated by only a limited group. It is learned, not usually inborn. Those who cope well frequently, if not usually, cannot say what they do and how they do it. The world is thronged, however, with people who claim to know exactly what someone else should or ought to do, or should have done. When people talk about themselves, especially with how they coped with problems that only get bigger with each telling, we should acknowledge and allow for 20/20 hindsight and the human capacity to inflate one's difficulties and accomplishments. Nevertheless, Dr. Vachon wisely lets them have their say, without looking too closely at reasons why. Self-esteem is valuable; all too difficult to defend under stressful conditions. It is often an accomplishment simply to come through dangerous situations. We notice, however, that good copers are somewhat independent people who are resourceful and diligent, conforming to social expectations yet refusing to knuckle under to unjustified demands. Good intentions, as usual, are not enough, but may provide the kindling for good practice. While flexible in many respects, good copers heed inner warnings and protect themselves from demands that drain away the will to live.

Let us make sure that good health care providers escape dead routine and find new sources of energy and appreciation. Humanity cannot afford to lose them. Let us study what it takes to successfully deal with vulnerability. Mary Vachon has provided much for us to consider and draw upon. This book may even teach us how to better instruct ourselves in coping effectively.

Avery D. Weisman, MD
Senior Psychiatrist
Massachusetts General Hospital
Professor of Psychiatry, Emeritus
Harvard Medical School

Preface

When Hannelore Wass first invited me to write this book, I had reached the stage in my own life where I was prepared to "slow down and smell the roses." I was nearing the end of two major research studies, had just completed my PhD, and had a second child. I had vowed to learn something about relaxing and enjoying my family and personal life while I decided where to next focus my professional energies. That vow lasted for about 2 weeks, when I received the call inviting me to consider writing an article on "Staff Stress in the Care of the Dying Child" and to then consider expanding my ideas into a book on "Staff Stress in the Care of the Dying." My ambivalence about refocusing my energies so quickly led me to reflect for several months before accepting the challenge.

During that time my invitations to speak and conduct workshops for health professionals and volunteers on subjects such as "Staff Stress," "Care for the Caregivers," "Stress in the Care of the Dying," "Burnout," and similar subjects began to escalate. Invitations to consult to hospitals and health-care agencies became more frequent. At the same time my colleagues in the Social and Community Psychiatry Department at the Clarke Institute of Psychiatry, building on work they had already been doing, began to concentrate even more of their research skills in the area of occupational stress in such groups as air traffic controllers and government employees. They too began to notice an escalation in their speaking engagements to teachers, people in business and industry, and women working at home.

Clearly the time had come when society was being sensitized to the problem of stress. Indeed, it has been said that stress is the disease of the 1980s. If it has not yet caught up with you at work or home, or with tight economic times, then soon it will. Stress, so the myth goes, lurks around every corner just waiting for the opportunity to put a viselike grip around your heart; reduce you to tears; cause you to burn out, divorce your spouse, have a nervous breakdown, or in some other way fall prey to its mysterious ravages.

Of all the people vulnerable to the symptoms of stress, certain groups, as another myth goes, are especially prone to difficulties because they are in what are considered to be high-stress occupations. What types of jobs are high stress? Jobs thought to have the potential to cause stress are those that involve: heavy responsibility for other people's lives (e.g., air traffic controllers, intensive-care nurses), responsibility for making major decisions affecting the future of many individuals or a company (executives, politicians), little control over the flow of one's work (secretaries, emergency room personnel), and tedious or boring work (factory piece-workers, the underemployed, e.g., university graduates in dead-end positions).

Clearly, however, not all of the people in each of these jobs experience a marked degree of job stress. Indeed, many seem to thrive in jobs that theorists would have us believe are incredibly stressful. Others exhibit all the signs of stress in a job that on the surface looks quite simple and straightforward. For example, the surgical nurse whose role is supposedly to circulate, pass instruments, and hold retractors may exhibit far more signs of stress than the surgeon who has the responsibility for life and death decisions.

What makes the difference in individuals' responses to stress? Are there certain groups that are more prone to stress? If so, can some type of intervention alleviate their stress? This book will clarify these issues for those providing care to the critically ill, the dying, and the bereaved; work that most people would agree is potentially stressful. After all, constant exposure to the critically ill and dying reminds us of our own vulnerability and mortality; threatens our sense of power, omnipotence, and omniscience; and confronts us with the repeated need to deal with feelings of loss and grief. In addition, there are often few guidelines for the "proper involvement" of professionals with the dying person. Whereas many of us were taught in our early professional training programs that the "good professional" does not get involved or have "bad" feelings like anger, disgust, depression, anxiety, or sexual urges toward patients or their families, the reality is that these issues may recur repeatedly in one's clinical practice until such time as one gains insight into their source and how to deal with such problems.

This book will attempt to clarify the sources of stress within our work settings and to discuss which attributes of our personality structure or personal life make us more or less susceptible to the ravages of stress. It will look at how stress is manifested—physically, psychologically, or in our behavior; more importantly, however, it will show how other caregivers manage to cope with the types of stress that may confront you.

◆   ◆   ◆

In this as in any other book there are many people to thank. Janice Dembo, Jo-Anna Greenhalgh, and Ann Spitzer provided valuable comments on earlier versions of specialty chapters. Drs. J. William Worden and Hannelore Wass were of great assistance in reviewing an earlier version of the manuscript. Jackie Creber, Carolyn Grant, Lorraine Milne, and Georgie Powis served as research assistants and typists and were ever-willing to be of help. My colleagues in the Department of Social and Community Psychiatry at the Clarke Institute of Psychiatry and Department Chief, Dr. S. J. J. Freeman were quite helpful in tolerating my preoccupation with the book. Particular thanks are due to my colleagues W. J. Lancee for research and computer assistance and Susan Erle for clerical help.

I am also most grateful to Mark Rochan and the Clarke Institute for providing financial support for this project, and to Kate Roach and Elizabeth Maggiora at Hemisphere for editorial help and support.

The members of my personal support system at a home, local, national, and international level have been a constant source of encouragement. Most particularly I deeply appreciate the sharing from the almost 600 caregivers who were willing to be interviewed or who spoke to me at meetings. Truly without them this book would never have existed.

Mary L. S. Vachon

OCCUPATIONAL STRESS
IN THE CARE
OF THE CRITICALLY ILL,
THE DYING,
AND THE BEREAVED

Occupational Stress and the Caregiver

For the last decade and a half there has been an increasing recognition of the needs of the dying patient and his or her family. Initially this interest evolved through the writing of pioneers like Feifel (1), Fox (2), Folta (3), Glaser and Strauss (4-6), Hinton (7), Quint (8-10), Sudnow (11), Saunders (12), and Weisman and Hackett (13). Their work began to sensitize small groups of professionals to the plight of those dying in a variety of settings. Directly and indirectly, these authors touched on the issue of caregiver stress as well, but the needs of caregivers were largely ignored. As a result of their work, small groups of professionals began to work in institutions and in the community trying to improve the care of individuals and small groups of dying patients.

However, more than just a few people had to be sensitized if the needs of the dying were really to be addressed. It is now part of the established history of the death movement that the work of Dr. Elisabeth Kübler-Ross (14) made the issue of the plight of the dying more of a concern to the general public as well as to larger professional audiences.

The movement as a whole, however, resulted from the juxtaposition of a number of societal issues beyond the work of particular authors. The late 1960s saw North America and the Western world in great conflict about the morality of the Vietnam war. The reality of war deaths was shown regularly on the six o'clock news. There was increasing disenchantment with the promises and the wonders of medical science and technology which sometimes resulted in increasing the dehumanization of patients. Women had begun to gain control over their fertility and the issue of abortion became a major public concern. The sexual revolution was in full swing. Since society had taken one taboo subject out of the closet and was attempting to gain insight into and control over it, the time was now ripe to deal with the other taboo subject of death.

Dying patients were urged to talk about their experiences from their hospital beds, at grand rounds, in community settings, and in the public media. Some professionals listened to what they said. Students and practitioners alike attended lectures and seminars, memorized the stages of dying, and tried to help patients work through their dying process so as to be able to move into a state of acceptance, overlaid with hope.

An attempt was made to try to humanize death within the hospital system, even on intensive care units where technology had hitherto been thought to reign supreme.

Professionals and lay persons from North America wandering in search of even better ways to die "discovered" the British hospices with which Dr. Cecily Saunders had been involved since the 1960s. Despite their fairly recent rediscovery, hospices themselves are not a recent innovation but can be traced back almost 2,000 years to the work of one of St. Jerome's disciples who built a hospice for pilgrims returning from Africa (15).

The hospice concept was taken up with great vigor and became almost a bandwagon phenomenon. Experts like Dr. Balfour Mount, founder of the Palliative Care Unit of the Royal Victorial Hospital in Montreal warned caregivers to proceed slowly so as to avoid a "Kentucky Fried" hospice movement with the feeling that there should be a hospice on every block or at least within every hospital, community agency, and with every interested group of volunteers.

With interest in the needs of the dying in particular and in client needs in general, caregivers began talking to patients in hospices and palliative care, intensive care, abortion, and oncology units, and in the various other places in the hospital and community where people grapple with the issues surrounding life and death. As they talked, these professionals experienced the risks of involvement with patients and their families. While caregivers have always cared about and talked with patients, there had previously been considerable pressure not to get "too involved", but to maintain a certain professional distance so as to protect oneself from overinvolvement with its risk of impaired professional judgments.

The death and dying movement, however, urged professionals to escape from their professional barriers and to extend themselves to become much more involved with patients and their families. Volunteers were brought into the hospital system to work more directly with patients—again, involvement was urged. While old standards were crumbling for some "enlightened" professionals, new guidelines were not quick to emerge. Caregivers began to give all they had to give to patients and their families, and then to give more than they had to give. Sometimes it almost seemed as though there were contests to see who could give the most, be most involved and grieve the most when patients died. This involvement initially felt good and was encouraged, in some settings at least, but gradually many caregivers began to experience symptoms that were variously defined as "staff stress," "burnout," etc. It became clear that caregivers, both professionals and volunteers were experiencing considerable distress from the work they were performing.

Meetings on death and dying began to feature the occasional lecture on staff stress. Later, workshops were organized to deal with the issue; books and articles on stress and burnout appeared in large numbers and caregivers were warned of the problems and pitfalls inherent in their work.

It was said that those most prone to burnout were enthusiastic, involved, committed types that were doing much of the work with the dying. Most of the data that emerged, however, was anecdotal in nature. Few attempts were made to study the phenomenon to identify who was at risk of developing a stress reaction. What was it in the environment that caused the difficulties? Why did it affect some caregivers more than others? How was stress manifest? What coping mechanisms did caregivers use that enabled some to become involved and work in the field for many years while others could last only a few months? Some studies were done but these generally focused on one professional group and often in a particular setting. For example, Quint (Benoliel) studied nurses in a variety of settings (16–18); Claus and Bailey (19) studied nurses in intensive care units and Harper (20) attempted to conceptualize the stress experienced by social workers in an oncology center. Bosk (21) looked at the career of the surgical resident and the ways in which the hospital system developed norms that determined what types of error and behavior were accepted and which were seen as incompatible with performance as a skilled surgeon in a prestigious teaching hospital. Fox and Swazey (22) studied physicians involved in transplantation and dialysis, pushing back the frontiers of medical science. Lyall, Vachon, and Rogers (23) looked at nurses on a new palliative care unit, while Marshall, Kasman, and Cape (24) studied caregivers in neonatal intensive care units.

This book is an attempt to go beyond the work of previous authors and to provide a working model within which to view the stress of caregivers of a variety of disciplines dealing with critically ill and dying patients and their bereaved family and friends.

I have set myself the broad, and perhaps naive task of drawing together my own research and clinical findings with some of the literature on stress to develop a model that can be applied across institutional and community settings, and which can seek to elucidate some of the stress experienced by both professionals and volunteers of various backgrounds. The basic premise of the model is that if we can understand stressors and stress, we can then more readily develop healthy coping mechanisms to deal with them.

This then leads us to a discussion of some of the literature and basic concepts that underpin the model.

STRESS THEORIES

The concept of stress is probably one of the most ill-defined in the biological and behavioral science literature. It has been used to cover a number of divergent dimensions ranging from stimuli or stressors that lead to changes in the organism, to the outcome of such stimuli, and the emotional state or experience accompanying a changing social or personal situation (25). Much of the current interest in the subject can be dated to the research of Hans Selye who, in 1936 (26) articulated his biological concept of stress as the "General Adaptation Syndrome," a set of nonspecific physiological reactions to various noxious environmental agents (27).

For the purposes of this book, the definitions used by Antonovsky (28) will be used. He sees stress as evolving from exposure to stressors. His framework distinguishes between stressors and other routine stimuli. A routine stimulus is seen as being one to which the person can respond more or less automatically. This is not to imply that the person has necessarily been exposed to the exact stimulus previously, rather that one can incorporate this new stimulus into an existing framework that allows the person to respond in a routine fashion. It presents no problem in adjustment. A *stressor,* however can be defined as a demand made by the internal or external environment of an organism that upsets its homeostasis, restoration of which depends on a nonautomatic and not readily available energy-expending action (p. 72). It is possible for a routine stimulus to become a stressor under certain circumstances and it is not always possible to determine when and why this is happening. It must also be acknowledged that one person's stressor is another person's routine stimulus. Whether a given phenomenon, experience, or stimulus is a stressor or not is going to be dependent on the meaning of that stimulus to the person at that point in time and on the repertoire of coping mechanisms readily available.

Antonovsky (28) says that stressors are omnipresent in human existence. They are impossible to avoid. Our response to a stressor is tension that can have pathological, neutral, or salutory consequences. In Antonovsky's model, "stress" refers to the strain that remains "in response to the failure to manage tensions well and to overcome stressors" (p. 10).

According to the work of Lazarus and his colleagues, stress can be observed at the physiological, psychological, and behavioral levels of analysis (29-31). Within Lazarus' model, stress "is viewed as an ongoing process, affected by individual personality factors and environmental variables. The individual is constantly responding to and interacting with the environment and whether the stress is a benefit or a harm to the individual depends greatly on the individual's cognitive appraisal of the stress and the subsequent coping process" (32, p. 6).

Stress is not always a problem, many people thrive on and enjoy stress, and no learning takes place without stress. Indeed, life itself is dependent upon the organism maintaining itself at the cellular level in a state of tension with the environment. In fact, stress only disappears when equilibrium is reached with the environment at the time of death.

Elliott and Eisdorfer summarized the opinion of several leading experts as being that stress "also may have desirable effects associated with successfully meeting physical or psychological demands. Among such changes might be increased physical stamina, more effective coping styles, or stronger social ties" (33, p. 17). The problem is when an individual perceives a stressor and the resulting stress as being more than she/he can cope with either because of the stressor itself, the meaning attributed to it, or the resources available to cope with it. In addition, it must be acknowledged that individuals do not normally function in a vacuum and with only a limited number of stressors. New stressors frequently impinge on the system under stress (34) complicating an individual's problems.

The stressors that impinge can evolve from the internal or external environment or both (28). An example of an internal stressor might be a caregiver's expectation that in one's professional role it would always be possible to cure disease and prevent death. An example of an external stressor might be the death of an important patient or a change in one's personal life such as bereavement, job loss, divorce, etc.

An individual's response to stressors is conditioned by certain "mediating variables" that might also be internal or external. Internal (personal) mediating variables might include inherited genetic factors, previous exposure to similar events (27), value-structure, actual ability, belief in one's ability to meet stress (35); skills, assets, resources, defenses, and previous experiences (36). External mediating variables include finances (28, 35), and availability or lack of social supports (35, 36). Certain factors such as social relationships may be both stressors and mediating variables (25). Finally, stressors, stress, and coping mechanisms must be viewed within a social-cultural perspective (28, 31, 34).

THE PERSON–ENVIRONMENT FIT MODEL
OF OCCUPATIONAL STRESS

The Person-Environment Fit Model is one useful way of approaching the specific study of occupational stress that integrates many of the concepts we have already discussed. This model will form the basis for the author's working model of occupational stress in caregivers. The Person-Environment Fit Model is derived from work done by the Institute for Social Research at the University of Michigan by French, Rodgers, and Cobb (37). The advantage of this model is that it looks at the fact that both job satisfaction and occupational stress are a result of the interaction between the person holding a particular job and the environment in which he or she is employed. The model is presumed to be dynamic. The fit between the person and the environment is not static but needs to be constantly reassessed.

Harrison gives an overview of the model and some of the research it has generated. He describes the model as accounting for two kinds of fit between the individual and the environment: (1) the extent to which the person's skills and abilities match the demands and requirements of the job, and (2) the extent to which the job environment provides supplies to meet individual needs. This is basically a supply and demand model that acknowledges that the individual comes into a job with certain supplies (e.g., marketable skills) which the organization wants to purchase. In exchange, the individual has certain demands that he or she makes of the job; these demands may be overt or covert. In turn, the organization provides the individual with certain supplies (e.g., pay) in exchange for certain demands which again may be overt or covert. With good Person-Environment Fit the job provides the supplies wanted by the individual (good salary and fringe benefits, social involvement, opportunity to achieve, a sense of self-worth) while the person provides the abilities required by the job environment (e.g., counseling skills, technical knowledge, good physical and mental health).

The concept of Person-Environment Fit can be used to define job stress. "A job is stressful to the extent that it does not provide supplies to meet the individual's motives and to the extent that the ability of the individual falls below the demands of the job which are prerequisite to receiving supplies" (38, p. 178).

Kahn et al. (39) say there is a need for us to acknowledge that we must think in terms of "goodness of fit" between person and job because individuals vary in their needs, abilities, and standards of judgement. "A job that is too strenuous or too demanding of vigilance or isolating for one person may be just right for someone else. To some extent, therefore, the quality of a job must be assessed in relation to the needs and abilities of the individual who holds it. Goodness [of fit] is not absolute . . ." (39, p. 13).

Job stress consists of a poor fit in the job environment which may lead to physical, psychological, or behavioral manifestations of stress. When the qualitative demands of a job are too great, an individual may be threatened by job loss or loss of the esteem of others, which in turn results in a decreased sense of competence. For example, the new intern who is assigned to the intensive care unit as his first clinical experience may find himself totally overwhelmed both by the complicated illnesses of the patients and by all the machines that surround them. He may fear that he will be unable to perform as a physician and may feel totally incompetent. This may cause him to become anxious, irritable with nurses who question his judgement, and may interfere with his ability to make decisions.

Too little job complexity may also be a problem, however, as it can prevent a person from gaining a sense of competence and the esteem of others because the work lacks challenge and meaning. The nurse who goes from the busy pace of an intensive care unit to working as an office nurse may find herself feeling under-utilized, unless she is able to find that her current job presents a different type of challenge or meets new needs, such as the need for a routine job in order to be able to go home more relaxed at the end of a day.

OVERVIEW OF THE STUDY

My original mandate in writing this book was to use the data I had previously gathered with my colleagues in the Department of Social and Community Psychiatry at the Clarke Institute of Psychiatry, and to add to that work some of my own observations about staff stress and its management to create a book that would look at the problem of stress in the care of the dying. As I began to think about this mandate I felt that I needed to gather more data on the subject. In addition, I realized that my natural instinct would be to talk about the stress associated in dealing with dying cancer patients who were being cared for either in teaching hospitals, at home, or in palliative care units or hospices. This is my greatest area of expertise. Yet maybe this was not what was needed.

As I thought about the requests that I had received for speaking engagements or consultations, and the groups I was asked to address or to work with, I recognized that obviously death is not limited to cancer patients and that caregivers in other specialties experienced stress as well. I also wondered if dealing with dying patients was really the major problem we confronted in our work situation.

In my own clinical work I have spent the last 15 years doing psychotherapy with patients and families with life-threatening illness and bereavement. When I first began this work, the people referred were on the verge of dying and often had experienced significant deterioration in their family situation. I felt that had they been referred sooner, their current problems would not be so great. Over time, my referral system has changed—people are usually referred earlier in their illness, and it is frequently possible to prevent family breakdown from occurring. While it may be a tragedy when an individual and his family are struck by disease, death itself, when it comes, is often not a particular tragedy—it goes "as well as can be expected." The family, other caregivers and myself often have a feeling of satisfaction with "a job well done, considering the circumstances."

When a patient dies, I as a caregiver may experience a feeling of loss or grief, but I have ways of dealing with this both personally and professionally so that dealing with death and with dying people generally does not, at this point in my career, leave me feeling terribly stressed. When I think about what does cause me stress, I can certainly relate to particular illnesses that I find to be especially difficult, such as amyotrophic lateral sclerosis or muscular dystrophy, and to patients or families with whom I could identify or with whom I had communication problems that left me feeling dissatisfied or frustrated. More often, however, I think of my stress as coming from the role I perform—a role that may well be unclear, from trying to do too many things at once, or from the institutions with which I deal wherein I may come up against policies I don't like. If these are problems for me, then presumably others share my difficulties.

Realizing then that people die in a variety of settings and from a number of diseases other than cancer, and recognizing that the stress of dealing with dying people comes from more than just being exposed to dying patients, I set out to ask experienced caregivers what caused them stress, how it was manifest, and how they coped with it. My goal was to describe what it is really like "in the trenches," to look at how people survive, and to discover what gives them pleasure and satisfaction in their work.

A more complete description of the study can be found in the Appendix. Realizing that many readers are not interested in the methodology of research studies, it is enough to note here that the sample consisted of data gathered in 327 interviews with close to 600 caregivers from a variety of professional backgrounds and specialty areas. The caregivers were from teaching and community hospitals, palliative care facilities, chronic care hospitals, and voluntary agencies. They were interviewed in Canada, the United States, Europe, and Australia.

In approaching caregivers I told them I was writing a book dealing with occupational stress in the care of the critically ill, dying, and bereaved. I showed them earlier versions of the model of occupational stress seen in Figure 1 and asked them to describe to me what caused them stress in their work, how this was affected by factors in their personal lives, how their stress was manifest, and what they did to cope with the stress they experienced. Most of the caregivers interviewed were experienced practitioners. The bias in favor of more experienced people is reflective of my attempt to discover how caregivers manage to cope and to survive within the system. By studying how people manage to continue to work it is then possible to teach some of their survival skills to other practitioners.

It seems appropriate to end this chapter with a caveat from one of the caregivers interviewed. Dr. Bob Tracey* said, "You are going to have to qualify the information you report so as not to substantiate as 'truth' people's subjective experiences. People's perceptions are not necessarily reality. You must avoid the propagation of false science built on false science."

I hope that I will be able to fulfill the mandate of not propagating false science by being very clear that what I am reporting are individual caregivers' personal perceptions of what constitutes a stressor for them, what mediates the impact of those stressors, how their stress is manifest, and how they cope. Another researcher, who chose to watch the same caregiver actually perform might report completely different data. Alternatively, a caregiver might report different information to a different interviewer.

One of the hypotheses of this book is, however, that occupational stressors do in fact result, at least in part, not only from objective stimuli but as well from the way in which certain stimuli are cognitively and emotionally appraised by caregivers as having certain meaning. The renowned sociologist, W. I. Thomas has stated: "If men define situations as real, they are real in their consequences." Robert Merton has described the Thomas Theorem meaning "that men's definitions of situations affect their consequences: 'What disturbs and alarms man are not the things, but his opinions and fancies about the things' " (40, p. 19; references in original).

---

*All caregivers' names are fictitious. Identifying data have also been changed.

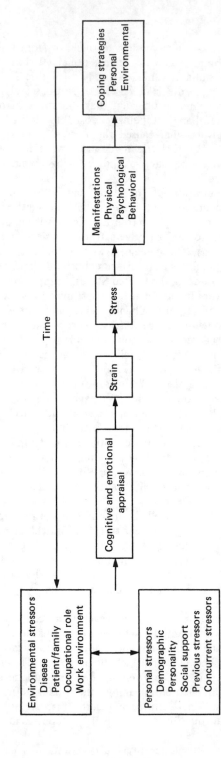

Figure 1 Occupational stress in caregivers

8

In this book we shall be discussing not only the "things" (stressors) but also our "opinions and fancies" (cognitive and emotional appraisal or perceived meaning) about these "things."

REFERENCES

1. Feifel, H. (1959). *The meaning of death.* New York: Blakiston Division, McGraw-Hill.
2. Fox, R. C. (1959). *Experiment perilous.* Glencoe, IL: The Free Press.
3. Folta, J. R. (1965). The Perception of Death. *Nursing Research, 14,* 233-235.
4. Glaser, B. G., & Strauss, A. L. (1964). Awareness contexts and social interaction. *American Sociological Review, 29,* 669-679.
5. Glaser, B. G., & Strauss, A. L. (1965). *Awareness of dying.* Chicago: Aldine.
6. Glaser, B. G., & Strauss, A. L. (1968). *Time for Dying.* Chicago: Aldine.
7. Hinton, J. (1967). *Dying.* Baltimore: Penguin.
8. Quint, J. C. (1964). Mastectomy-Symbol of cure or warning sign? *G. P. 29,* 119-124.
9. Quint, J. C. (1967). When patients die: Some nursing problems. *Canadian Nurse, 63*(12), 33-36.
10. Quint, J. C. (1966). Awareness of death and the nurses' composure. *Nursing Research, 15,* 49-55.
11. Sudnow, D. (1967). *Passing on: The social organization of dying.* Englewood Cliffs, NJ: Prentice-Hall.
12. Saunders, C. (1959). Care of the dying. *Nursing Times* (Reprint). London: Macmillan.
13. Weisman, A., & Hackett, T. (1961). Predelection to death. *Psychosomatic Medicine, 23,* 232-256.
14. Kübler-Ross, E. (1969). *On death and dying.* New York: Macmillan
15. Stoddard, S. (1978). *The hospice movement.* New York: Vintage.
16. Quint, J. C. (1967). *The nurse and the dying patient.* New York: Macmillan.
17. Quint, J. C. (1968). Preparing nurses to care for the terminally ill. *International Journal of Nursing Studies, 5,* 53-59.
18. Benoliel, J. Q. (1976). Overview: Care, cure and the challenge of choice. In A. Earle, N. T. Argondizzo, & A. H. Kutscher (Eds.), *The nurse as caregiver for the terminal patient and his family,* pp. 9-30. New York: Columbia University Press.
19. Claus, J. T., & Bailey, J. T. (1980). *Living with stress and promoting well-being.* St. Louis: Mosby.
20. Harper, B. C. (1977). *Death: The coping mechanism of the health professional.* Greenville, SC: Southeastern University Press.
21. Bosk, C. L. (1979). *Forgive and remember: Managing medical failure.* Chicago: The University of Chicago Press.
22. Fox, R. C., & Swazey, J. P. (1978). *The courage to fail.* (2nd ed., revised). Chicago: The University of Chicago Press.
23. Lyall, W. A. L., Rogers, J., & Vachon, M. L. S. (1976, October). Professional stress in the care of the dying. In *Palliative care service report.* (pp. 457-468). Montreal: Royal Victoria Hospital.
24. Marshall, R. E., Kasman, C., & Cape, L. S. (1982). *Coping with caring for sick newborns.* Philadelphia: Saunders.
25. Levine, S., & Scotch, N. A. (1973). *Social stress.* Chicago: Aldine.
26. Selye, H. (1974). *Stress without distress.* Philadelphia: Lippincott.
27. Selye, H. (1956). *The stress of life.* New York: McGraw-Hill.
28. Antonovsky, A. (1979). *Health, stress and coping.* San Francisco: Jossey-Bass.
29. Lazarus, R. S., Cohen, J. et al. (1980). Psychological stress and adaptation: Some unresolved issues. In H. Selye (Ed.), *Selye's guide to stress research.* Vol. 1, (pp. 90-117.) New York: Von Nostrand Reinhold.
30. Lazarus, R., & Launier, R. (1978). Stress related transactions between person and environment. In L. Pervin & M. Lewis (Eds.), *Perspectives in international psychology,* (pp. 287-327). New York: Plenum.
31. Lumsden, D. P. (1981). Is the concept of stress of any use anymore? In D. Randolph (Ed.), *Contributions to primary prevention in mental health.* Toronto: Canadian Mental Health Association (National Office).

32. Hawk, J. (October, 1982). *Sources and levels of stress in family practice residents: A descriptive study*. Unpublished Doctoral Dissertation, Berkeley: The California School of Professional Psychology.

33. Elliott, G. R., & Eisdorfer, C. (Eds.) (1982). *Stress and human health: Analysis and implications of research*. New York: Springer.

34. Lumsden, D. P. (1975). Towards a systems model of stress: Feedback from an anthropological study of the impact of Ghana's Volta River Project. In I. Sarason & C. Spielberger (Eds.), *Stress and anxiety*. Vol. 2 (pp. 191–228). Washington: Hemisphere.

35. Dohrenwend, B. S., & B. P. (1973). Class and race as status-related sources of stress. In S. Levine and N. A. Scotch (Eds.), *Social Stress* (pp. 111–140). Chicago: Aldine.

36. Rabkin, J. G., & Struening, E. L. (1976). Life events, stress, and illness. *Science, 194,* 1013–1020.

37. French, J. R. P., Rodgers, W., & Cobb, S. (1974). Adjustment as person-environment fit. In G. Coelho, D. Hamburg, & J. Adams (Eds.), *Coping and Adaptation.* (pp. 316–333). New York: Basic.

38, Harrison, R. V. (1979). Person-environment fit and job stress. In C. L. Cooper & R. Payne (Eds.), *Stress at Work* (pp. 175–205). Chichester: Wiley.

39. Kahn, R. L., Wolfe, D. M., Quinn, R. P., & Snoek, J. D. (1981). *Organizational stress: Studies in role conflict and ambiguity*. Malabar, FL: Robert E. Kreiger (originally published 1964, New York: Wiley).

40. Merton R. K. (1967). On the history and systematics of sociological theory. In R. K. Merton (Ed.), *On Theoretical Sociology.* (pp. 1–37). New York: The Free Press.

2

Caregivers as People

The Effect of Demographic
and Personality Variables

Caregivers to the critically ill, dying, and bereaved must be aware that much of the stress we experience is the result of the interaction between who we are as people and the environments in which we work. Because aspects of our personal lives mediate our response to occupational stressors, it is imperative that we understand the effect of these variables before we can begin to understand our response to the stressors to which we are exposed as professionals. Therefore, we shall start the discussion of the data on which this book is based with a view of caregivers as people. Chapter 2 will look at the impact of demographic variables—age, sex, marital and family status, social class, and religion; and personality variables—motivation for entering the field, personal value system, and personality and coping style on our perception of stress.

Elliott and Eisdorfer (1) put the study of personal variables into perspective when they reflected that even the most chronic work stressor is self-limiting in that most of us give up our work roles at least temporarily each day to take on new roles outside of the work place. They comment that it is only by understanding the interrelationships among our different life roles that we will be able to come to understand the health impact of work stress. It is this understanding of the relationship among our various life roles that will be one of the crucial tasks of this book.

The factors that provide support or protection against life stressors are still poorly understood (1). These factors, called mediators, can be seen as filters or modifiers that provide for individual variation in response to stressors. "Mediators help to explain why many people seem to experience many potential stressors without having any apparent consequences while others react markedly and have many consequences" (1, p. 22). There are two major categories of modifiers—those that are "relatively enduring properties of the individual, which can be thought of as characteristic vulnerability or resistance to any specific stressor, and properties of the context or situation in which that stressor is imposed. That context may be supportive and stress-buffering or threatening and stress-intensifying" (1, p. 105).

"Relevant social, physical, or economic contexts may be as broad as the economy or as narrow as the family unit" (1, p. 107).

Some of the modifiers that may determine individual vulnerability may include genetic and developmental factors, age (which although not constant, changes slowly), personality, previous experience, preparation for the event, as well as personal and cultural values and aspirations. According to Elliott and Eisdorfer (1), individual vulnerability varies within each person as well as between persons. While some individuals might have characteristic vulnerabilities to particular stressors these might well vary depending on moods, daily events, and other concurrent experiences. "These less enduring personal properties would then act to moderate or exaggerate responses to stress, much as do more stable characteristics. The accumulation of stressful events also can be thought of in terms of individual vulnerability" (1, p. 106).

DEMOGRAPHIC VARIABLES

Age

A large questionnaire survey of nurses' attitudes toward death and dying found that the age of nurses had little effect on their response to issues surrounding death and dying (2). While the current study did not find very many marked differences amongst the age groups studied, some interesting trends were noted that deserve further study. Of the caregivers surveyed, 14% ($N = 45$) were under 30, 50% ($N = 162$) were between 31 and 45, and 36% ($N = 115$) were over age 45.

For all of the age groups studied, stressors related to the work environment were the major area of stress. Caregivers over 45 reported equal stress from their work environment and occupational role with patient/family stressors close behind. Their younger colleagues, however, found their work environment stressors to be more problematic than any other stressor.

The major occupational stressors for the younger two groups were problems with their colleagues as reflected in team communication problems. For all age groups, dealing with patients and families with personality or coping problems were among the top five stressors. This would seem to indicate that regardless of age, we have difficulty either when our colleagues or our patients and families do not act the way we would like or expect. Further evidence for this is the difficulty the middle and older groups had with communication problems with patients with different ethnic backgrounds and value systems.

Both the youngest and the oldest groups had identification with patients and families among their top five stressors with it being the single greatest stressor in the oldest group and the fifth stressor in the youngest group. This may be surprising to the reader who might tend to think that increasing age and experience causes less feeling for patients. It might be understandable that the neophyte would identify with patients but the experienced practitioner "should" not feel this way.

A middle-aged obstetrician reflected on some of the reasons for the increased sensitivity that more experienced practitioners might have towards identifying with patients, when he commented:

Recently I was reminiscing with one of my colleagues about the days when we were residents and we said, "Remember, as residents, the more blood and calamity, the better we liked it?" We loved to deal with any complication that we hadn't created ourselves. There was the feeling that if there was a placenta previa, let's go to it.

It's a lot easier for residents because they have no relationship with the patient. The private physician has a personal relationship, often built up over years of caring for this woman, and he has an appreciation of what this particular complication means to this person. Having had your own family, and having had some of your own life experiences also makes it different.

For those caregivers over 30, there were also difficulties with role ambiguity and role conflict. By this point they had become reasonably experienced practitioners and were able to perform a multitude of roles. They frequently became frustrated because they felt they did not have the independence that they needed and as well they were more apt to have difficulty in dealing with the conflicts that emerged amongst their various roles. The youngest group was more apt to report difficulties with their work environment, having inadequate staffing resources and being in a high stress work situation. They were still at the point in their lives when they did not have the power to influence their work environment and felt very much at the mercy of the environment.

All of the age groups reported that their major psychological manifestations of stress were depression, grief, and guilt. The age groups were also similar with respect to their behavioral manifestations of stress, with staff conflict and job-home interaction being their primary symptoms.

Here it is worth noting however that the oldest group was the most likely to report problems with job-home interaction and they were also almost twice as likely as their younger colleagues (32% vs. 17%) to report that they were currently having marital problems. Many of the caregivers within this group had well-established professional reputations and were being called upon from many directions to perform not only their clinical work, but to do research, teaching, traveling, writing, etc. While this can be rewarding it can also be an additional stressor. Many were at the point in their lives when they were seriously reconsidering job-home interaction and the amount of home life they were prepared to give up for their work life. Some had gone beyond the point of marital trouble to divorce and had developed new relationships in which they were exploring the possibility of divesting themselves of some of their professional commitments and concentrating more on interpersonal closeness, which seemed to be more important to them at this point in their lives. Sometimes as caregivers did this, either within or outside of their marriage, they found that the people in their social support system had in fact changed so much over time that they were no longer as interested in spending time with the caregiver.

The age categories of caregivers were similar with regard to the personal coping strategies they developed and the primary strategy for all groups was that of developing a sense of competence, control, or pleasure in their work situation and developing some sense of control over their work environment. Younger colleagues were more apt to report either feeling tempted to leave or actually leaving the work situation when under stress than were their more mature colleagues. This might have been both a reflection of the fact that those over 30 felt that they had more power to change the work environment, or it might also have reflected the fact that they felt committed or "stuck" in their work environment because of financial and familial pressures.

With regard to environmental coping strategies, the two older groups were more apt to cope by developing a sense of team philosophy, team support, and team building; whereas the younger group was more apt to approach particular colleagues at an individual level. The younger group did not seem to have either the sense of belonging or the ability to plug into a team for support. This then was apt to leave them isolated and much more vulnerable to coping with their job stress by simply leaving the work situation.

The younger group rated the most important coping strategy as being adequate time off to pursue other areas of their lives. This of course is quite logical in view of the fact that many of the younger caregivers would either be single and interested in active social lives, newly married, or just beginning families.

There were also trends that seemed to vary with age. The number of work stressors and the reported symptoms of stress were highest in the youngest group and decreased with age, whereas the reported number of coping strategies increased with age. These findings lend support for the hypothesis that people who stay within the system do gain control over the stress they experience, through a variety of mechanisms. A number of caregivers commented on how they matured with age. Dr. Patrick Nelson, an experienced oncologist, reflected on the changes that had come with his professional maturation:

> I used to get very depressed in my thirties. I used to agonize and take everything very seriously. At that time there was less likelihood of success than there is with the patients I am working with today. Then I worked with patients with acute leukemia who were my age and they were all going to die. They became my brothers and sisters and I grieved their deaths.
>
> Recently, a colleague of mine who was running a leukemia unit and had a good wife just blew and split up with his wife. It was all the stress he was experiencing. In retrospect I realized how difficult it had been for me in my thirties, but I didn't realize it at the time.
>
> There's an inability to communicate what you do. You work 8 a.m. to 8 p.m. and come home and just settle into a funk. I couldn't explain the depth of emotional involvement in this emotionally draining situation.
>
> I don't feel the same now. I've matured and can care for patients without letting it destroy me.

A 42-year-old social worker working with children with cystic fibrosis reached out to her 28-year-old nurse colleague who was feeling quite depressed, and attempted to put her experience into perspective and to provide the younger woman with a philosophy of practice. "The difference between the two of us is age. I remember when I used to feel as involved as you do and when I had to right every wrong. Eventually you develop a philosophy and realize that you can't right every wrong in the world. You can only just do what you can to try to make it better. It makes it easier when you reach this stage."

While it has been noted that older and younger colleagues can be quite supportive of one another, this was not always the case, and a number of respondents, particularly physicians, referred to the rivalry that occurred between caregivers of various ages, each attempting to show the greater knowledge.

In a major longitudinal study of Harvard students who were followed into middle age, Valliant (3) made some observations that seem particularly germane to the understanding of this problem. He stated that whereas a young boy may enjoy membership in a cub pack, his 30-year-old counterpart, fighting to be a success in his job, must attempt to differentiate himself from his peers. He suggested that during their twenties and thirties professionals often adopt mentors to help with career development and establish a solid career identification. After forty, mentors ceased to be important. The process of seeking, developing, and outgrowing mentoring relationships is probably more common amongst the physicians surveyed and accounts in part for the rivalry they experienced. First they battled to set themselves apart from their peers, to attain limited rewards, and to develop a mentor relationship; they learned from their mentors and assumed the power of becoming an independent practitioner, only to then become involved in rivalry with their previous mentor or with other younger threatening colleagues, even those whom they mentored. Organized medicine has the most clearly developed mentoring system of the groups studied—hence, perhaps, the most potential for rivalry, but these dynamics will become more common in the other professional groups studied as they eventually develop more effective mentoring systems.

Sex

According to Haw (4), for every study of women in the work force there are six studies of men. In her very thorough review of the literature she has found that while one-third of the studies done on women looked at the proliferation of role demands of work and home for working women, very few of the studies on men looked at a similar overlap between work and home roles. Reviewing a number of research studies she found that employed married women had greater life satisfaction, greater self-acceptance, and fewer psychiatric symptoms than house-wives, but reported more daily stress than housewives. In general, professional women had fewer problems than clerical women. When compared with working men, however, working women were found to experience greater physical and emotional distress than men—they were nearly twice as likely to express negative attitudes toward their work, and when compared with men at similar occupational levels the women reported more symptoms of stress, such as feeling depressed and overwhelmed, experiencing nightmares and stomach distress. Reviewing studies of dual-career families she found that wives but not husbands experienced strain between their work and home roles. In addition, she reported on a study of physicians by Nadelson (5), noting that one-third of the female physicians but none of the male physicians reported that marriage and family responsibilities provided impetus for them to change directions. Multiple role demands did not seem to significantly affect the mental health of working women except when they received little support from others or rated their role performance negatively.

In the present study sex differences were somewhat confounded by the fact that females formed the clear majority of the subjects (71%), and of the males studied 65% were physicians. A few differences did, however, emerge between the two sex groups. For example, females were almost twice as likely to report trouble dealing with disfiguring illnesses (23% vs. 12%). This was not due to a difference between physicians and nurses reflecting greater or lesser contact at the bedside as might be thought, but appears to be a true sex difference. Males reported more trouble with unpredictable trajectories (35% vs. 13%)—again not a difference between professional groups but between sexes, perhaps reflecting the males' greater need for control.

Males also reported more difficulty with role overload and decision-making, while females had more difficulty with role conflict. These three variables were linked with professional roles, with male physicians reporting more role overload and difficulty with decision-making and female nurses or social workers experiencing more role conflict. What is probably of more interest, in view of the literature on females having more difficulty balancing roles, was the fact that males were somewhat more apt to report more concurrent stressors with their marital relationships than were females (31% vs. 21%), and males were also more likely to report job-home interaction as the major behavioral manifestation of their occupational stress (30% vs. 19%). The first finding of marital relationship problems was not associated with physician role, while job-home interaction was.

Despite the fact that the literature shows differences between males and females in response to psychological manifestations of stress, the present study did not confirm this. More differences were reported on behavioral manifestations of stress where an equal number of responses were generated from men and women, but women were more apt to report staff conflict (37% vs. 23%) while men, as already noted, reported job-home interaction more often. Men reported slightly more personal coping mechanisms (6.9 vs. 5.6) but there were no differences in the personal coping mechanisms employed by the sexes. With regard to environmental coping, however, while there were equal responses on strategies, females were more likely to report team building, support, and philosophy as being helpful, although these were the most important strategies for both groups.

Marital and Family Status

The caregivers interviewed for this chapter agreed that their marital status often had a significant impact on their capacity to deal with the ongoing stressors of their jobs. Marital status itself, however, is too narrow a concept to define exactly what influences caregivers' responses. The critical variable is probably not so much marital status as the presence of a confidant. In a large community survey of women, Brown et al. (6) found that those who had a confidant (defined as a person, usually male, with whom the woman had a "close, confiding, intimate relationship") were at less risk of developing psychological impairment when exposed to a serious life stressor. They found that those women who experienced severe life events and who lacked a confidant were roughly ten times more apt to be depressed than were the other women in the study. A more recent study (7) found that nonmarried women, but not married women, had a lower rate of psychiatric morbidity if employed—this was true regardless of occupational status or income. They postulated that employment may protect women who lack social support in other areas, such as in a marital relationship, by providing an opportunity to develop social bonds.

Miss Barbara Thompson, a single nursing supervisor in her late forties, spoke of the unrealistic attitude of some of the single nurses she worked with regarding future plans. "Young nurses say they don't need to worry about career progression because they're just working until they get married—despite the fact that there's no one on the scene yet. They don't pay any attention to the fact that their colleagues who have married often aren't happy, are divorced, and/or have to work."

Caregivers who mentioned their marital relationship described how it mediated their response to occupational stressors in a variety of ways. Dr. Stu Innes, an internist, described the maturing process it facilitated for him: "I'm a lot different now from when I was a second year resident when I was easily horrified or judgmental. Marriage, fatherhood with five children, growing expectations, and gestalt couple groups through my church have really matured me."

Despite the advantages some caregivers found in being married, many felt they had to make compromises in their professional lives to accommodate their family responsibilities. This was not always regarded as a problem—some saw it as a way to maximize their option to enjoy many facets in their lives. Dr. Ruth Nelson, a general practitioner with a young family who works part time and specializes in palliative care remarked: "I had been offered a residency in oncology but I like the homemaker role. I can't rely on my husband to do stuff at home because of his hectic schedule so I keep mine more flexible. To meet my own standards I have to be the best palliative care doctor, the best mother, the best homemaker—it's all very demanding."

A survey of 757 Canadian physicians found that married physicians appeared to be better adjusted than their single counterparts, and that the most contented group of physicians were those who spent as much time as possible with their families. In that survey the physicians who rated their marriages as the best, rated being away from home too much as their number one problem (8).

The Townes were a couple interviewed for this study. Dr. Eric Towne is an oncologist and his wife Ingrid a nurse. She remarked:

Eric was never there. I didn't expect anything different but it occurred to me a couple of years ago that he really never was there when I heard one of his colleagues talking about bathing his kids—Eric never did.

Eric replied:

Ingrid could always entertain herself. That was always one of her endearing features. A couple of years ago she decided to work because she decided she'd done enough volunteer work, it was time she started getting paid. Now when I want to go to the Art Gallery she can no longer drop everything to go.

Ingrid responded:

Now that Eric can spend more time at home I don't really want him there as I'm too busy doing other things.

Marital partners were often regarded as important sources of social support. Such a person can serve a number of functions—from the psychological, "He draws me out when I get quiet and mopey"—to the practical, "If I've had a bad day he'll cook even if it's not his turn." However, not all spouses were equally helpful. One psychologist working with critically ill children said, "It would be hard to do the kind of work I'm doing without a spouse, but no spouse at all would be better for me than one I'd have to protect."

Lois Meier commented that her husband, like many of the spouses of other caregivers, had an inordinate fear of death. "While he's proud of my work we don't talk about it at all, while I know everything about his work."

For caregivers who have unhappy marriages, work can provide an important source of relief. A nurse who directs a chronic care hospital commented that many of the nursing assistants in her hospital were older women "who have limited lives without much joy or meaning. Many are widows or have sick or elderly husbands. What happens in the hospital is very important to them. This is their life. They stay here for many years."

Caregivers with children spoke about feeling a particular vulnerability because of the nature of their work with its constant exposure to death. Mrs. Rita O'Neil, a volunteer coordinator commented: "I get upset at the thought of something happening to my kids. I'd be at risk if my kids were to die. I ask myself how I'd cope if my husband were to die—that's in part why I went back to work to be an independent, self-contained person, not just his wife. I think I could cope if he were to die but my kids are a different story."

Dr. Ruth Nelson said that she became more aware of her own vulnerabilty to death from her work, but her anxiety focused specifically on how her children would cope if she were to die.

Such feelings of vulnerability can even influence family planning. Kevin Nash, a young, single funeral director observed: "In this business you become aware that kids can die. I wouldn't have more than 3 or 4 kids because I don't know how you look after more than that—but I wouldn't have just one. I can't help it. In this business you're always aware something can happen. I'd talk it all out before marriage. . . but I've made up my mind."

Caregivers with children found that they often experienced multiple role demands leading to role conflict—problems that require some working out but which can be solved, as witnessed by Dr. Helen Ulysses:

> When it comes to my kids I find that my expectation of myself is that I can do all things at the supermom level. I feel guilt that I don't spend enough time with my kids. The time I do spend with them isn't always so hot because I'm overtired. Recently I had a big speaking engagement in London which meant I had to miss my son's play. I couldn't give up the speaking engagement which was booked nine months before—but it was a real problem.
>
> My salvation is that I have a fantastic husband. He takes a much more active role than most other husbands—he's the classic mother image. So it works for us.

Religion

While religion had the potential of being an important mediating variable, for most of the caregivers surveyed however, their specific religious faith was not as important as the impact that religious beliefs had on their personal value system, so this will be discussed in the section on personality.

In other instances however, religious values prove to be quite important. A surgeon who came from a family with a strong tradition of church involvement said: "You have to have a religious background. I find colleagues without a religious background don't want to get involved in stressful decision-making. It's given me a sense of conviction from deep within my family roots that the golden rule is very important to deal with the stress of a situation."

An oncologist with a strong Christian faith struggled somewhat with how he might integrate his religion with his medical practice in such a way as to be true to his religious belief system while maintaining his credibility as a physician.

> I will share my religion with people but I don't push it. Maybe it's a lack of guts when I don't get up on a pulpit or soap box to preach to those who are dying. After all I have an opportunity to save someone. But I use it as an excuse that I can't do all these things.
>
> Sometimes I feel guilty about making my religious beliefs too widely known—I've seen it happen to others. It reduces their credibility.

Religious beliefs proved to be quite important with caregivers working in the area of abortion. Bourne (9) suggests that of all the personal factors an individual brings into the abortion situation, religion is the most obvious, but not always the most important of personal factors. In general, Catholic caregivers are thought to have the most difficulty in dealing with abortions and abortion patients but Bourne says that in the actual clinical situation, Catholic caregivers have resolved the issue in a number of ways. Some work in abortion units despite censure from the church, while others provide warm and humane pre- and postabortion care, abstaining only from participating in the procedure itself. She suggests that fundamentalist Protestant caregivers may have at least as much difficulty with the abortion issue as their Catholic colleagues.

Stewart found that Catholic physicians were generally more resistant both to doing abortions and to referring patients for abortions (10). Other authors have found that Catholics and Mormons hold more negative attitudes towards abortions than do Protestants, agnostics, and atheists (11, 12).

Dr. David Evans, a gynecologist from the midwest described the difficulty he experiences dealing with the abortion issue based on his religious background, age, and personality characteristics.

As a Catholic I had been raised with the idea that abortion was a nondecision. I knew when I entered residency training that I would have to deal with the consequences of illegal abortions but I never thought that I would have to perform abortions. In the middle of my residency training the law changed and abortions became legal.

I never considered myself to be an orthodox Catholic but I'd always conceptualized myself as a Catholic—all my spiritual rituals were Catholic and in my mind I'm still a Catholic. I had to make a decision so I ran for help to the only two sources I had—a very bright agnostic philosophy professor and a priest. I called the philosopher and asked if I could discuss the issue over a drink. I said I didn't know what to do. He listened and said he didn't either. I felt really upset—if he couldn't make a decision with his background, then how could I?

Then I went to a priest who told me that I had no decision to make. He said, "When you raise your hand to do this you will be excommunicated." I guess this dogmatic approach presented me with a challenge. Immediately I became involved. I became the best damn abortionist in the city. I became a highly successful pregnancy terminator.

Then I had to accept the balance. I had to look at total ambivalence, at the total disregard for human life involved—not only in the abortion procedure but in creating women as victims.

Social Class/Ethnic Background

In previous work by the author and her colleague, Dr. Ed Pakes (13), the problems of staff stress in the care of the critically ill and dying child were reviewed. In that work, the issue of social class was discussed; it was suggested that significance of the social class of caregivers had not received much recognition, other than the acknowledgement that the superior social status of the physician may cause communication barriers with families of a lower social class.

In that article a few of the issues related to social class that might tend to increase the stressors involved in the care of the dying child, and that might apply to other situations as well were mentioned. It was suggested that these might include the fact that caregivers might identify with those of a similar social class and tend to either overtreat or withdraw from such a client. The threat of superior knowledge or high expectations of educated consumers may serve to threaten the caregiver's sense of competence and lead to withdrawal.

One group of caregivers who reported stress that often went unrecognized were those who served as translators for members of their own cultural group. Nurses, nutritionists, nursing assistants, housekeepers, and social workers noted some of the problems inherent in this role. A nursing assistant mentioned the issues that this ill-defined involvement could present in that it could lead to role conflict and communication problems with colleagues and family:

> Patients of the same cultural background that I come from are referred to me in the hospital. They often then call me at home and my husband objects strongly. Very few people know it but I can't read or write and I get really embarrassed when patients give me documents to translate. I make lots of excuses.
>
> I was translating for one of my countrymen and he grabbed me and said, "My wife can't die. I need her too much."
>
> He started hugging and kissing me and took the doctor's hand and started hugging and kissing him too. The doctor just looked at me and said, "What's going on here?"

PERSONALITY VARIABLES

The three mediating variables of personality, social support, and life events are closely interrelated. There are many discussions in the literature related to this interaction as authors debate such issues as whether one is better able to cope with stressful life events because of having a good sense of self-esteem which is derived from a stable social support system, or whether social support systems serve simply to buffer us against stressful life events regardless of our personality structure.

Personality variables that serve to mediate stress responses will be discussed under three major categories: conscious motivation for entering the field, personal value systems, and personality and coping style.

Motivation

An individual usually enters into a job situation with certain conscious goals. In addition, there may be other goals or motivating factors that are not completely conscious which one may be seeking to attain through the job. There are numerous factors, both conscious and unconscious, that might lead a caregiver to seek to work with the critically ill or dying. Job stress might well develop when there is a discrepancy between the individual's motivation for seeking a particular job and the supplies for meeting that need existing within the job environment (14).

Several years ago I sought to identify factors that might motivate a caregiver to work with the dying, especially in an oncology or hospice setting, and to identify how certain motivating factors might then lead one to develop job stress.

These motivating factors were:

- Accident, convenience, or a part of one's caseload.
- A desire to do the "in thing" or to affiliate with a charismatic leader.
- Intellectual appeal, that is, the desire for control and mastery over illness, pain and death.

- A sense of "calling" in religious or humanistic terms.
- Previous personal experience, either with oneself or with those close to him or her.
- The suspicion that one will some day develop the disease (15).

Each of these motivations can potentially lead to occupational stress. That is not to say that either the motivations are poor or that occupational stress is necessarily bad. Rather, the caregiver should reflect on what motivated her to choose her current position and to decide whether this motivation is in part contributing to the stress she might be experiencing. For example, the person who happens to be working with terminally ill patients by chance may work quite hard at what is simply regarded as being a job. Such a person might have chosen to work in intensive care because of the excitement and challenge—the fact that patients are dying there may not have been previously acknowledged. However, sometimes such a person begins to become more emotionally involved than initially intended, and problems may develop.

Susan Jones, a 22-year-old nurse working on a pediatric intensive care unit remarked:

> I came here because I liked the challenge of mastering equipment and never knowing what was going to happen. After about 6 months when I became comfortable with the place, I looked around and realized that all of these machines were in fact attached to children and that all of these children were connected to families. When I realized this and began to get close to the children and families and became aware of their tragedies I came to realize that I could no longer work here and be exposed to this stress.

"With increased involvement came increased risk. When one has not anticipated such involvement and perhaps even tried to avoid it, unexpected difficulty may result when certain patients with whom the individual is involved deteriorate or die" (15, p. 116).

Working with the dying became quite "trendy" in the 1970s. Many caregivers were attracted to the field because it was fashionable and because, particularly in the hospice movement, it sometimes gave them a chance to be in the presence of charismatic leaders. All too often such charismatic leaders turn out to be only too human and to have a tendency not to practice what they preach. The caregiver can then find herself feeling abandoned and resentful. This may then lead to games such as "Let's dethrone the leader." This issue has been particularly crucial in hospices where the person who has started the unit frequently has been fired or urged to resign. This phenomenon which I have observed in various settings throughout the world is due to many factors including the fact that people who have the motivation and charismatic leadership necessary to start hospices do not necessarily have the personalities and/or skills to run hospices. In addition, however, hospice work often attracts people with a strong sense of themselves as individuals. Strong rivalries and power struggles may then develop. In this situation when one leader is away, another will often emerge to depose that person and claim the leadership role. That such struggles are masked as "what is best for the patients or the organization" should not mask the fact that what is happening often reflects a motivation to gain considerable power in this new movement. It is seldom that such a new movement has evolved that has allowed people without clear-cut expertise in a given area to rapidly gain power and be catapulted into local, national, or even international prominence.

Caregivers may also be motivated to begin to work with the critically ill or dying in order to gain a sense of control and mastery over illness, pain, and death. Feifel, Hanson, Jones, and Edwards (16) have suggested that physicians may seek out their profession as a way to control their personal concerns about illness and death by acquiring mastery over disease. In a study of over 15,000 nurses, Popoff (2) found that some subjects deliberately chose to work with dying patients in order to come to terms with the reality of their own personal death. Mount and Voyer have suggested that "at the very least, giving terminal care may provide a way to control the power of death by controlling its attendant symptoms" (17, p. 461). In addition, they hypothesize that those working with the dying, especially in a hospice unit may experience the ultimate denial of death—"It keeps happening to thee, but never to me."

Reverend Edward Connors commented that he came into his work with the dying because of a sense of religious calling. "I came into this business hoping to get some richness in my spiritual life, but find that if I'm not careful I don't have any time for my spiritual life."

Reverend Connors' comment reflects the fact that many of those who enter into this work because of their own spiritual needs have a tendency to become quite involved, and to approach their jobs with missionary zeal. No demand is too great for such people—they have a tendency to remain on call 24 hours a day, 7 days a week. In addition, if they are clergy or physicians, the hospital often holds the same expectation that they will be constantly available. Such involvement leads to emotional and physical depletion unless one is able to learn to set some limits and also to have an outside source of replenishment—spiritual, interpersonal, or preferably both.

Those with a sense of religious calling can also appear to have a surfeit of virtue that may lead to colleagues feeling guilty and useless as well as hostile and resentful. There is also the risk of imposing one's own value system on patients whose belief system may well be quite different.

Previous personal experience can also influence one's choice of specialty. Rita O'Neil, a volunteer coordinator on a palliative care unit commented:

> Anyone who wants to do volunteer work has a need—we all have needs. They do it because they've had a spouse die; to do something challenging; because they have a sense that they've taken from life so long that they now want to give back, or because they've watched a family member die badly and want to give something different to those dying now. . . People want to feel good about themselves.

The motivation for choosing to work with the dying because of previous personal experience can be admirable, and such people often have considerable insight to offer. However, it is suggested that insofar as possible, previous grief experiences should be resolved before beginning to work with seriously ill people. Otherwise it is possible that one might be motivated by guilt to do more for patients than one did for one's own relative, or to prove oneself to be a better caregiver than were those who cared for the deceased relative.

Motivations may at times overlap, as was the case for Reverend Deborah Jones who decided to become a pastoral minister in a hospital because of her own personal illness experience. "I said, 'Lord, what did you want me to learn from this?' I listened and He said, 'Go and do likewise.' So I began my training for chaplaincy." Reverend Jones says she is always careful to try to avoid talking about her own experience with patients unless it seems to be appropriate. Caregivers must always be careful, however, lest what they feel is appropriate use of their experience seems intrusive to patients.

The final motivating factor from my earlier work is the belief that one might one day develop the disease. Caregivers with a personal or family history of a particular disease may well be attracted to working with patients with the disease as well as with those dying of it. This too, causes problems. A social worker said: "I have breast cancer and I've always enjoyed working with people with the same disease, but now that I have a recurrence I feel differently. It seems that everyone in the ward either had cancer many years ago and I get resentful because I suspect I won't have a lot of years with mine—or else the patients are dying and I'm reminded of what my fate might be."

An additional motivation is the belief that in one's previous job one was unable to effectively utilize one's real skills. Thus one might be attracted to a new position in order to show that one really is a competent professional and not the unhappy and dissatisfied person one has come to see oneself as being. Thus caregivers may be attracted to areas such as hospice, oncology, or abortion work where it is believed that there will be the opportunity to really get to know patients and to utilize the skills one feels she or he has. In such a situation one might be desperately driven to prove one's own competence and thus might tend to become overly involved, be particularly vulnerable to rivalry with colleagues, be particularly vulnerable to criticism (because of one's secret fears of inadequacy), and be desperate to prove one's competence. This leaves one quite vulnerable to a severe depression if the satisfaction of the job turns out to be less than hoped. In such a situation one may then have to confront a low sense of self-esteem and may come to seriously question one's professional competence.

Many caregivers reading this section might believe that none of the above described motivations apply to them. If so, they are encouraged to take a few minutes to reflect on what did motivate them to begin their current work and how this motivation may affect the stress they experience. Other caregivers might feel that while they may have been motivated to choose their work for one reason, there are other factors that have caused them to continue in the work.

For example, Dr. Sarah Barlowe, a 50-year-old internist and oncologist said that she first took on a job in oncology by chance between her written and oral fellowship exams. Because of a family illness she stayed in the position longer than anticipated. She found that the role demands of caring for cancer patients enabled her to put into practice some of her basic beliefs about medicine. Dr. Barlowe said:

> In medical school I was never taught that I had to cure to get satisfaction. I was taught that caring was important too. I realized that lots could be done to alleviate the symptoms of cancer patients. I remember one patient I saw who was bedridden with bone pain from metastatic breast cancer. We gave her hormones. She got up and walked out of the hospital and had a good year to live at home. I decided that this wasn't too bad compared to a disease such as multiple sclerosis. Cancer patients also seemed "special" to me in the way in which they seemed to face what was happening to them. These were the main reasons that made me stay in oncology.

It is also important to be aware that in the Person-Environment Fit Model, many needs or motivations may be met simultaneously. As Harrison (14) notes, contacts with co-workers may lead to social interaction that may meet one's needs for affiliation; accomplishing challenging tasks may directly fulfill one's needs for personal growth; and recognition of accomplishment by one's employer and others fulfills one's need for esteem and security.

Personal Value System

Davis and Aroskar state that values "may be considered to be a set of beliefs and attitudes for which logical reasons can be given. Values are significant as they influence perceptions, guide our actions, and have consequences . . . values are basic to a given way of life and serve to give direction to life" (18, p. 199). Yet values are often taken for granted and individuals are frequently unaware of the extent to which their personal value system influences their decision-making, unless their ideas are challenged in one way or another. According to Davis and Aroskar, the values and mores that govern our behavior are deeply embedded in cultural patterns, but they are also fact dependent as well. In addition, they suggest that there can be a difference between the values we think we have and those we actually have.

The value system described by the caregivers interviewed had an important impact both on the ways in which they perceived potential stressors and in providing them with a way of coping with such stress.

Caregivers described their own value systems and what they perceived as being their colleagues' value systems in a number of different ways. For some, a value system was a philosophy of life that did not necessarily involve religious values, while for others, their value system was fairly heavily influenced by religion.

Dr. Stu Innes, an internist in his late forties who is very active in his religious community reflected:

> The faith position of the professional and the degree and kind of self-awareness one possesses has a lot to do with how he or she copes. I was brought up with a concern for others. My father's influence was quite strong in my life. I was brought up rather like Linus feeling that there's no heavier burden than a great potential. I was very accepting of this belief and my potential but they were a burden.
>
> I was brought up with a concern for others—basic Christian modeling on my father's behavior. He was opposed to ventillating feelings, however, as that didn't indicate a concern for others—that included not being allowed to express my feelings when my mother died when I was a young boy. It took me a long time before I could really confront grief.

One's value system can also reflect personal beliefs about the way one should function as a professional. A few examples of such beliefs that may consciously or unconsciously undergird one's professional practice and possibly lead to stress might be the following:

• That all caregivers are beyond the normal human emotions of depression, anger, frustration, and despair and are always patient and understanding.
• That all caregivers should be able to relate equally well to all patients and families.

- That all caregivers are capable of separating the stressors of their personal and professional lives.
- That all caregivers will always be completely up to date with the most recent technological advances (13).

Personality and Coping Style

An individual's personality style may well play a part in determining whether one is attracted to work with the critically ill and dying, and whether one stays in such work or chooses to leave it.

Pearlin and Schooler state that in looking at stress and coping one must be carefull to distinguish between social resources, psychological resources, and specific coping responses. They define psychological resources as "the personality characteristics that people draw upon to help them withstand threats posed by events and objects in their environment. These resources, residing within the self, can be formidable barriers to the stressful consequences of social strain" (19, p. 5). They distinguish personality characteristics from "the specific coping responses: the behaviors, cognitions, and perceptions in which people engage when contending with their life problems" (p. 5). They state that: "The psychological resources represent some of the things people *are,* independent of the particular roles they play. Coping responses represent some of the things that people *do,* their concrete efforts to deal with the life-strains they encounter in their different roles." (19, p. 15).

Type A Personality

Doctors Friedman and Rosenman, defined a Type A Behavior Pattern as an "action-emotion complex that can be observed in any person who is *aggressively* involved in a *chronic, incessant* struggle to achieve more and more in less and less time and if required to do so, against the opposing efforts of other things or other persons" (20, p. 84). Type A personalities are characterized by free-floating aggression and hostility, a sense of time urgency, excessive drive or competitive enthusiasm, polyphasic activity—or a tendency to carry out two or more activities simultaneously; a tendency toward stereotyped responses rather than creative thinking; a preoccupation with money and accomplishments without a real sense of pleasure in them; a frenzy to gain the esteem of their peers and of those in authority; a basic sense of insecurity requiring them to pace themselves so as to accomplish a maximal number of accomplishments in a minimal amount of time. Type A personalities are contrasted with Type B personalities who only rarely have a sense of time urgency and then only in relation to work, have no free-floating hostility, and no need to speed things up. In some studies, Type A personalities have been found to have a greater risk of heart attack. Type A personalities can be difficult to live and work with.

A physician leaving work at 4 a.m. after spending the night with a critically ill patient bumped into a colleague arriving to start his day. The physician said to his overweight diabetic colleague who was nibbling on a chocolate bar, "Hey, if you keep up this pace you'll be dead of a heart attack by the time you're 40."

His colleague's response was, "I know that, but I would rather be dead at 40 having written 100 papers, than alive at 60 and a nobody."

The physician went on to describe the environment in which he worked. The physicians' offices were situated along a hallway and everyone knew who was leaving early to go home for dinner with his or her family—anyone who left early was labeled as not being serious enough about his or her career, while the last to leave achieved a certain amount of status.

A good Person-Environment Fit may well occur when an individual with a Type A personality works in such an environment. Indeed, some authors have suggested that Type A behavior is not so much a personality characteristic as a reflection of the interaction between the work environment and a personality variable (4).

The Type A Personality may well experience a person-environment misfit when placed in a position that does not involve sufficient challenge, responsibility, or independence. However, a Type B person would prefer a more tranquil work environment and would be unduly stressed in a fast-paced, challenging position (21).

Family relationships of Type A persons can also suffer as they tend to place work above family which frequently leads to marital breakup. A nurse who was married to a physician said that she had waited for many years for her husband to finish one degree or paper after another, always feeling that once a particular project was completed, her husband would have time for her. She gradually came to realize that each project or challenge was followed by another, and that there was never going to be any time for her and their family, so she set career goals of her own to occupy her interest.

A study by Burke and Weir found that Type A men in senior administrative positions in correctional institutions reported more occupational demands, more concrete stressful life events at work, greater interference of work with home and family life, and less marital satisfaction, but they also reported more self-esteem at work, greater job involvement and organizational identification, and greater life satisfaction, a fact which indicated that they would not likely change their behavior (22).

In the present study, while Type A personality was not studied directly, physicians as a group were much more likely to report the characteristics commonly associated with this personality type. Role overload was their second most commonly reported stressor, they were more likely than the other groups to report difficulties with job-home interaction, marital and family problems, and they coped with their work stress by developing a sense of competence that often reinforced their sense of self-esteem.

Self-esteem and Mastery

Other personality characteristics also play an important part in the perception of job stress. Perlin and Schooler studied self-esteem—the positiveness of one's attitude toward oneself, self-denigration—the extent to which one holds negative attitudes towards oneself; and mastery—the sense that one regards life chances as being under one's control as opposed to being fatalistically ruled. These authors found that "freedom from negative attitudes toward self, the possession of a sense that one is in control of the forces impinging on one, and the presence of favorable attitudes toward oneself" (19, p. 12) were helpful in vitiating stress, although somewhat less so in the work situation than in the other areas studied—marriage, parenting, and household economics.

Pearlin, Lieberman, Menaghan, and Mullan (23) further suggest that protection and enhancement of the self are fundamental goals for which people strive. More competent people appear less likely to perceive given objective conditions as stressful (24). However, the presence of chronic noxious stimuli such as those that can be found in role strains often strips away the insulation that protects one against threats to self-esteem and confronts people with evidence that they cannot always alter the circumstances of their lives. Under the situation of chronic role strain caregivers might then become vulnerable to the loss of self-esteem and the erosion of mastery (23).

In a study of newly graduated nurses Schmalenberg and Kramer (25) found that the nurses' self-esteem was decreased if they felt that they could not live up to their own personal values and aspirations; were incompetent in their role performance; and received negative input from fellow staff members. These factors combined to lead to low feelings of self-esteem. It is quite possible and indeed probable that some caregivers will be more vulnerable to feelings of low self-esteem than will others. Much will depend on whether the person sees herself as responsible for the problem or whether she sees the problem as being outside of her control.

Locus of Control

The concept of control is often discussed in terms of external and internal locus of control, a concept initiated by Rotter (26). The basic hypothesis is that people vary in their expectations about the extent to which they control rewards, punishments, and other aspects of their lives. Those with an internal locus of control expect to be in control of their lives while those with an external locus of control expect to have little control (1).

One difficulty with respect to the personality characteristic of an internal locus of control is that the work environment may not allow one to fulfill one's innate need for control and this may result in considerable stress and a person-environment misfit.

A nurse with a strong internal locus of control took a new job as a head nurse, a position that she had held in two other settings. After a short period of time she attempted to make some changes but found herself in a situation where each attempted change was blocked by her staff. Within a few months her stress level increased to the point where she was no longer able to perform in this role. Being in a front-line, decision-making position without control, recognition, or authority may be a particularly difficult position for a caregiver with a high internal locus of control.

Self-efficacy

Another important personality trait in mediating occupational stress is a sense of self-efficacy. Coyne and Lazarus (27) describe this as a tendency to perceive a situation as a challenge rather than a threat—presuming of course, that this does not represent a gross distortion of reality. They state that a firm sense of self-efficacy "can lead one to appraise transactions as benign or irrelevant that would otherwise be threatening; in contrast, if one believes that his coping resources are depleted, then he may perceive a transaction as threatening where it otherwise would not be" (27, p. 153).

The Pseudo-independent Personality

The pseudo-independent personality (28) is one with which many caregivers can identify. Such a person often had early childhood experiences that led the person to believe that it was not safe to trust that one's needs would be met. Such persons come to believe that they are the only ones upon whom they can rely to meet their needs. Often this type of personality develops because of a feeling that parental love was withdrawn early: for example with the birth of a sibling when one was going through the dependence versus independence stage of development (29); or because a parent (usually a mother) withdrew because of depression, illness, or difficulty with parenting.

With the feeling that love and attention were withdrawn, the person comes to feel that it is only possible to trust in one's self and to depend on one's self. In typical 2-year-old fashion this is best expressed by the philosophy, "Me do it me self." The pseudo-independent person is quite independent from about age two and goes through life relying on others as little as possible. In addition, however, such a person may have a great need to show that, "Not only can I take care of myself. I can take care of others; indeed I may be able to nurture the world." This type of personality structure might then well be attracted to work within the helping professions where there is an opportunity to care for others. Such a person often has difficulty saying "no" to any requests that show that others need them because it is only by being needed and having others depend on them that they have a sense of value or purpose in life. Such a person might well have a real "missionary zeal" to care for others.

This behavior is, however, a reaction formation against a desperate need to be cared for and to be dependent on others. The caregiver gives to others the unconditional love that he or she needed to receive at an earlier stage of development. Problems arise when these unresolved dependency needs come to the fore. This may happen if the caregiver enters into the patient role. In such a role, the caregiver may fight desperately against becoming dependent on other care providers because of a basic feeling that they "cannot be trusted to meet my needs." If such a caregiver is then forced into a dependency role then many of the unmet earlier dependency needs emerge and may threaten to overwhelm the person's sense of integrity. In such a situation one can get the very demanding behavior which is almost anticipated when a caregiver becomes a patient or the caregiver-patient may be quite hostile and resistant to the patient role, demanding to be quite involved in treatment decisions, refusing to follow the treatment regimen and refusing to have anything to do with anyone other than the ultimate authority figure in his or her treatment. Such personality characteristics can also lead to difficulty with authority figures within the team.

Caregivers who see themselves in this profile would do well to gradually seek some healthy expression for their unmet dependency needs—such as putting themselves into positions where they build up trust by letting themselves rely on others for at least a few small things. This might involve allowing others to do you the favor of doing something you might ordinarily do yourself; or by forcing oneself to put at least some trust into other caregivers in one's professional role and/or if one is in the patient role.

The Hardy Personality

Suzanne Kobasa and her colleagues have added to these concepts and proposed what they call a "hardy personality style." Hardy personalities tend to have considerable curiosity and find experiences interesting and meaningful. They feel they can be influential and see change as being the norm and an important stimulus to development. Thus they can cope effectively with stressful life events.

Kobasa et al. define the three components of hardiness as commitment (as opposed to alienation), which reflects the hardy person's curiosity about and a sense of meaningfulness of life; control (as opposed to powerlessness), which reflects the belief that one has the power to influence the course of events; and challenge (as opposed to threat), epitomizing the expectation that it is normal for life to change and for development to be stimulated. In a number of studies Kobasa and her colleagues have found that personality-based hardiness functions prospectively as a resistance resource in decreasing the constitutional predisposition to disease and as well to stressful life events (30-32). Persons low in hardiness find themselves and the environment boring, meaningless, and threatening. They are frightened by change and see themselves as being incapable of growth (30).

Fear of Death

It has been hypothesized that fear of death is another personality trait related to stress. One of the most renowned of the early death researchers, Dr. Herman Feifel, carried out a research study of 40 physicians, which is often quoted in the literature. He found that physicians thought less about death than did control groups of patients and nonprofessionals, but were more afraid of death than any of the other groups (33). More recently, Schultz and Alderman measured physicians' death anxiety and then looked at the length of the final hospital stay for their patients who died. They found that patients of doctors having a high death anxiety were in the hospital an average of 5 days longer than patients whose physicians had low or average death anxiety. These authors suggest that physicians' behaviors may be influenced by personal attributes and previous experience which may then influence their response to patients (34).

An oncologist, Dr. Lauren White, has suggested that caring for a patient who is going to die has all the elements of threat, failure, and helplessness so often associated with the process of dying itself. White suggested that when in the presence of a dying patient a physician may well feel a threat to his sense of mastery, which may in turn lead to feelings of frustration and defeat (35).

White also comments that clergy and nurses may also have their own unresolved fears of death. In a large study of nurses' attitudes it was found that nurses who had not worked through their own fear of death were much more likely to report feeling anxious or uncomfortable when patients spoke of impending death (36).

REFERENCES

1. Elliott, G. R., & Eisdorfer, C. (Eds.) (1982). *Stress and human health: Analysis and implications of research.* New York: Springer.

2. Poppoff, D. (1975). About death and dying. Part 2. *Nursing, 5*(8) 16-22.

3. Valliant, G. E. (1977). *Adaptation to life.* Boston: Little, Brown.

4. Haw, M. A. (1982). Women, work and stress: A review and agenda for the future. *Journal of Health and Social Behavior, 23,* 132-144.

5. Nadelson, C., Notman, M. T., & Lowenstein, P. (1979). The practice patterns, life-styles and stresses of women and men entering medicine: A follow-up study of Harvard Medical School graduates from 1967 to 1977. *Journal of the American Medical Women's Association, 34*(11) 400-406.

6. Brown, G. W., Bhrolchain, M. M., & Harris, T. (1975). Social class and psychiatric disturbance among women in an urban population. *Sociology, 9,* 226-256.

7. Finlay-Jones, R. A., & Burvill, P. W. (1979). Women, work and minor psychiatric morbidity. *Social Psychiatry, 14,* 53–57.

8. The time-out survey. (1981, May). *Physicians' Management Manuals.*

9. Bourne, J. P. (1972). Influences on health professionals' attitudes, *Hospitals, 46,* 80–83.

10. Stewart, P. L. (1978). A survey of obstetrician-gynecologists' abortion attitudes and performance. *Medical Care, 16,* 1036–1044.

11. Allgeier, A. R., Allgeier, E. R., & Rywick, T. (1981). Orientations toward abortion: Guilt or knowledge? *Adolescence, 16,* 273–280.

12. Such-Baer, M. (1974). Professional staff reaction to abortion work. *Social Casework, 55,* 435–441.

13. Vachon, M. L. S., & Pakes, E. (1984). Staff stress in the care of the critically ill and dying child. In H. Wass & C. Corr (Eds.), *Childhood and death.* (pp. 151–182). New York: Hemisphere.

14. Harrison, R. V. (1978). Person-environment fit and job stress. In C. L. Cooper and R. Payne (Eds.), *Stress at work* (pp. 175–205). Chichester: Wiley.

15. Vachon, M. L. S. (1978). Motivation and stress experienced by staff working with the terminally ill. *Death Education, 2,* 113–122.

16. Feifel, H., Hanson, S., Jones, R., & Edwards, L. (1967). Physicians consider death. *Proceedings 75th Annual Convention of the American Psychological Association.* Washington, D.C.

17. Mount, B., & Voyer, J. (1980). Staff stress in palliative/hospice care. In I. Ajemian & B. Mount (Eds.), *The R. V. H. manual on palliative/hospice care.* (pp. 457–488). New York: ARNO Press.

18. Davis, A. J., & Aroskar, M. A. (1983). *Ethical dilemmas and nursing practice.* (2nd Ed.). Norwalk, CT: Appleton-Century-Crofts.

19. Pearlin, L. I. & Schooler, C. (1978). The structure of coping. *Journal of Health and Social Behavior, 19,* 2–21.

20. Friedman, M., & Rosenman, R. H. (1974). *Type A behavior and your heart.* Greenwich, CT: Fawcett.

21. Rohan, P., & Dolan, S. L. (1979). The management of occupational stress. Paper presented at the 2nd International Symposium on the Management of Stress, Monte Carlo, Monaco: November 18–22.

22. Burke, R. J., & Weir, T. (1980). The Type A experience: Occupational and life demands, satisfaction and well-being. *Journal of Human Stress, 6*(4) 28–38.

23. Pearlin, L. I., Lieberman, M. A., Menaghan, E. G., & Mullan, J. T. (1981). The stress process. *Journal of Health and Social Behavior, 22,* 337–356.

24. Pearlin, L. I., & Johnson, J. S. (1977). Marital status, life strains and depression. *American Sociological Review, 42,* 704–715.

25. Schmalenberg, C., & Kramer, M. (1979). *Coping with reality shock: The voices of experience.* Wakefield, MA: Nursing Resources.

26. Rotter, J. B., Seeman, M., & Liverant, S. (1962). Internal vs. external locus of control of reinforcements: A major variable in behavior theory. In N. F. Washburne (Ed.), *Decisions, values and groups.* London: Pergamon.

27. Coyne, J. C., & Lazarus, R. (1980). Cognitive style, stress perception and coping. In I. L. Kutash & L. B. Schlesinger and Associates (Eds.). *Handbook on stress and anxiety.* (pp. 144–158). San Francisco: Jossey-Bass.

28. Nemiah, J. C. (1963, May). Dependency: Normal and pathological. *Journal of Kentucky State Medical Association.*

29. Erikson, E. (1963). *Childhood and society* (2nd Ed.). New York: Norton.

30. Kobasa, S. C., Maddi, S. R., & Courington, S. (1981). Personality and constitution as mediators in the stress-illness relationship. *Journal of Health and Social Behavior, 22,* 368–378.

31. Kobasa, S. C. (1979). Stressful life events, personality and health: An inquiry into hardiness. *Journal of Personality and Social Psychology, 37,* 1–11.

32. Kobasa, S. (1982). The hardy personality: Toward a social psychology of stress and health. In J. Suls & G. Sanders (Eds.), *Social psychology of health and illness.* (pp. 3–32). Hillsdale, NJ: Erlbaum.

33. Feifel, H. (1965). The function of attitudes towards death. In *Death and dying: Attitudes of patients and physicians.* Group for the Advancement of Psychiatry: Vol. V, Symposium 11. New York.

34. Schultz, R., & Alderman, D. (1978). Physicians' death anxiety and patient outcomes. *Omega, 9,* 327-332.

35. White, L. P. (1977). Death and the physician: Mortui vivos docent. In H. Feifel (Ed.), *New meanings of death.* (pp. 92-106). New York: McGraw-Hill.

36. Poppoff, D. (1975). What are your feelings about death and dying? *Nursing, 5*(9) 53-62.

3

Social Support and Life Event Stressors

Before beginning the discussion of social support and life event stressors, it must be noted that in the model of occupational stress which we are using, certain variables are discussed in more than one category. For example, social support is viewed as being both a mediating variable and a coping mechanism, while marital and family problems can be a concurrent life event stressor or a manifestation of stress. As far as possible, when we discuss mediating variables, we will describe aspects of a person's life that are relatively independent of one's work role, although over time they may have been influenced by one's work situation. Manifestations of stress will be viewed as being in direct response to particular occupational stressors; coping techniques may be in response to particular stressors, or manifestations of stress, or may have developed over time and serve a protective function. Obviously, if a caregiver is under chronic work stress and has continued difficulty with job-home interaction, this can eventually lead to significant marital and family problems that may lead to decreased resistance to occupational stressors and increased job-home interaction.

If, on the other hand, one has a good preexisting social support system and is experiencing occupational stress, one can draw on people within that support system to cope with job stress—or one can use one's experience with a good personal support system as a basis for deciding if it is worth trying to develop a good support network at work to help deal with specific occupational stressors. Cobb defines social support as "... information leading the subject to believe that he is cared for and loved, esteemed and a member of a network of mutual obligations" (1, p. 300). He suggests that social support begins in utero, continues at the mother's breast and as life continues, involves other family members, peers at work and in the community, and perhaps, members of the helping professions.

"... [People] may be said to have social support if they have a relationship with one or more other persons which is characterized by relatively frequent interactions, strong and positive feelings, and especially perceived ability and willingness to lend emotional and/or instrumental assistance in times of need" (2, p. 79). A second important concept in the area of social support is the term "social support system" or "social network." Despite the fact that these two terms differ somewhat they will be used interchangeably in this book. A social support system "May be defined as that set of personal contacts through which the individual maintains his social identity and receives emotional support, material aid and services, information and new social contacts . . . This network may include relatives, friends, neighbors, fellow employees, or professionals paid for their services . . . " (3, p. 35).

For many years psychiatrists, psychologists, and sociologists have maintained that social support is a crucial variable in determining how an individual adapts to stressful life events; but the exact role of this variable has yet to be determined.

Some authors feel that social support primarily serves as a buffer against life's stressors. Schaefer has stated that "Social support as a buffer is often described as if it were an invisible shield, like fluoride for teeth, except applied to those areas of the psyche and soma otherwise vulnerable to stress" (4, p. 98). Social support has been seen to buffer response to illness (1, 5-8); stressful life transitions such as separation and bereavement (8-15); and stressful life events (16-23).

Other authors contend that social support has pervasive effects on one's general sense of well-being, even without life's stressors. This corresponding general sense of well-being, self-esteem, and social support may then increase one's ability to deal with life's stressors (24-27).

The contention in this book will be similar to the findings of Turner (25) that social support does have an effect on psychological well-being, in and of itself and that it may be most important when one is experiencing stressful circumstances.

The social relationships we have may however, not only provide us with social support, they may also prove to be a significant stressor. Levine and Scotch (28) point out that many stressors have their original source in social relationships—family, work setting, and social class position. One of the crucial concepts in this book is that social relationships and social supports can be the cause of stress as well as serving to buffer the individual from the impact of stress.

In addition, as Cobb (1) has pointed out, social support is dynamic—support systems change over time and one's need for social support may also vary with time. In a very interesting article, Gribbons and Marshall (29) traced the ways in which the support system of neonatal intensive care nurses changed over time. In the early stages of initiation to the system, the nurses tended not to verbalize their stress within the work situation, but to take it home to husbands and boy-friends. After the orientation period was over and during the nurse's first year on the unit, she was found to be likely to share her problems with other nurses and then, because her stress had not completely dissipated before leaving work, she was apt to bring her problems home to discuss them with her husband or boyfriend. After the first year, discussing stressors with fellow workers was seen as the most effective coping mechanism. By now the complexities faced by the nurse were probably beyond her husband's understanding. By venting their feelings to fellow nurses, the nurses managed to alleviate some of their stress. But by not taking their stressors to administrative staff, they negated the possibility of being able to make changes to actually alleviate the source of their stress. Finally, after a few years of working on the neonatal intensive care unit the nurses came to limit their venting to a few close nursing friends and developed the 'detached concern' referred to in the sociological literature.

During the process in which caregivers mature in their professional roles, the other members of their social support system are also undergoing their own growth and life experiences. The simultaneous changes that may be occurring within members in a support system may result in the fact that previously helpful members of one's support system may no longer want to play the supportive role they once willingly assumed. Hayden (30) has noted this to be the case with new physicians. McCue (31) has cautioned against the physician's tendency to use his or her family primarily as "a professional support system" and Sargent, Jensen, Petty, and Raskin (32) have warned that physicians who do this run the risk of this support system withdrawing under particularly stressful situations, thus leaving the physicians open to psychological problems and even to suicide.

The final concept regarding social support has to do with the fact that not everyone seeks or needs equal amounts of social support in times of life stress. In one study for example, it was found that people confronted with a stressful life event who did not seek help from their social support system could be divided into two categories: *Self-reliant respondents* who had well-integrated networks from which they could seek help if it was required, but who chose not to seek it, and *reluctant nonseekers* who were dangerously handicapped and had the least effective coping repertoires and the lowest self-esteem of any group studied. This group had comparatively unsupportive and unreliable informal networks and strong reservations about discussing their problems with others (33).

CAREGIVERS AND SOCIAL SUPPORT

The relationships with people within one's social networks and the support or lack of support received, prove to be important variables in the present study. Social relationships were seen to be potential stressors, important mediating variables, a major area in which stress was manifest, as well as a major source of help in coping with work stress. Social support appeared to be reflective of personality and self-esteem as well as serving to buffer job stress. In addition, the ways in which social support function were seen to vary with age.

Social relationships were the major stressor for the total group in that team communication was the most frequently mentioned stressor for the group. Furthermore, staff conflict was the major behavioral manifestation of stress for the group, with job-home interaction in second place. This latter manifestation of stress was also reflected in the fact that when caregivers commented on the role of personal social relationships in mediating their work related stressors, they were more apt to comment on their lack of social support or problems in their personal social support system (60%) than on finding their home relationships to be helpful (40%).

An oncology nurse noted: "I feel that I can't verbalize some of the problems I face at work to my family and sometimes that I have to support all my friends and family, as well as patients and co-workers."

For others, the need for social support at home might have altered over time. Dr. Patrick Nelson, a well-respected and quite thoughtful middle-aged oncologist observed that:

Social support is less important with age. I don't articulate as much at home. I don't feel that no one understands me—that's selfish and egotistical to think that you must be understood by others.

Father Edward Connors, a priest in his late thirties, provided an illustration of one caregiver who found deficiencies in his social support system and managed to remedy them but not, as it will be noted, without some difficulty. Father Connors said:

One of the things that's been most difficult about my job is the loneliness of the celibate. I go home to my own place and in this I guess I may be similar to people who live alone. There's the stress of going home and finding that the people within my religious community are not really interested in my work. They don't really want to hear what I've been doing. Priests in religion are very nervous dealing with death and the concept of dying. I find that they can work out a whole theology of death until 5 a.m. with a few drinks but until they have to face it face to face, they tend to avoid its reality and hide behind a sacramental ministry.

I've worked out a social support system for myself now in that I've developed lots of good friends outside of my religious community. I have four or five doctors and nurses that I can really share things with. They're my confidants. I've found it really necessary to have them. I've also found that it's particularly helpful to have a woman to confide in, that gives me a new perspective and insight on my problems. This has been different women at different times. Using a woman as a confidant started without my realizing it and then I began to sense over time that it was a real need that I had. I find talking with a woman gives me a new perspective which I don't have myself. There would be a danger of misinterpretation of this if my community knew about it and this is part of my ongoing struggle. There used to be the old idea that as a priest you didn't miss fraternizing with women. You became "a man on an island." I found that for myself, I had to stop that.

LIFE EVENT STRESSORS

Not only does one's personality and presence or absence of social support influence an individual's response to job stressors, so too do the stressful life events that a caregiver has experienced, either previously or at the moment. According to Thoits, "Life events are typically defined as experiences that cause the individual to substantially readjust his or her behaviour patterns" (27, p. 148).

There has been much debate in the literature regarding the measurement and assessment of life events and the subsequent impact such stressors have on physical, psychological, and social well-being.

These research issues will not be discussed in this book because it is assumed that they are of little interest to most readers. Those who wish to pursue the issue further will find many references quoted in this section that should be of help in the perusal of that literature. In this book it will be assumed on the basis of literature findings, plus the data gathered from the caregivers surveyed, that the stressful life events we have experienced in the past as well as those we are experiencing at the moment (concurrent stressors) may serve to make us more or less vulnerable to occupational stressors. Not surprisingly factors such as personality and social support have also been found to interact with life events to influence their perceived meaning for individual caregivers. As we have already seen, not all life events are equally stressful for all individuals; indeed, even events such as the death of a spouse may not produce stress (15), but may primarily produce a sense of relief (12). The perceived meaning that a given event has for an individual will in a large measure determine whether or not one will experience a life change as a stressful event and in turn may well determine whether this life change then makes any kind of impact on one's perception of the occupational stressors to which one is exposed.

Life events can be seen to be divided into three major categories: benign/ positive, irrelevant, or stressful. Stressful life events can then be seen to be primarily of three main types—harm/loss, threat, or challenge (34). For a given individual, for example, marriage might be seen as a benign/positive event; moving to a new apartment closer to work as an irrelevant life event; parental death as a harm/loss situation; problems with an employer as a threat; and the birth of a first child as a challenge. Not surprisingly life event stressors may be seen as growth enhancing or potentially destructive.

Life event stressors can be further divided into four major categories according to their duration:

- *Acute time limited stressors* such as awaiting surgery or meeting with a particularly difficult patient/family.
- *Stressor sequences* or a series of events that occur over an extended period of time as a result of an initiating event such as separation, divorce, or bereavement.
- *Chronic intermittent stressors* such as problems with an employer or employee or sexual problems that surface only occasionally.
- *Chronic stressors* such as chronic illness, marital difficulties, or chronic job stress that may or may not be initiated by a discrete event and that may persist continuously over a long period of time (35).

An example of the way in which potentially stressful life events may interact to lead to either physical, psychological, or social difficulties was provided by Terry Katz, an experienced head nurse on an intensive care unit. Ms. Katz said:

We have a new staff man on our service now who had previously been here as a resident. He was everyone's favorite resident and we looked forward to his coming back from the West Coast where he had been having some extra training. We expected him to bring back his new ideas and great personality to help us to make some changes and get things going around here. He returned in July and by September we were having major confrontations. We had a huge fight which was totally unlike what would have happened with him previously in that he was insisting that he was going to put in a balloon pump on a patient and I had to tell him that we couldn't do this as there was not staff to cover for it. He was insisting and screaming that it had to be put in, regardless.

As I tried to figure out how come we were getting into more and more conflicts, I began to realize that at this point in time, he has a new position as a staff man, he's beginning a new practice in cardiology, his wife is pregnant with their first child, he has a new house that he just bought which needs all kinds of repairs done to it and because he doesn't have the financial resources to do this, he's having to renovate his house on his own minimal off-duty time. He arrived here to find that the job that he thought he was coming for did not in fact exist, and he was going to have to work at least twice as hard as he thought he was going to; he just finished putting together his first research proposal; and he's trying to set up a new office. Our explosion happened right after he had been informed that he was going to have to be on duty for Thanksgiving weekend. He had been promising his wife that he would take her away for a weekend before their baby was born and now all of a sudden he finds that because he's junior man on the totem pole, he's on call for Thanksgiving weekend. He's walking around here now with his head held down and he's obviously really depressed. We really care about him and we're not sure what to do about it.

One of the questions that emerges in the study of stressful life events is the issue of how life events actually come to be seen as being stressful. This may happen through a variety of ways:

1. The life event may not impinge directly but may in fact exert influence through the wider context of life strain. For example, the fairly minor life event of finding out that you have to be on call for a holiday weekend (as happened with the physician above) added to the fact of having numerous chronic strains going on in his life, led to the development of a fairly severe stress reaction.

2. Life events may create new strains or intensify preexisting strains. These new strains may then create stress. For example, in the case above, the birth of the new child and impatience with the house which is in disrepair might create both new strains and exacerbate preexisting strains. Difficulties with job stress such that the physician is not able to get enough sleep at night, may lead to his having even less energy to cope with the ongoing problems of work stress and so preexisting stress is intensified.

3. Life events can intensify more persistent preexisting role strains. Then the combination of life events and the residual strain can combine to lead to a source of stress. The fact that the physician above is obviously experiencing role strain in his new position added to the fact that his colleagues have decided to put him on call for this particularly important weekend, can lead to the development of a fairly significant stress reaction.

4. Life events and role strains together may generate stress when they result in a diminishment of self-concept, especially with regard to a sense of mastery and self-esteem. Again to use the above example, it is clear the physician who had seen himself as being quite competent and was aware that people were anxious to have him back on staff and an integral part of the work team, may well have found his sense of self-esteem and mastery decreased when he was in obvious conflict with his medical colleagues and simultaneously experiencing difficulty in exerting his new role with his nurse colleagues (36).

From the above analysis it can be seen that much of the potential stress from life event change can come not necessarily from major changes such as bereavement or illness but from the accumulation of a number of purportedly minor changes.

For example, Ilfeld (37) noted that while only 3% of respondents who reported no social stressors had high depression, 34% who had three or more social stressors reported a high number of symptoms. If one looks at the case study of the physician listed above, it is clear that with the number of life stressors that he was experiencing, he was a potential candidate for the amount of depression that in fact he seemed to be exhibiting.

In the present study data were gathered regarding the impact of previous and concurrent stressful life events. The caregivers who reported familial life event stressors spoke of previous issues such as the presence of retarded siblings, chronically ill relatives, or the illness and death of their relatives. An illustration of the way in which one caregiver's interaction with her retarded sister affected her as a professional was given by Norma Diamond. Norma, the second born of four siblings, had a sister who was 2 years older. When her sister was age 3, she was diagnosed as being severely mentally retarded. Norma stated:

I knew my sister was different and because I was 2 years younger than she was I was put into the position of being her guardian from an early age. I'm from a small town and I began taking care of my sister first, but then this extended to taking care of animals and friends with problems. I seem to have a need to care for other people that others in my family don't have. My friends call me whenever they have problems and generally I prove to be fairly helpful.

A few female physicians also spoke of having mentally retarded sisters and stated that they felt this gave them the maturity to be able to speak up for stigmatized groups. While they sometimes reported difficulty initially in adapting to this family problem, in general these caregivers felt that it had strengthened them in the long run.

With regard to personal life event stressors, caregivers sometimes reported having been seriously ill and close to dying themselves which gave them a new understanding of what patients experienced. They also reported having gained from their own personal experiences with bereavement when family members died but they also could see that this could sometimes cause problems. Dr. John Nielson is an oncologist who has experienced both his sister's and mother's death from cancer within the last 3 years. He stated both of these deaths were quite different and each had a separate impact on him.

My mother was 80 and quite fulfilled at the time at which she was diagnosed as having cancer. We probably had the best time in our lives together two weeks before she died, when it became clear to her that she had cancer and was going to die. She was very calm in response to this. In contrast my sister's death was quite different. She was a very active go-getter who was quite successful and ignored the fact that she was sick for half a year. She died within two months of her admission to the hospital and within just 6 weeks of her diagnosis.

It hits close to home with you when you go through this kind of experience with a family member. You begin to have a better feeling for other people's families and begin to spend more time with them, being more sympathetic to relatives in the same situation. I find I'm apt to take more time now if families want to talk and I try to find the time to talk. Having been through this situation with my sister also makes it clear that while as a physician it is easy to say to a family member that there's no active treatment of this disease, to really explain this and get people to accept it can sometimes be very difficult.

Other times caregivers found that they were apt to use their interactions with patients as a way of working through their own feelings. A funeral director who had had a stillborn said that he became very interested in working with other families with stillborns because he felt that he would be able to handle their grief better than any of the other funeral directors. He stated:

I really unloaded on other unsuspecting families for about two years. My first child was a son with spina bifida who was stillborn. There was no expectation that there would be any difficulty until just a few hours before his birth. We coped with his death although it hurt like hell and we felt cheated but because of the spina bifida it was easier to say "for him, he's better off." For us, after a few months we were able to say "for us, we're better off." With honesty, the hurt was still there but it wasn't as much on the surface. Suddenly I felt I could really understand the men who had come in to make arrangements for their stillborns and I decided that I was going to handle all of them.

After a while I did some reading and it struck me that one of the authors said that when you're working with people who are bereaved, you have to make sure you're not just dumping your own grief onto them. I had a sudden thought, "gee, I really understand what they're talking about" and I began to realize I was doing more for myself than for the families involved. At that point I was able to back off and now will only sometimes say "I have some idea of what you're going through. My wife and I had a stillborn as well." Then if the families want to come back and discuss it they can or they can leave it. The choice is now theirs instead of my dumping on them.

Concurrent stressors also had a significant impact on caregivers' responses to occupational stressors. They reported more concurrent stressors than previous stressors. These fell into four major categories:

- Illness or bereavement in family or friends (38%).
- Problems within marriage or relationships (23%).
- Personal problems including health problems, concerns regarding infertility and pregnancy, divorce and separation (22%).
- Family problems including problems with children, in-laws, parents, one's role as a single parent, unemployed spouses, etc. (18%).

Problems with family illness or bereavement were found to increase with age and were most commonly reported by physicians. Of the concurrent stressors mentioned by physicians 46% had to do either with illness within their own family or with their own bereavement. One of the more common experiences that caregivers noted was the problem of working with patients with a particular illness and then having one's family members develop the same disease. An ICU nurse found that when her father was critically ill on the ICU she was unable to work there as she felt completely unable to have any sympathy for other family members as she was going through her own particular turmoil. Other caregivers found that they had increased sensitivity to the needs of other family members; but this sometimes involved an overidentification with the problems experienced by patients and families and was not always helpful. Some caregivers felt that they were completely able to separate the problems that their own family members experienced and those experienced by their patients, but more often than not, this was not the case. Caregivers spoke of occasionally feeling angry at their family members for becoming ill. One nurse said that when her mother called to tell her that she was critically ill on the intensive care unit, her immediate response was "How dare you get sick in the middle of my exams." The resulting guilt from such feelings sometimes led to caregivers getting into significant conflict with the physicians and nurses caring for their family members. The caregivers interviewed spoke of being accused by caregivers caring for their family members of being unrealistic in their expectations of what should be done. They also sometimes felt that their own experience was used against them. One nurse said that a physician told her, "You're making it hard for me to treat your mother. You're used to big town CCUs and what you have to realize is that in smaller communities we don't have the money needed to expand our hospital to give people that kind of service."

Obviously this discord sometimes reflected the discomfort of the nurses or physicians who were treating the family members of other nurses and physicians. Caregivers frequently talked of removing their family members from the particular hospital system in which they were being treated in order to give them better care.

At other times caregivers who were upset with the way in which a family illness was being handled felt that given their professional role, they could not let their anger be known. A particularly stressful situation was mentioned by a social worker whose brother was diagnosed as having cancer at age 25: "He never even had it out. He was in therapy where they did a lot of talking about people's right to suicide. He went out and jumped off the balcony of my mother's apartment his first day out of the hospital. I'm very angry at the doctor involved and his smugness about the right to suicide, but I can't say very much because I'm in the field."

When a family member was critically ill with the same kind of disease with which caregivers worked, it was frequently difficult to make decisions about what kind of treatment should be used. An oncologist whose child was diagnosed as having leukemia said that she was uncertain whether or not her child should be treated or whether she should simply avoid treatment and enjoy whatever time was left. She said:

> I know my son is going to die but I keep hoping that something might be done to change the inevitable. Many would detach and become a physician in this situation and feel that since the child isn't going to survive, there's no sense attempting to treat him. As a physician parent, however, I have to try at least once but I know that I won't treat if there's a recurrence.

Caregivers said that clinically there were sometimes family problems when one of the parents was a physician or nurse and the other partner was not medically trained. The partner would frequently want to try just one more kind of treatment, whereas caregivers were frequently cynical about using the same kind of treatment on their own family members that they sometimes prescribed to patients. Other times of course there was a tendency to over-treat one's family members. This kind of conflict clearly shows the ambivalence that we frequently have about the kind of treatment that we give to patients.

Caregivers had difficulty if they felt that their family members turned away from them during the time of illness. Sometimes family members became quite demanding and wanted the caregiver to assume a very active role, but at other times they very much withdrew and didn't even let the caregiver know what was going on. A nurse whose sister was dying said: "It's very frustrating. As a nurse, I want to do a particular job with my sister but I can't very well if she won't let me know what is going on, or even meet me half way. What really hurts however is when you find that they've talked with someone else about the problems that they've been experiencing."

An oncologist who had been through several illness and death experiences within his own family spoke of the great difficulty he had in coping with family illness. He stated: "In general, the problems in my family cause me more problems than anything else. When someone in my family is very sick, I find that I have trouble working and pulling my load. It takes me so long to concentrate that I find it very difficult to make decisions and I just don't function as efficiently as I usually do."

When family members or friends coped with stress in a way that was not consistent with the way in which caregivers anticipated they might have coped, there was also some trouble. An oncology nurse who was having difficulty in her own job situation decided to go to her family home at Christmas time to see a family friend who was critically ill with cancer and yet was coping very well. She states that she went over to see this woman and was shocked to find that the woman's husband had recently attempted suicide. She was even more shocked when within a fairly short period of time the man did in fact manage to kill himself. The nurse found it particularly difficult to deal with this stressor because of the fact that a few of her friends had cancer at the time and simultaneously, for her own reasons, she was questioning whether she should be working in oncology. Seeing the tragedies operating within the lives of her family friends as a result of the disease served to further increase her personal difficulties.

When a family member died, caregivers found that this made an impact—sometimes unexpected—on both their personal and professional lives. A physician who works with people who are terminally ill said:

> People working with the terminally ill, as with any other kind of work, may have some need to examine their own psychodynamics. One of the areas that may trigger this need is when our own family members die and we find that unknown psychodynamic issues begin to surface. When my father died I found that I began to examine what I was doing with my life. Working with the terminally ill served to intensify for me the importance of getting on with my life and with wanting to live my life with a certain degree of freedom. I decided that I wanted to write, become more involved in religion, become a better photographer, and begin to create something. I began to question whether in fact I wanted to stay within the marriage that I had been in for the past few years.

Marital difficulties were the second concurrent stressor experienced by care-givers. These were twice as common in caregivers over 45 as they were in caregivers of younger ages. It was interesting to note that despite the fact that most of the physicians interviewed were over 45, and physicians frequently reported marital difficulty, that this high rate of marital difficulty in the over 45 group was not primarily due to physicians, but went across all professional disciplines. A physician in the over 45 category commented on the rate of marital disruption that he had been seeing amongst his colleagues. He stated:

> We're seeing a high divorce rate amongst many of my colleagues. This happens in the upper 40s and later. It hasn't happened in my particular subculture because these were my friends who are academic men who married academic women, and they're still satisfied. With physicians who've led a more traditional life however, they often find that they want to change partners as they begin to get into their middle years.

In some instances this desire to change partners may come about because of an awareness of one's own mortality and the mortality of one's spouse. A nurse spoke of a surgical colleague whose wife developed a benign breast lump and 6 weeks later they separated. The surgeon had been completely unable to deal with his wife's upset and with her feelings of what he would do if in fact she had cancer. During the time she waited for her biopsy, she came to see her husband, not as her husband who happened to be a surgeon but as a "mutilating beast" who had "mutilated" countless other women. He found it hard to deal with her anxiety and began to treat her as a surgical patient. By the time she was diagnosed as having a benign lump, there was little left in the relationship.

Caregivers from a number of disciplines spoke of the many marital difficulties that they experienced. Some decided to stay within less than perfect marriages while others decided that they were not prepared to live this way. One physician found that his wife was spending huge amounts of money in order to get back at him for not giving her time. He stated, "I never thought I'd hear her admit it. I always knew she did it, but didn't know that she knew she was doing it until we went into couple therapy together." An administrator said that she found that working in a stressful situation had helped her to deal with the stress that she experienced in her marriage.

> I decided to get a job because I was seriously considering separating from my husband. This has been coming on for a while. I had begun to change my personality, previously I had been timid but I became independent with a better sense of my self-worth and was no longer satisfied to stay at home. Being in a situation which takes a lot of my energy and thought, has let me forget my own personal situation and concentrate on work.
>
> Now I feel that I can probably carry on in my marriage. Sure, I know it's not utopia but I have come to realize, from working with people who have a lot less than I have, that in fact it's not all that bad. It's not utopia but I can live with it.

Not everyone decides to stay in this kind of marriage, however. A physiotherapist said that she had heard a physician tell a patient that he was going to die within a fairly short period of time. The physician said, "You must look at what you've done with your life. You must be really happy with the family that you've had." The patient paused and said, "I've had a shitty life. I have nothing to be thankful for." The physiotherapist said, "I thought to myself 'I don't want to be in this situation when it's my turn to die.' Maybe it's selfish of me but I want some personal happiness, so I decided to get a divorce."

Other caregivers who were not married found that their career had an impact on their relationships, and they had to decide how they would integrate relationships and career. A nurse said that she frequently found that when she was advancing in her career, the men in her life would abandon her. "It gets to be that I come to expect this abandonment around times of crisis or growth and I have to be careful to avoid setting it up or looking for it where it doesn't exist."

Personal problems that caregivers carry into the work situation ranged all the way from getting married through having major personal illness, through the upsets of divorce. One nurse on an intensive care unit said: "The place has been crazy lately because three of the staff are getting married. They're running around not sleeping, feeling pressured about decisions and they come in and dump on all the rest of us. It gets to be too much dealing with all of them dumping their anger and frustration." Another nurse observed: "If you have problems outside of work, it makes you feel that you don't want to work. That's when I'll come in but I don't want to have to see or talk to doctors or families."

One of the health problems that kept resurfacing in caregivers that may be worth further research, was difficulty with infertility. A social worker said that "I'm a person first and then a woman. Therefore I didn't have problems with making a decision to have a career, but because I have conflicts about myself as a woman, I had a great deal of difficulty dealing with the fact that I was infertile."

A nurse said that she found the infertility testing that she was going through to be quite humiliating and that it was really beginning to bother her. Given her very strong desire to have a child she found it quite ego depleting to find that she was infertile. She stated: "I find that I feel the remorse for my husband and parents ... almost more than my remorse for myself. I don't think it's created personal problems or problems within the work situation, but it has certainly added to the problems which already exist within my work environment."

When staff members were awaiting tests for the same kind of illness that they were treating, they also often had extreme difficulty. A nutritionist talked of having a polyp removed from her nose at the same time she was counseling head and neck patients. She knew that because of her cultural background she had a high risk of having a naso-pharyngeal carcinoma yet at the same time she tried to deny this. She said:

> It made a real difference in the way that I was working with patients. I watched the symptoms in the naso-pharynx patients and I kept looking at the pattern that they followed subconsciously thinking that I'd be following the same pattern. Every symptom you get, you worry. I'm going for a scan on Monday so it's really on my mind. They tell you not to worry while you're waiting five weeks for a scan, but you've seen so many other patients told not to worry and you know what has happened to them that you don't really believe that you're going to be any different.

Caregivers going for surgery or investigations frequently were quite anxious at the thought of whether in fact the professionals could be trusted to take care of them. A nurse spoke of her physician colleague who was going for a hysterectomy. The physician had a great fear of developing a pulmonary embolism and never coming out of the anaesthesia. The nurse specialed her at night because the physician felt that the other nurses couldn't be trusted to care for her. The nurse said: "I said to my physician colleague, 'Perhaps this will give you some insight into what patients go through after the chest surgery that you do,' because she's not very sympathetic to her patients. Her response was, 'Oh no, abdominal surgery is much more painful than chest surgery.' "

When caregivers actually had physical or psychiatric illnesses, they frequently found that their colleagues were not terribly helpful to them in dealing with these problems. A nurse spoke of a colleague of hers who was on dialysis and working in the intensive care unit. She attempted to switch to a day job in order to be able to regulate her life more effectively, but the hospital administration was unwilling to allow her to switch. This nurse spoke of the concern that she had, feeling that it must have been extremely difficult for her colleague and stated that, "She was absolutely gray some days." When caregivers were acutely ill their colleagues sometimes had great difficulty in acknowledging and dealing with this. A priest who worked with dying patients spoke of his experience.

> I began to have chest pain a few days after surgery when I was at home. The pain started to hit me at 11:00 at night. By midnight I was down in Emergency and by 3:00 a.m. I was told by a resident that it was muscle pain, even though the ambulance drivers had already told me it was probably an embolism. In this confusion I kept getting flashbacks of a person who had died with an embolism. I thought myself that I was dying and I thought "this can't be right. I'm only 37." Three of my colleagues were around me—a couple of ministers and a surgeon that I'm quite close to—and they were all crying. I said to them, "Will you please go away, I'm the one who's dying, you three cheerful bastards!"
>
> I really appreciated a female resident who came in and told me exactly what was going on. She said, "We can do nothing for you for the next 48 hours so I'm going to put you out. You won't be able to do anything during this time, so if there's anything you want, ask for it now." Having said this, she left me on my own. She went and spoke with her colleagues in the corridor and I overheard their conversation about what was apt to happen to me. I desperately wanted someone with me at that point in time and I was left alone.
>
> I should have dealt with that young resident who had told me it was a muscular problem, right then and there. I know now that he was overworked and doing someone else's job but I needed to deal with my anger right then.
>
> I got in touch with the fear that people have around death with that experience,

and I also learned the importance of being with people and telling them what's going on with them. When I came in with chest pain, they took an ECG and I was sure I was having a heart attack and thought I'd die young like my father. They never came back to tell me what showed up on the ECG, so I never knew what was going to happen.

Caregivers with physical illness problems are not the only ones who sometimes feel abandoned by colleagues. A minister who had a severe psychological problem spoke of difficulty that he had in getting any support from his colleagues. He stated:

It's not easy to say how it happened, but as I started going into this break I began to lose my perspective on life. I became depressed, suicidal and frightened. Even now I can't separate out the social, professional and work factors which interacted. I know that I had a rotten marriage from the beginning and I know too that my predecessor had a nervous breakdown, which was the reason that I got the job in the first place. He too had a bad marriage, but he too was subject to the same unrealistic job pressures. I was trying to do the work of six or seven chaplains and trying to do everyone's job plus carry a full teaching load. I went into acute depression when my marriage broke up and found that I was beginning to overcompensate. It got to be a vicious cycle. You know that you're constantly being exposed to death and you're a part of it. I began seeing a psychiatrist because I found that I wasn't holding together and I begged for hospitalization. I began doing things that were totally against my personal value system and seemed unable to get any kind of closeness with anyone.

I found that my professional colleagues seemed almost joyful to find that I was falling apart, and I found that none of them were available to help me. Some of them in fact seemed to engage in a personal vendetta which continues to this day.

I guess part of the problem has always been that I'm not a conformist, and that's probably why they lifted my certification so that I can no longer practice.

The symptoms that I had were of hyperactivity and an exaggeration of all the normal pathology that has always existed in me; I was very irritable and angry much of the time. I guess this was just my ego's way of trying to hang on in a difficult situation. During this depression I stayed away from suicidal patients, but as I came out of the depression I found I could be very helpful to them as I now feel that I know a lot about depression. The thing that's so sad is that with all the people I've helped over my professional career, only two people that I had helped got in touch with me during the bad time. The fact that we too need people and no one came through, was the hardest thing to take. I found that I got only criticism from people and never got any support. Now when I know someone else is in trouble, I try to get through to them because I'm much more aware of the stress that other people experience. I've gone and sat with them now when they're in distress and I'm very attuned to it.

I was also upset that I didn't get the time that I felt I need from the psychiatrist that I was seeing. I went in Monday very suicidal and felt that if someone came to me that upset, I would have given them more time and seen them every day. But she seemed to be very much scared off by me and I felt guilty because I had scared her.

The minister who had gone through a suicidal depression felt that he was in a position to help other people experiencing similar feelings. However one must always be careful to question whether this is true. A nurse who had cancer felt that she too had great insight into what her patients were experiencing, but her colleagues felt the need to speak with her and to suggest that in fact her own personal experience with cancer was a very powerful tool and needed to be used very carefully. They told her, "You know about your own feelings and that's all you really can assume."

Feedback from colleagues was extremely important when caregivers were experiencing personal stressors. Many caregivers spoke of the importance of having other people who served as a barometer and told them whether in fact they were coping adequately during their particular stressful period. One physician said that she went through a 3-year-period with an incredible number of personal stressors. During that period of time she was aware that her stress caused stress with her colleagues. "I reassessed frequently whether or not to resign and had considerable input from a panel of my friends that I spoke with regularly."

A secretary working with a physician who was having considerable difficulty said that on an especially rough day that he was having following his divorce, she suggested to him that he not see any patients that day. "When the patients came in I said, 'He's in a bad mood because he had to go to court today. How about coming back tomorrow?' They were glad to. They don't want to have to see him in a bad mood, and have to be poked a few times because he can't get the needle in. They'd just as soon come back tomorrow."

In the literature on selection of caregivers to work with the dying, it is frequently said that anyone who is currently experiencing a major life event should probably not be hired until such time as they seem to have resolved this particular problem (38). A volunteer who went to work in a hospice at the time when she had recently separated from her husband and children found that she was able to function, albeit in a fairly minimal role.

> I was the first person in the midst of a life crisis that they took on, so we all had to be careful. I came to them ready to die—now I no longer feel that way because there's so much to live for. I was aware that my life stress might cause problems and aware that I could do certain other things, so I volunteered for one hour a day instead of four. I realized that I couldn't serve meals here because that was too much like the things I had left and I felt physical pain if I tried to do it. I could comb one woman's hair because she understood my sorrow and celebrated my joy.
>
> My guideline was that I felt centered and in touch, not flying or depressed so I thought that I'd probably be okay. I have to acknowledge that it was very risky for them to have someone like me there in my state of crisis, but I'm more in touch now than I've ever been in my life.

One must also be careful of a tendency when a caregiver is going through a major stressful life event, that he or she does not presume that such crises should be the norm. A physician spoke of the difficulty that he was having in the set up of a new clinic because the head nurse was currently going through a major personal crisis: "She seems to have collected together the 'palace revolt' group who've all shed their spouses and led revolts elsewhere. She seems to find it difficult to select a phenotype other than her own and this is causing us problems."

The family problems that people were dealing with included problems with unemployed spouses, difficulties in relationships with family members, and problems with children. One physician who directs an intensive care unit said that when he and his colleagues are having family problems, it can cause difficulty at work because decisions don't get made as quickly.

> If you're spending time at home dealing with problems like sick children, then you're not spending time in the unit talking about problems that are there. The problems don't get ignored, but decisions just aren't made as quickly. It hasn't been a big problem with us because none of us in the department have had the family problems—maybe that's because we're careful with making sure that we get enough time off to spend with our families. Maybe that's why we haven't had big problems.

One group of caregivers who were having family problems were nurses whose husbands were unemployed because of the current economic situation. One large group of nurses in a community with a high unemployment rate were in a situation wherein many of them had not wanted to work full time and had been very pleased to either stay at home or work part time. When their husbands were then unemployed and the nurses had to go back to work full time, they found themselves fairly ambivalent in that they were pleased that they could at least support the family, but they were very angry that they were being forced into doing it.

Occasionally family members complained about not having enough attention from caregivers and this caused additional stress. One nurse said, "My mother and mother-in-law say to me that I'm not seeing them enough and I shouldn't be working but should be spending more time with them and giving them some of what I give to my patients. It seems that the men in my family die off early and leave lonely women who then expect their children to care for them."

Other caregivers found that when their colleagues brought a lot of family problems into the work situation with them, they were more than ambivalent about being able to give a lot of support during work time.

Severe family stress was mentioned by one physician who felt that his family stress contributed to his work stress. He said:

> I projected unrealistic expectations onto my children and then I wasn't around to implement them, but would get shattered when they didn't turn out the way I wanted. I have a strong religious value system and my kids completely abandoned it. I find when I'm feeling pressured at home that I just can't cope with my work situation. I generally enjoy work and love to go to work. I like to go home but things pile up and I find myself not wanting to be there. I have seven dependents and my income is dropping these days. I'm then profoundly depressed with my income dropping and feel that I'm going bankrupt. It's most threatening and fearsome to realize that my financial status is going down when it should be going up. I've been considering changing jobs. Sometimes I get the feeling that I'm just finished; business is dropping off and I'm looking for some kind of job doing something other than clinical medicine. When I start feeling this way and look around, I begin to realize, however that there's no way I could afford to take the salary cut that I might get if I were to go into university teaching or something else that might interest me.

REFERENCES

1. Cobb, S. (1976). Social support as a moderator of life stress. *Psychosomatic Medicine, 38,* 300–314.

2. House, J. S., & Wells, J. A. (1978). Occupational stress, social support and health. In A. McLean, G. Black, & M. Colligan (Eds.), *Reducing occupational stress: Proceedings of a conference* (H. E. W. [NIOSH] Publication No. 78-140). Washington, DC: U. S. Department of Health, Education and Welfare.

3. Walker, K. N., MacBride, A., & Vachon, M. L. S. (1977). Social support networks and the crisis of bereavement. *Social Science and Medicine, 11,* 35–41.

4. Schaefer, C. (1982). Shoring up the "buffer" of social support. *Journal of Health and Social Behavior, 23,* 96–98.

5. Croog, S., Lipson, A., & Levine, S. (1972). Help patterns in severe illness: The roles of kin network, non-family resources and institutions. *Journal of Marriage and the Family, 34,* 32–41.

6. Finlayson, A. (1976). Social networks as coping resources: Lay help and consultation patterns used by women in husbands' post-infarction career. *Social Science and Medicine, 10,* 97–103.

7. Vachon, M. L. S., Lyall, W. A. L., Rogers, J., Cochrane, J., & Freeman, S. J. J. (1981–

1982). The effectiveness of psychosocial support during post-surgical treatment of breast cancer. *International Journal of Psychiatry in Medicine, 11*, 365–372.

8. Vachon, M. L. S. (1986). A comparison of the impact of breast cancer and bereavement: Personality, social support and adaptation. In S. Hobfoll (Ed.), *Stress, social support, and women* (pp. 187–204). New York: Hemisphere.

9. Maddison, D., & Walker, W. L. (1967). Factors affecting the outcome of conjugal bereavement. *International Journal of Psychiatry, 113*, 1057–1067.

10. Glick, I., Weiss, R., & Parkes, C. M. (1974). *The first year of bereavement.* New York: Wiley.

11. Weiss, R. S. (1976). Transition states and other stressful situations: Their nature and programs for their management. In G. Caplan & M. Killilea (Eds.), *Support systems and mutual help: Multidisciplinary explorations* (pp. 213–232). New York: Grune & Stratton.

12. Vachon, M. L. S. (1979). *Identity change over the first two years of bereavement: Social relationships and social support in widowhood.* Unpublished doctoral dissertation, York University, Toronto.

13. Vachon, M. L. S., Lyall, W. A. L., Rogers, J., Freedman-Letofsky, K., & Freeman, S. J. J. (1980). A controlled study of self-help intervention for widows. *The American Journal of Psychiatry, 137*, 1380–1384.

14. Vachon, M. L. S., Rogers, J., Lancee, W. J., Sheldon, A. R., & Freeman, S. J. J. (1982). Predictors and correlates of adaptation to conjugal bereavement. *American Journal of Psychiatry, 139*, 998–1002.

15. Vachon, M. L. S., Sheldon, A. R., Lancee, W. J., Lyall, W. A. L., Rogers, J., & Freeman, S. J. J. (1982). Correlates of enduring distress patterns following bereavement: Social network, life situations and personality. *Psychological Medicine, 12*, 783–788.

16. Nuckolls, K. B., Cassel, J., & Kaplan, B. H. (1972). Psychosocial assets, life crisis and the prognosis of pregnancy. *American Journal of Epidemiology, 95*, 431–441.

17. Brown, G. W., Bhrolchain, N., & Harris, T. (1975). Social class and psychiatric disturbance among women in an urban population. *Sociology, 9*, 225–254.

18. Henderson, S. (1977). The social network, support and neurosis—The function of attachment in adult life. *British Journal of Psychiatry, 131*, 185–191.

19. Henderson, S. (1981). *Neurosis and the social environment.* Sydney, Australia: Academic.

20. Henderson, S., Duncan-Jones, P., McAuley, H., & Ritchie, K. (1978). The patient's primary group. *British Journal of Psychiatry, 132*, 74–86.

21. Gore, S. (1978). The effect of social support in moderating the health consequences of unemployment. *Journal of Health and Social Behavior, 19*, 157–165.

22. D'Arcy, C., & Schmitz, J. A. (1979, June 2). Some social parameters of disease in a provincial population. Paper presented at session on Sociology of Psychiatric Care at the Canadian Anthropology and Sociology Association of the Learned Societies Meetings in Saskatoon, Saskatchewan.

23. Antonovsky, A. (1979). *Health, stress and coping.* San Francisco: Jossey-Bass.

24. Andrews, G., Tennant, C., Hewson, D. M., & Vaillant, G. E. (1978). Life event stress, social support, coping style and risk of psychological impairment. *The Journal of Nervous and Mental Disease, 166*, 307–316.

25. Turner, R. J. (1981). Social support as a contingency in psychological well-being. *Journal of Health and Social Behavior, 22*, 357–367.

26. Williams, A. W., Ware, J. E., & Donald, C. A. (1981). A model of mental health, life events, and social supports applicable to general populations. *Journal of Health and Social Behavior, 22*, 324–336.

27. Thoits, P. A. (1982). Conceptual, methodological and theoretical problems in studying social support as a buffer against life stress. *Journal of Health and Social Behavior, 23*, 145–159.

28. Levine, S., & Scotch, N. A. (1970). *Social stress.* Chicago: Aldine.

29. Gribbons, R. E., & Marshall, R. E. (1982). Nurse burnout in an NICU. In R. E. Marshall, C. Kasman, & L. S. Cape (Eds.), *Caring for sick newborns* (pp. 131–144). Philadelphia: Saunders.

30. Hayden, W. R. (1982). Support systems for caregivers: The physician. In R. E. Marshall, C. Kasman, & L. S. Cape (Eds.). *Caring for sick newborns* (pp. 66–81). Philadelphia: Saunders.

31. McCue, J. D. (1982). The effects of stress on physicians and their medical practice. *The New England Journal of Medicine, 306*, 458–463.

32. Sargent, D. A., Jenson, V. W., Petty, T. A., & Raskin, H. (1977). Preventing physician suicide. *Journal of the American Medical Association, 237,* 143-145.

33. Brown, B. B. (1978). Social and psychological correlates of help-seeking behavior among urban adults. *American Journal of Community Psychology, 6,* 425-439.

34. Coyne, J. C., & Lazarus, R. (1980). Cognitive style, stress perception and coping. In I. L. Kutash & L. B. Schlesinger and Associates (Eds.), *Handbook on stress and anxiety* (pp. 144-158). San Francisco: Jossey-Bass.

35. Minter, R. E., & Kimball, C. P. (1980). Life events, personality traits and illness. In I. L. Kutash & L. B. Schlesinger and Associates (Eds.), *Handbook on stress and anxiety* (pp. 189-206). San Francsico: Jossey-Bass.

36. Pearlin, L. I., Lieberman, M. A., Menaghan, E. G., & Mullan, J. T. (1981). The stress process. *Journal of Health and Social Behavior, 22,* 337-356.

37. Ilfeld, F. W. (1977). Current social stressors and symptoms of depression. *American Journal of Psychiatry, 134,* 161-166.

38. Vachon, M. L. S. (1979). Staff stress in the care of the terminally ill. *Quality Review Bulletin, 5,* 5:13-17.

4

Dying Patients Are Not the Real Problem

The Work Environment

Having received the mandate to write about staff stress in the care of the dying I must admit that I expected to find that much of the stress caregivers experienced would be related to their interactions with patients. Such was not the case. An analysis of the 3,101 environmental stressors reported showed the following distribution: illness variables (15%), patient/family variables (23%), occupational role (26%) and work environment (36%). It seemed clear that caregivers felt that more of their stressors emerged from their work environment and from their occupational role than from their direct work with dying patients and their families.

The next four chapters will present a detailed overview of the occupational stressors identified by the total group of caregivers. The data within each category will be presented in order of descending importance as reported by the individuals surveyed. Varying across specialties, 43 environmental stressors were identified. A rank ordering of the top ten environmental stressors reported can be seen in the Appendix in Table 4. These ten variables accounted for 51% of the environmental stressors mentioned. The two most frequently reported stressors were team communication problems and dealing with patients and families having personality or coping problems in response to the disease. Of the top ten stressors, six were unrelated to direct difficulty experienced in dealing with dying patients and had to do with the work environment and occupational role. Those stressors related to patients concerned "problem" patients or families, e.g. those with personality or coping problems, those with whom caregivers experienced communication problems because of social class or ethnic differences or conflicting value systems, and those with whom caregivers identified. Only the final stressor of unexpected illness was directly related to death.

It can of course be argued that caregivers may displace their anxiety regarding dying patients onto system problems. I, too, have argued this on previous occasions, but having spent many hundreds of hours listening to caregivers I am less inclined to believe the displacement theory. The basic reality that those who work with the dying must confront is that the individual clients with whom they work do die, although they may live on in our minds. However, problems within the system, especially communication problems with our colleagues do not die off but tend to outlive patient problems. Such system problems may then decrease our tolerance for dealing with the additional stressors imposed by dying patients, while the stress of dealing with dying patients may make one less tolerant of systems problems. Nevertheless, the systems problems would probably remain even if the patients were all to be cured tomorrow.

Organizational environmental stressors accounted for 36% of all work stressors mentioned and were the major stressors in all professional groups. Environmental stressors were the major stressors in the following specialty areas: emergency room (53%), palliative care (48%), intensive care (42%), and chronic care (33%).

There were also differences between the two types of hospital environments in which most caregivers worked—university teaching hospitals and community hospitals. Those working in university hospitals reported more difficulty with radical or disfiguring surgery, iatrogenic illness or the threat of a lawsuit, unpredictable trajectories, and team communication problems. Those in community hospitals were more likely to report difficulty dealing with accidental or unexpected death and the artificial prolongation of life.

TEAM COMMUNICATION PROBLEMS (17%)*

As already noted, team communication problems were the single biggest stressor reported. A physician and nurse palliative care symptom control team noted: "The stress related to staff relationships is more of a problem than patients ever are." Certainly this proved to be true amongst many of the caregivers surveyed. Team communication problems were the greatest environmental stressor in intensive care, chronic care, and oncology. (See also references 1–8 for further information on this subject.) They were rated as somewhat less of a stressor by physicians than by any other professional group.

Team communication problems can result either because members do not know one another well enough and therefore do not acknowledge and recognize each other's areas of expertise, or because the members are quite close. It has been suggested that an almost incestuous relationship may develop between members of a team. The staff physician, who is frequently male, can often become the father figure, and the head nurse, the mother figure. Rivalries can build up amongst the various siblings on the unit, and semi-incestuous sexual liaisons can also develop. Parent-child conflicts may result with challenges to authority and attempts to "dethrone" the leader. It has been suggested that this type of incestuous team relationship is most apt to occur in units that see themselves as set apart from other groups within the hospital, much the same way the families who are involved with incest are often socially isolated from their communities (8). Palliative care groups or milieu therapy groups in psychiatry are particularly vulnerable to this problem. Both groups tend to regard themselves as being quite unique within the hospital system and see a need to develop good team relationships, and open communication. Both groups are also apt to socialize together

*Percentages in parentheses represent the percent of the work environment stressors for which this subcategory accounts.

outside of work time. Frequent contact with one another and intense interchange in the absence of outside stimuli may precipitate this problem.

Team communication problems also result from a lack of team stability, intragroup conflict, and intergroup conflict. In analyzing the underlying sources of team communication problems, it appeared that most of the problems could be traced back to questions of control. Who is actually in control and who should be in control?

Often there were problems in assessing who was in charge, who actually knew the most, who was the most competent, and who had the right to make decisions. Inherent in this stressor was the underlying concern that whatever decision might be made, might prove to be the wrong decision and as a result a patient might die. Campbell has in fact suggested that death anxiety is the major stressor in intensive care units and hypothesized that much of the communication difficulty that caregivers complain about is in fact a reflection of their own personal death anxiety. He suggests that such anxiety "... may be the hidden cause behind the sense of professional inadequacy and conflicts in working relationships among the staff of intensive care units" (9, p. 127). While death anxiety is a real issue for caregivers working in a number of settings, we must also be aware of the fact that to simply ascribe all of the stress to caregivers' death anxiety is too simplistic. Death anxiety exists as a reality that must be acknowledged within these settings. However, all of the team communication problems that exist cannot simply be ascribed to death anxiety.

The team communication problems which will be discussed in this section need to be differentiated from staff conflict which will be discussed as a manifestation of stress in a later chapter. Here an attempt will be made to show team communication problems as a chronic stressor rather than as a direct manifestation of stress in a specific situation.

Lack of Team Stability

Staff turnover, whether of nursing staff or of rotating residents can be a major contributor to team communication problems. In part, of course, this is because the deletion or addition of any member essentially means that the team as it existed no longer exists and must be reconstituted. Although the issue seldom is discussed, this may require that team members need to grieve for what has been lost before being able to become involved in relationships with new colleagues. When this does not happen, the new team member may be resented if he or she is seen to be replacing a highly regarded colleague, or treated with relief or great caution if replacing a colleague who was disliked. There may be constant comparisons made between the new person and the person who has left and until the newcomer establishes a personal relationship and history with the team, it is easy to feel that one is being seen simply as an object and not as a real person.

In some teams where rapid turnover occurs for whatever reasons, newcomers may never feel integrated into the group. A nursing supervisor commented:

> Turnover in itself is a source of stress and it's hard to know what precedes what. There's a lack of stability on a unit when you're working with people who don't know what's going on, and a lack of cohesiveness can result. Sometimes there are also pressure groups within units which determine how the unit goes. They develop negative sanctions and frequently get other members of the team to do less than they normally would. I've

seen units where one person who had significant influence on the service will pull every-one down to her level. Even fairly sophisticated people have succumbed to being pulled down by a particular person, and then they often wind up leaving because of their unhappiness.

Intragroup Conflict

Intragroup conflict and rivalry was seen amongst a number of professional groups. An oncologist said that he had observed senior staff being envious of bright junior staff, and putting them down. A resident spoke of the difficulties he encountered with differing objectives in care between physicians, and the problems that resulted with respect to the development of appropriate intervention and treatment, especially when these concerned issues like bed availability, and the decision as to whether particular patients should be treated as being chronically or acutely ill. He also commented on the disagreements that sometimes resulted between staff and residents regarding such issues as drawing arterial gases on patients dying of cancer.

In nursing intragroup conflict often involved issues of authority and respon-sibility. Staff nurses frequently refused to cooperate with one another if for example one of them was put into a temporary position of authority. In one recovery room staff nurses spoke of what happened when the system of rotating team leaders was used.

Someone different is acting team leader every week because the head nurse is always away. If you're team leader then you say, "Sue, there's a ventilator case coming in, and I'd like to you take it." Sue says, "No I don't feel like a ventilator this week. I won't take it." You can't pull rank on her because her rank is the same as yours and everyone does this to everyone else.

I've left the unit. I couldn't take it anymore. I was constantly bringing problems home and dumping them on my husband. It got to be too much. It's like you say, there's a group of people who've been on the unit for a long time and they're pulling everyone else down and making everyone else want to leave because they won't cooperate.

Frequently there is envy within a group as some members experience the success that eludes others. A surgeon commented:

It's the politics of medicine that is my greatest problem. It's dealing with the person-alities of other people who don't understand what you're trying to do. It's dealing with lightweights with lots of professional jealousy at a time when I can't work any harder and I'm getting along with my own research.

Intergroup Conflict

Intergroup conflict was described by Dr. Sam Toomey, a resident, who stated that he felt quite pessimistic in his current rotation because he found that the two professions which

... should be cooperating are just bitching—house staff and nurses are at each other all the time. It's hard to make the extra effort to understand each other, especially with the fast turnover. I find that for the first week or two that I'm on a new service, the nurses test me out. They call me and show me things that they don't need to show me. If I challenge what they're doing and ask them why they're doing it, most will deny that it goes on, but there really is a lot of testing. The nurses seem to need to know that you'll be around if they really need you... I guess the implication is that a lot of people aren't.

A hectic environment, such as may occur in an emergency room may also lead to interdisciplinary team communication problems.

> With a lack of communication problems arise leading to stress. It's easy to have interstaff conflicts because one person doesn't explain what he wants done, and someone else goes and does it in a different way. We don't take the time to communicate to each other and pretty soon you get yelling, loss of control and doctors and nurses upset with each other. With this lack of communication, then the nurse frequently doesn't explain to the doctor that she gets upset when he yells at her in front of other people. Instead we tend not to speak with the person who did it, and bad feelings begin to mount up. We're still handling all the garbage and then in a new emergency situation we may be particularly prone to having difficulty.

Major problems also developed when caregivers were not available to communicate with other team members when critical decisions had to be made. Norma Diamond, a staff nurse, described a situation in which she had been involved the week before our interview.

> An 18-year-old girl went for fairly minor surgery. When she returned she was intermittently nonresponsive all night. She appeared to be a "street-liver," that is, she was emaciated and unkempt. I called the intern and said, "This girl doesn't seem quite right. She seems to be hallucinating and there seems to be something really strange about her. I think she's too sick to be here." The intern said, "Clearly she's coming off drugs." I said, "I already asked her if she used drugs and she told me she never touched the stuff." The intern said, "She's full of shit."
> Early the next morning I called the intern again and said, "This girl is really too sick to be here. She needs to be transferred to the ICU." He said it wasn't convenient to transfer her then because Grand Rounds were starting. I went off duty.
> When I came in that night I asked how she was. My colleagues told me she had died. The family became very violent and upset when this happened, and the head nurse had to deal with them for hours. The doctor seemed quite abashed and much less cocky than he had been early that morning. He said that by the time she was transferred, her condition was much too critical and she wouldn't have made it anyhow.
> I wonder, if we had communicated better, if they hadn't been having rounds on ICU, and if he had been there, would she be dead?

This type of situation is most apt to develop when team members have not had the time to get to know one another and come to trust one another's professional judgements.

Rosemary Young is a head nurse on an intensive care unit where she has worked for the last 15 years. She looked at the issue of stress which occurred between nurses and residents in general and observed the impact of a stressful life event on a resident's role performance and subsequent team communication problems.

> Residents may be threatened by intensive care unit nurses until they're there for a while. Once they get to know the routine and what they need, then if you suggest something they'll generally back you up. There are others, however, who as soon as you suggest something they will say no. We know that the staff men on our unit will come and order things if we think that it's indicated and they agree; so with a difficult resident, we'll often short-circuit him and go directly to the staff man.
> Recently however we had a resident who's usuually fairly good with us, refuse to get up to deal with a patient one night. The nurse called him a couple of times but he kept saying, "Everything's all right, just leave it, I'm not getting up." The nurse couldn't

figure out why he wouldn't get up, but the patient was bleeding 900 CCs an hour and the resident not only wouldn't get up, he wouldn't even order blood. We found out that he had just failed his fellowship exams but he just shouldn't bring this into the unit. Because of this difficulty, things are at the point where some of the nurses are almost prepared to refuse to be in charge when this physician is on. We know that we can call a staff man at night, but lots of the junior nurses are uncomfortable calling one of the senior men at home at night. Even when you do call, some of the staff men wouldn't believe that the resident would be that bad.

Issues around decision-making often get team conflict out in the open and cause tempers to flare. Fran Douglas said: "The medical director on our ICU is young, aggressive and on his way up. He makes a big deal about how we're all peers on a team together. He says that nurses are equal to doctors and we're all buddy-buddy, until you disagree with him and then he comes down hard and you find out where you really rate."

From the physician perspective however, Dr. Chuck Cartwright says: "Nurses don't have control over decisions and decision-making and that can be a stress for them. We try to talk to nurses but they don't have the ultimate control."

Other team communication problems between nurses and physicians involve the treatment of dying patients. Nurses frequently felt that family members were not involved in the decision-making about dying patients or they felt that family members were not being given enough information. One nurse summed it up with "We're caught in the middle. We don't know what the family has been told. Most physicians are uncomfortable with death. With one of our physicians, no one dies with him unless they arrest. He's a big chicken with death."

Nurses became very upset when the physician's apparent fear of death kept him/her from allowing families to see a patient who had died. One group of nurses from a coronary care unit came to me after a workshop to ask what to do with a physician who routinely tells the family, "I don't want you to see the body" when the family really wants to see the person who has just died.

There are also communication problems when members of one professional group do not share information with other groups. This is not always a purposeful hiding of information; rather it often reflects a lack of realization that more than one professional group feels the need to have explanations for what is going on or what has happened.

Nurses on a perinatal unit for example, spoke of their need to have some kind of closure and explanation of why certain babies died. If they did not have a good communication system with the physicians on the unit, then they often did not have this kind of information. A nurse on a perinatal unit said:

> The doctors don't talk to us and tell us what's caused the death. We're like the parents though, we need to know why a baby died. The consumers that we work with are such that they want to know what has happened to cause the problem, and this concern hangs on until the next pregnancy, or even beyond. We as nurses also need to know what's gone on in order to be able to help the patients deal with their conflicts.

NATURE OF THE UNIT/SYSTEM (14%)

The nature of the unit or system was the major environmental stressor in pediatric chronic care, obstetrics, and emergency rooms. The systems problems of which caregivers spoke related to the hospital system as an organization and discrepancy between the values of certain community members and the hospital as an institution. Stressors within one's unit reflected difficulty with the type of person or illness that was dealt with on the unit, the pace of the unit, the physical environment, and stressors inherent in the particular setting in which caregivers worked.

Systems Stressors

Caregivers who worked in both community and teaching hospitals compared the two types of institutions.

Dr. Ken Walters, a physician who had left the teaching hospital system to work in a community hospital spoke of how pleased he was with the change: "You get trapped into the teaching system and a lot of guys would no more think of quitting the teaching hospital than of jumping off a bridge."

Another physician, Dr. Cam Collins, who had left a small community practice to work in an intensive care unit of a teaching hospital commented:

> The advantage of being in a teaching hospital is that I can say to the family that everything possible is being done, and I'm not giving a false impression. Out in a smaller community, like the one I used to practice in, you know there are places that can do more. I couldn't do in a general practice what I can do here. Here I can say, "Everything that can be done is being done." In a smaller community I'd have to say, "If she gets any worse we may have to transfer her to the big city." You wonder, and the family wonders, if the patient really should be transferred today.

A funeral director contrasted his setting with that of a hospital and commented: "In a general hospital there are balances—for deaths there are births—in a funeral home there are no balances. Every time someone comes in to access you, it's because of something negative. Someone has died, and it may be someone you know."

Sometimes systems problems extend to an entire institution and caregivers may respond with stress symptoms, especially if the systems problems keep them from being able to give the care they feel they want to be able to provide to people with life-threatening illnesses. A physician experienced considerable stress in response to the systems problems that existed in the hospital in which she worked. She commented:

> We have leadership problems here in that most of the department heads don't know how to run a department at an administrative level. They have no long-range vision for growth; no game plan and bad leadership skills. With a new director there was great optimism but.... It seems sometimes that they deliberately choose weak people to head departments.
> The whole management and organizational system is bad. The Out-Patient Department is awful, the number of patients is excessive—all factors, instead of alleviating the stress we might experience in working with seriously ill patients, serve to compound it. This leads to great morale problems so they suggest we meet to plan for the future of each department. We do but they tell us we've worked too quickly so we'll have to wait—so morale goes down again. It's like they're saying, "OK kids, we'll let you play." After a while you just become detached and cynical.

In addition, there may be problems within the larger community within which caregivers work. For example, units for chronically ill children may have a basic treatment philosophy that the children would do well to be cared for at home, but it may be difficult to find physicians who are willing to treat them in the community, which then increases the stress caregivers feel as it appears that the "system" won't let them give patients the best care. Dr. Charles Eastbrook, an oncologist said: "We want our kids to die at home and not here on the oncology unit, but their family doctors are afraid and won't come to see them and aren't willing to pronounce them dead at home. Therefore, we have to find someone who will and by the time we've done this, it's too late."

Pediatric units were not the only settings that had to confront societal values that were at odds with the role the unit expected to perform. Caregivers working with women having abortions spoke of the stressors to which they were exposed because of society's ambivalence in dealing with this issue.

Society as a whole is not yet certain how the abortion issue should be treated. While both Canada and the United States passed laws legalizing abortion in 1969 and 1973 respectively (10, 11), the 1980s have seen groups working for the repeal of such laws (11). Recently a United States Congressional subcommittee investigating public attitude towards the legal status of the unborn and abortion found both the scientific community and the public as a whole to be deeply divided on these issues (11). In the United States funding has been cut off for some abortions, and in both countries members of religious groups and the Right-To-Life movement have fought to keep hospitals and clinics from performing abortions even to the extent of using illegal methods such as burning buildings to do so. This has caused considerable difficulty for caregivers who may or may not themselves be ambivalent about the issue. Caregivers spoke of having to cross picket lines to come to work and of fearing for their safety and that of their clients.

Other systems problems may result from the fact that some large city hospitals are used as referral centers which sometimes means that the women who reach them are in the advanced stages of pregnancy. This then may cause more stress for staff (12). This problem has been noted to be particularly acute in Canada where abortions can legally be done only in accredited hospitals and only after approval by a three-person board, on the grounds that the pregnancy is dangerous to the mother's health and life. This process can cause delays in a woman being referred to the proper institution, and thus make the timing of the abortion later, increasing her risk of complications (10), and causing increased difficulty for the staff.

> We get the bigger fetuses. We've become a "dumping ground." People get to us later as it is known that we'll do abortions up to 20 weeks. Lots of the problem is with the system and women not knowing where to go.

Obviously, given the kind of ambivalence found in society and in the hospital system, caregivers working with abortion patients often feel misunderstood by administration. This may lead staff to feel that administration does not understand the needs of caregivers or clients. especially when the systems designed put abortion patients with other obstetrical and gynecological patients, thus increasing role conflict for staff members and contributing to staff stress.

In some institutions the nature of the system was such that caregivers were expected to rotate to a number of different areas within obstetrical and gynecological services. As physicians would be expected to do gynecological surgery, abortions, and normal deliveries, so too were the nurses often expected to work in labor and delivery, postpartum, gynecology, and the nursery. Some nurses felt they did not receive sufficient preparation for these roles and they felt incompetent dealing with these multiple role demands. For some this presented a major problem.

Linda Eaton stated that she was on duty one evening in the nursery when a new baby was admitted. She said the baby was grunting and didn't look right, and she was told by the nurse who brought the baby down that the pediatrician knew that the baby had been admitted. After a few minutes the baby started looking "strange":

> The baby wasn't jaundiced or cyanotic but just looked strange, so I called the doctor. I had no real preparation for working in the nursery and I didn't really know what might be going on with this baby. I wanted the doctor to come in to see the baby and called him, but he said just to start oxygen, and he'd be in later. The baby didn't look any better when I started the oxygen, and at 5:00 a.m. I had to start feeds of 15 other preemies with just the other nurse and myself on duty. I couldn't watch this other baby that I was concerned about. Eventually the doctor came in and yelled at me, "This baby's septic. Get it to the children's hospital." The baby then started having seizures. I am not adequately trained to know what a sick baby is, and he started screaming at me, "How could anybody be so stupid as not to know a septic baby when she sees one?" He then went in and told the mother, "Don't worry, everything will be fine."
>
> He treated us like shit and said it was our fault; why in the hell were we here if we didn't know a septic baby from a normal one? I felt guilty enough about my lack of knowledge, and I had tried several times to get him to come in. The other nurse and I who were on duty are both leaving. We've decided we're not going to work in a place which expects us to take responsibility without training us in order to be able to do it.

Unit Stressors

The type of person or illness that may be dealt with on a unit may also be a stressor. For example, caregivers in obstetrics may expect that to be a happy environment in which to work. Many caregivers have chosen this environment because of the expected pleasure inherent in working there, but as one nurse said, "When my friends ask me, 'Isn't delivery a happy place to work?'—I have to say yes, but when it's sad, it's sadder than anyplace else. All you have to do is see an obstetrical emergency with a healthy young woman and what should be a healthy baby winding up with a severely brain-damaged child or a stillborn to understand what unhappiness is." In other units where perinatal deaths are somewhat more common, caregivers commented that patients often seemed to die in cycles. When they have five or six deaths of infants within a week, the environment can become a very sad place in which to work.

In emergency rooms the type of patient and the illnesses with which they present may involve the potential for a legal suit. Caregivers there felt they had come to regard each patient who walked in as a potential law suit in part because of the change in consumer expectations and the increased rate of law suits and in part because of the nature of their illnesses. Caregivers in a large urban area emergency room spoke of the fact that they were frequently confronted with dealing with cases that might then turn out to be medical-legal inquests. They described a particularly difficult day that they had recently.

> We are constantly aware that each patient could be a medical-legal case and we were dealing with a man who came in with an attempted homicide. The police were looking for evidence in his clothing about what had happened and we were trying to resuscitate him without ruining the evidence. (Since that time we've learned not to tear the clothes

off of a homicide victim because then you have to identify to the police which tears are yours and which might have come from the attempted murder. Now we use scissors to cut the person's clothes off.) We were trying to resuscitate the man and things weren't going well at all. The people who brought him in were tearing up the department and we weren't certain whether in fact they were the ones who had attempted the murder. Then the relatives came in and a battle insued with relatives pulling couches over themselves to protect themselves in the waiting room.

In the middle of all of this, the helicopter arrived with a new trauma case. One of the physicians who was busy with a patient looked around and said, "This place is a zoo." A patient who was coming out of a drug overdose punched the doctor in the face and said, "Don't call me an animal."

The pace of a unit may also prove to be a stressor for some caregivers. In part the stress that may result in response to the pace of a unit may be the result of person-environment misfit. The caregiver with an internal locus of control may feel helpless and stressed in an environment in which it seems impossible to exert control. Others may find they can maintain a sense of control in the most hectic of environments, while still others with an external locus of control may be able to function well in an environment in which they are responding to a number of external stimuli. Intensive care units and emergency rooms were both settings in which the erratic pace of the environment could prove to be a challenge to one caregiver and a nightmare to others.

Nurses in a community hospital emergency room described the trauma they felt one morning close to Christmas when they went from having no one in the emergency room to suddenly having five children who were burned beyond recognition coming in from a family home that had suddenly caught fire. These same nurses spoke of the difficulty in going from a particularly traumatic death to dealing with someone with a minor problem.

It's really hard when you have to deal with someone who's seriously ill when you push yourself to the extreme trying to keep him alive, and then you turn around and have to go back and deal with someone with a general sore throat who's moaning because he's had to wait an hour and a half. Things were really tense one day like this and when the patient with the sore throat started complaining. I felt that I wanted to strangle him. The doctor took the man by the hand and led him in to see the code that was in process and said, "That's what we're doing; that's why we've kept you waiting." This was a real mild-mannered physician and we were really shocked to see how he handled it.

The physical environment may also be a stressor. Sometimes there were significant design errors. Other times there was a real lack of privacy for patients and families. For example, emergency rooms can become very public places at times of disaster. Nurses spoke of a hotel fire in which ten victims were brought to one hospital.

The press were there demanding to photograph the bodies and photographing everything and everyone in sight. We started camouflaging the bodies to get them to the coroner because we felt that relatives shouldn't be exposed to seeing their dead relatives on the front page of the newspaper the next day. We put guards on all the doors and snuck the bodies out a side entrance so that the press couldn't get pictures. The next day our public relations department complained that we weren't being nice to the press; but we feel that our major obligation should be to the patients and the families.

An additional stressor is the issue of dealing with family members within a hectic environment. A social worker who worked with pediatric oncology and intensive care unit patients contrasted the pressures he felt in these two environments.

> With our intensive care unit the death rate is only about 5% so we're not really dealing with death and dying, but whatever I do with the family there always seems to be a real sense of urgency involved. Within that technological environment I found it very difficult to relate to parents and felt that I was constantly under pressure to have a great deal of medical information and technical knowledge myself, in order to be able to try to translate it into layman's terms for the parents. I found that I could very often wind up getting sucked into focusing primarily on the environment and the technology. The pace in our unit is very fast and I found that this fast pace created a tension that was contagious both for me and for the parents. I easily got sucked into that and I'd wind up responding in that same sort of fast-paced way.
>
> I found that the caregivers also always expected things done quickly. A family would come in and I'd be called to come and see them right now. This was perhaps realistic because they may have needed help quickly, but I wound up always having an "on-call" feeling. I work in oncology and there there's the feeling that the kids are in the hospital and their parents are around. If I miss them this time I'll get them the next time that they're in because these kids will be in, but with the ICU you never know. The framework seems to be much shorter and that creates a tension all of its own.

Even clinicians who are comfortable in hectic environments often do not like the fact that these settings can be very public places. They feel that much of their activity is "on stage." This can become particularly problematic during an emergency or when staff members engage in the black humor so common amongst health care providers. When this occurs in front of parents or visitors, the behavior can be easily misinterpreted. Caregivers also mentioned the lack of private physical facilities for family members. Often there was no family room or not enough space for families who needed privacy.

> The family gets really ripped off here when a patient dies in that there's no family room anyplace. You're told that you should put the family in a room where they have privacy, but the only room we have is right off the nursing station and they hear us on the phone saying, "hurry up and get respiratory therapy down here" and they know it's for their relatives. We can't ask them to wait in the waiting room when they're waiting to hear that their relative has died and yet putting them in this room is incredibly difficult. They need a quiet, comfortable place where they can't hear anything and I get bothered because here I have to put them in a small room where they have no place to talk, the computer terminals are located here, and everyone is in and out all the time.

The final aspect of the setting has to do with the *nature of the deaths* caregivers experience because of the type of unit, and multiple deaths. A group of pediatric intensive care unit nurses met to discuss the stressors inherent in the environment in which they worked. They spoke of the number of deaths they experienced over the course of the year: "gory deaths"—that is children dying as a result of accidents, hemmorhage; "patients who are vegetables with green stuff pouring out of all orifices"; experiencing several deaths together, e.g. eight to one week; and extreme deaths—that is, children being brought from the oncology unit in the terminal phases of leukemia to be hitched up to ventilators to have their lives prolonged. They commented on the impact these situations had on them, saying, "If you lose six or seven kids in a row, you know you're in trouble. This kind of trouble is much worse than staff vacancies."

One nurse summed up her philosophy regarding the stressors of the PICU in which she worked: "There's always the next day. If the next day is bad for long periods it makes you want to quit. You can't look forward to getting to work when you know you're going to face chaos, death, and hysteria. It's hard to get here but once I do, I find that I really want to be here."

INADEQUATE RESOURCES/STAFFING (14%)

Reports of inadequate staffing or resources could be seen to derive from several lacks within the system. This variable included such issues as fiscal restraint in the current economic climate; the lack of an adequate number of caregivers; a lack of adequately prepared staff; a limited availability of medical coverage; and limited resources.

Fiscal Restraints

Caregivers from the United States, Canada, Australia, and Great Britain all mentioned difficulty obtaining funding for their programs, inadequate staffing resources, some staffing cutbacks, and increasingly heavy workloads. There were also some complaints that issues such as education, training, and psychosocial programs were the first to be sacrificed. Social workers in the United States complained that both Proposition Thirteen and "Reaganomics" eliminated many social work positions in the country, while DRG (Diagnostic Related Grouping) financing threatened other caregiver's positions or methods of practice. As one director of nursing stated, "There is the problem of continuous uncertainty on many units and in many hospitals with today's fiscal restraints.

Dr. Norman Thomas, a Canadian psychiatrist, discussed problems of underfunding in that country. He suggested that the fairly liberal funding patterns which previously existed led to unrealistic consumer expectations. He was upset by patients who failed to show any kind of gratitude to the caregivers working to serve them and felt that this was particularly obvious in the emergency room where, with the free medical care provided, patients sometimes showed "ingratitude for the care they're given." He suggested that caregivers in the emergency room in particular could find themselves recipients of client hostility because the current lack of funding sometimes meant that the services patients had come to expect were not necessarily available to them. When caregivers are the recipients of client hostility they may then become angry at their own administrators, blaming them for deficiencies in the system.

Lack of Adequate Staff

Several studies in the literature also report finding that inadequate staffing or resources is a major stressor for caregivers, particularly in intensive care units. A review article by Gentry and Parkes (13) looked at studies of stress in intensive care units over the last decade. They found that the primary source of stress in ICU work was work overload which in most cases, resulted from inadequate staffing. They stated that, "If adequate staffing is maintained, nurses are able to take all other frustrations in their stride; conversely, inadequate staffing over a long period of time seems to increase the nurses' sensitivity to all other stress" (13, p. 44). Hanna Foster an ICU nurse in her middle twenties spoke of the community hospital in which she had recently worked. She left that environment because of feeling that it was unsafe.

> That community hospital did the best of all of the hospitals in the area at keeping its budget down and so the government was very pleased, but they did that by not having enough staff. At the teaching hospital where I work now, I'm only allowed to look after one ventilated patient at a time and I can't leave the room. At that hospital I was looking after patients on both sides of the room with ventilators. I felt that I had to leave because the environment was totally unsafe. I spoke with the head nurse who agreed that the environment was totally unsafe but said that with the lack of staff she had, due to budgeting restraints, she felt it was impossible to give patients proper care.

Part of the difficulty with staffing certain units also evolves from the nature of the units and their lack of predictability. Particularly in emergency rooms and critical care units, it is impossible to predict when an emergency admission will occur or when crises will happen with patients already in the unit. This frequently means that it is difficult, if not impossible, to do effective staff forecasting. As a result, nurses are often asked to work extra hours, staff physicians may be called in at odd hours, and house officers often get no sleep when they are on call (14). Mrs. Nadine Tierney, a pediatric ICU head nurse said: "I'd rather have the staff nurses working normal shifts for a year and half than to burn out with overwork and working overtime and over-investing themselves over a period of 7 months. They become quite strung out when this happens and sometimes we cause it to happen because of our problematic staffing."

Nurses also commented that staffing shortages forced them to bring in registry nurses who did not understand the unit and had considerable difficulty in working with the patients. This caused them to question whether the environment in which they functioned was actually safe. On the other side, the relief staff who are called in are often clear that the environment is not safe.

A young nurse who had recently graduated spoke of a university classmate of hers who was doing relief work to put herself through school. Although she was not trained to work in an NICU she was sent there to relieve one day. The unit was quite busy and no one seemed particularly helpful. She was told that Baby Smith's drugs were ready to be given and that she was to administer them. She was unaware that oral drugs were placed in syringes on that unit. When she saw a syringe she gave the drugs intravenously. The baby died almost immediately.

When staff shortages result in the use of untrained people, the environment becomes one in which errors can easily be made. The nurse in the above situation readily admitted that she and her colleagues did not know what they were doing and that they felt that the other nurses were too busy to supervise them.

Limited Availability of Medical Coverage

Medical coverage was also difficult, particularly in community hospitals. "In the emergency room, shiftwork is a lot different. Days are okay because you can at least page the doctor and the anesthetist is always there; but at night the doctors are only on call and they may live half an hour from the hospital which makes for a rough time if you have a real emergency."

Caregivers in community hospitals also had problems with medical coverage on their ICUs. Sometimes this was the result of inadequately prepared physicians and other times it seemed to be the result of a lack of sufficient physicians to cover the unit. Nurses in one community intensive care unit said that they found that there were different stressors at different times of the year. They commented that it was particularly difficult in July when they had:

> . . . new interns—fresh out of medical school, real fresh out of medical school. We have two new interns in the ICU every month but in July, they're fresh out of medical school in June and immediately go to the ICU where they're responsible for half the patients and writing orders for them. There's no junior resident covering them; they're only covered by the staff pulmonary physician who has such a huge practice that he can't cover the interns properly. They're responsible for writing orders and lots of them come in gung ho and then write crazy orders. Some of them are good enough to listen to us when we tell them that the orders are crazy, but some are rather arrogant and say, "Who do you think you are as a measly nurse to tell me?"
>
> When you add to new interns the fact that we also have lots of new nurses who don't know •vhat's going on and then you find that the new interns are going to the new nurses, you get a sense of the kind of stress that we're under.

While nurses may give advice when physicians are uncertain what to do, the nurses often become fairly anxious. Diane Young, a young ICU nurse said:

> One resident we had—an anesthesia resident—I didn't trust as far as I could throw her. A patient was on a ventilator and we were trying to wean him down and she was giving all kinds of orders. She asked me, "What do you think I should do?" It's nice to be asked, but her questions were because she didn't really know what to do.

While nurses can be thought to be overly critical of physicians and perhaps not understand the types of stressors to which doctors are exposed, some of the problems which nurses mention still do seem to need to be resolved, particularly those related to competence and effective coverage. "You'd have to ask how many of them know how to intubate a patient. Or to do a cardiac massage. This isn't something they do all the time. You have to realize that here it's not like working in a big teaching hospital. It may have been years since some of these staff men had to deal with a cardiac arrest."

In my travels I met on several occasions with groups of nurses who worked in intensive care units. In one city the nurses contrasted the various intensive care units on which they had worked. At this point in time they were all working on a small intensive care unit in a community hospital. They commented that in a community hospital they felt that they had to have more knowledge than they had when working in a teaching hospital because the medical resources for decision-making were not always close at hand.

A male nurse spoke of the fact that he used to work in a 150-bed hospital in a small community. Here there was a 10 bed intensive care unit staffed by three registered nurses with no physician present for 16 hours out of the 24.

> At times we'd have two codes at a time and I remember once bagging two patients for more than 4 hours with no physician present. If one doctor was on the case you couldn't call in someone else because the patient wasn't white and the other doctor would only see white patients.
>
> I was a new graduate and within one year I was 20 pounds lighter with a hole in my belly from making decisions all the time. You have to be able to learn quickly in an intensive care unit but this was just too much.

Limited Resources

Finally, the physical resources available to caregivers could also be a problem. For example, physicians who trained at teaching hospitals and then went to practice in community hospitals found availability of resources to be a stressor. They often wanted to practice the same type of medical care that they had been trained to perform but found this to be impossible due to the decrease in available resources. An administrator commented on this problem:

> A new young surgeon wanted to do a certain sophisticated procedure on a patient. The chief said, "Don't do it—sure it may be justified to do it, but it's just too risky. We don't have the resources of the big teaching hospital from whence you came—there just isn't the back-up if you get into trouble.
> He went ahead anyhow. The operation was a success but the patient died. He's ruined his career. It follows him around now. No one will refer the difficult cases—they just don't trust his judgement anymore. Sure they'll refer the straightforward ones, but as far as the career he wanted in surgery, he's screwed.

Dr. Bob Tracey commented on the lack of adequate resources in an intensive care unit in a manner that put the problem within an interesting perspective. He stated:

> In an intensive care unit, one generally feels that there is a limited ability to deliver care. Previously on our first intensive care unit we felt that we lacked the proper equipment, personnel, funds, and space to provide the care we felt we could provide. Even with a fairly sophisticated new intensive care unit this is still true. It seems no matter what you have on an intensive care unit, you always have the feeling that you need to have someone else there, you need more space, an improved machine, or better staff. There's always something forcing you to ship out patients before you feel they're really ready to be shipped out, or you're feeling too crowded, or the unit is having to look after two patients with only enough to care for one.

Finally, a somewhat amusing anecdote about the lack of resources available in a hospital setting came from a supervisor working in a small nursing home. She had recently transferred to the nursing home from the public health department and was quite surprised at the lack of coverage that was provided on the weekends. She stated:

> Here on the weekend we have no maintenance, no ward aides. At night it's just me and the security man on duty. It's the role of the nursing supervisor at night to take the mice out of the mouse trap, and to check the boiler room for problems. It was really tense one night when the boiler was making funny noises and I didn't know what to do. On nights I also have to defrost the refrigerator and serve any meals that people want. It seems as if we have to do more and more these days. When I first started in nursing I was the doctor's handmaiden—now I'm everyone else's handmaiden as well.

COMMUNICATION PROBLEMS WITH OTHERS IN THE HOSPITAL OR OUTSIDE THE SYSTEM (13%)

Communication problems with other people within the hospital system were most pronounced within palliative care, and were the single biggest stressor of all for physicians. These stressors could be divided into three groups—communication problems with the rest of the hospital; problems of communication with other specialties; and a lack of support for others in one's own discipline.

Communication Problems within the Hospital or Outside System

Communication problems with other people within the hospital were related by several caregivers. Dr. John Nielson, an oncologist who directs a bone marrow transplant team remarked:

> I don't mind the stressful job that I have—but to write an order and get flak—"why do you need it right now?" To order an X-ray at midnight and have the X-ray technician say, 'Do I really have to show up now?" It's the lackadaisical method of so many staff members, be they nurses, lab technicians, or whatever. To make this whole thing run requires dedication—time—it's an around-the-clock job which requires extra effort. In this hospital it's so institutionalized that it's difficult to ask for extra effort. My colleagues on the team, on the other hand, are often very dedicated. If I tell my technician that something has to be done now, he'll be here until he does it. The head nurse will stay until the work is done as well.

Palliative care teams often experienced significant difficulty with their colleagues both within the hospital and in the outside community. Often this was because the original idea for the program did not come about because of an acknowledged need within a system, but rather because a small group of people saw that there was a need and/or felt the desire to develop a program. There is often a basic assumption that the idea is good and that others should therefore fall into line behind it. Frequently however, the others who were not consulted in the early stages sabotage the program in its later stages, either deliberately or because they simply do not understand what is to happen. Not unexpectedly it is dying people and their families who then become the victims of these internal wars.

A palliative care team in a medium size city had been formed by administrative decree. Some of the team members were known to hospital staff but others were hired for the team without the support of members of their professional disciplines within the hospital. The model for the team was that anyone from within the hospital could initiate the referral and then any team member could then go in and do an assessment and begin to work with the family. This type of model of course presumes a great willingness on the part of all hospital staff to be flexible in their roles. Such was not always the case. For example, if a nurse asked for a consult on a patient, the social worker involved might be quite resistant to having the palliative care social worker speak with the patient and family. Tempers might flare and the patient's treatment might well suffer. Team members gave the following example of the type of problem that might evolve.

> We were asked to consult recently on pain relief for a man who was a surgical patient whose family physician referred him to medicine. We knew what needed to be ordered but we couldn't find out who was the physician in charge who could write the orders. It became a matter of "Would the primary physican please step forward." The patient was in extreme pain. The surgical resident was in the operating room with a consultant and wouldn't be out for several hours. His family physician was not available and was covered by someone else who also wasn't available. Our physician cannot write orders but can only suggest. Eventually the resident came up and wrote the order but put

the wrong dosage because he didn't realize that in converting injectable morphine to oral, he had to change the dosage.

In the meantime, the patient is very depressed, worried about his family. He is afraid of dying in pain as his father did and is now threatening to jump out the window. There's just no support. We can help with the pain but it's a lot harder to deal with this mess. We walk back into the room to see what is going on and feel so guilty to see the distress this man is in. It's the problems of dealing with the system, with upset staff, with units with horrendous communication problems.

Problems in communication with others outside of the hospital system also served as a stressor, especially for those in palliative care. Norma Martin, a visiting nurse who worked with dying patients in the community commented that as hard as they tried to have things go well, there were often complications:

We try to find out what the patient and family wishes are regarding dying at home and make sure that the family doctor will make house calls at intervals and at the time of death. We discuss with the family that the patient can return to the hospital if they can't handle things and we're able to ease readmission when it's necessary by helping the family to feel that "It got so bad we had to send them back." We prepare the family about what might happen around death and what the person might look like. We also tell the family that at the time of death they should call the family doctor and not the emergency phone number.

Recently though we had a person dying. The family doctor didn't want to make house calls. He said, "Maybe you think I'm a terrible person but I deal with the living and not the dying." He did agree, however, that he would come to pronounce the person dead.

I was coming to do a home visit one day and saw the fire engine, ambulance, and police cars in front of the house. A neighbor had called the emergency number when the patient died. Because they were called it became a coroner's case. The police saw the morphine ampules and treated it like a "drug bust," seizing the morphine. The coroner wanted to talk with the nurses involved and the family was all upset.

You go through all the preparation and this is what happens. You try but you don't always succeed.

Problems in Communicating with Other Specialties

Problems in communicating with other specialities were noted by a number of different physicians. A family physician, Dr. Marvin Mendelson, complained of a lack of communication experienced by his colleagues when dealing with specialists.

There's a lack of early involvement with family doctors. We're not really considered a part of the team—we're really outside of the team. Now family doctors won't touch cancer patients because they don't feel a part of the team. It's only when the oncologist gives up that the patient arrives back on your doorstep—there's a lack of communication from early on. It's an insensitive team that doesn't recognize the family doctor's skills—we're used as instruments, not as people. This is especially stressful around dying.

As a family doctor you run that risk with anyone that you refer off—you have to refer, but you learn to refer to specialists who communicate with you. Too often specialists don't refer back. They just keep referring to other specialists and you never find out what's happened.

Lack of Support for Others in One's Discipline

The lack of effective communication was often a problem. A nurse who had transferred a patient from one unit to another found that when she tried to explain some of the patient's problems to the head nurse on the new unit, the head nurse seemed to constantly cut her off and not allow her to express her concerns. She stated, "That's what I hate about nurses—they treat you with such disdain when they don't really know what's going on. Doctors treat you okay, but other nurses—sometimes they represent everything I hate about the profession."

UNREALISTIC EXPECTATIONS
OF THE ORGANIZATION (10%)

Unrealistic expectations proved to be somewhat more of a problem for the people most intimately involved in psychosocial issues such as social workers, clergy, and psychologists than for nurses or physicians. It was also a problem in palliative care where many caregivers volunteered many extra hours a week beyond their paid job time and this was expected to continue with funding cutbacks. One chaplain who eventually had to leave the teaching hospital system, commented on what he regarded as totally unrealistic expectations of the organization.

> I started off as an easy-going person working with a lot of stressors. I came into the hospital and immediately I experienced a lot of broken promises. I had been told that I would have to do no teaching and that I would have a large group of chaplains working with me. Immediately there were budget cuts and administrative changes and it became clear that I wasn't going to get the staff that I was expecting. I wound up being the only chaplain, trying to do everyone's job, and carry a full teaching load in addition.
>
> I've gone two nights in a row without any sleep, just lying down with my clothes on and being called up again. I know that I personally can handle only two or three deaths per day, and then I try to get out. This is possible with more staff but with no other staff it's impossible to get away. In addition, there's a lack of appreciation on administration's part of any of the paramedical services, be they chaplains or social workers. With budget cuts there's a lot of apathy and actual overt hostility towards us.

Residents also commented on the stress they experienced due to being required to work incredibly long hours. One commented on staff physicians and their unwillingness to listen to interns and residents as they talked about the stress that they were experiencing. The staff man would say, "We went through it and took more calls for not as much money." To this the interns would reply, "But the reality is they didn't go through this. They didn't have to know as much as we do. They had much simpler care. Their patients weren't as old as ours are, and didn't have as many diseases simultaneously wrong with them."

Dr. Ken Walters described his experience:

> During my surgical residency there was never time to sit back and think. You worked 90 to 100 hours a week. You came in on Saturday morning and worked straight through until Monday at 6:00 p.m. Then you came back Tuesday morning and worked through till Wednesday at 6:00 p.m. Then you'd be off for a couple of nights. Out of 14 days, you'd spend 7 nights and 11 days in the hospital.
>
> Many of my colleagues seemed able to cope with this, but I was a different breed. They didn't have avocations like me. I was trying to get published and be involved with sports. Running, skiing, playing racquetball kept me sane, and I wasn't about to give them up.

The same physician talked about unrealistic expectations of the teaching hospital, but stated that many of his colleagues were very hesitant to leave this kind of environment.

> In the teaching hospital you get trapped within the system. Recently a patient showed up in the emergency room of the community hospital where I work. I looked at him and here was my former professor of internal medicine. He was the one we all went to when we wanted to know how to really examine a patient and do a differential diagnosis. I hadn't seen him in a few years and here he was with his first heart attack. He was no longer at the medical center, but had set up a practice in a local community. It seems they got a new chief who said, "If you don't publish and do research, you're out." They let him go after 25 years. He told me the story as I examined him. He said, "What does clinical medicine mean anymore?" This was a vibrant, active excellent clinician the last time I saw him 10 years ago. He lay there in front of me, a different man saying, "Can you believe they let me go after 25 years."
> You read the garbage in journals and you know a lot of it doesn't say very much. Is it worth it to just sacrifice these people?"

Staff members in other units, especially intensive care units complained of the unrealistic expectations of organizations that they had with work loads that seemed to be excessively heavy and which seemed to stretch their capabilities. A middle-aged nurse who worked in obstetrics in a community hospital told the story of her daughter who worked on the intensive care unit of another community hospital.

> With the unit that my daughter works on they had 10 patients recently, several of whom were on respirators. There was almost no staff to care for the patients and for 4 days in a row my daughter found herself unable to force herself to go to work. She felt that when she was there, there was not time even to turn patients. You know the level that you should be able to function at as a nurse and when you have too many patients and you don't have enough time to deal with patients, you know that you're potentially in trouble. She had two patients with Swans Ganz catheters. How can you attend to them when you're not sure of the equipment and you know you're missing things? You just don't want to come in.
> I know she feels that the pay she gets is good as an incentive to motivate her to go to work, but beyond a certain level of being pushed you just can't do it. She finally had to leave this ICU because of all the stress she was experiencing. She found that the work load was so heavy that even as she was leaving work on one day, she'd already be uptight about how she was going to cope the next day. She finally said, "I can't take one more day." She was just so concerned regarding her own professional and legal liability because of the inadequate staffing.

COMMUNICATION PROBLEMS
WITH ADMINISTRATION (10%)

Communication problems with administration were often related to the lack of recognition of expertise in a particular area. Nurses in a community hospital emergency room stated:

> Administration tries to tell us what to do and how to do it without input from us. They never listen to nurses, nor do they consider what we think, our problems, or the solutions that we would propose. The head nurse said, "I'm always called to meetings so I can't do the clinical work which I like, but when I go to the head nurses' meetings they don't listen to me there either.

A physician working in the same emergency room validated the nurses' feelings of a lack of respect of their expertise when he said:

The nurses here are called professional but are given no responsibility for independent judgement. They have to punch in and out, the supervisor looks at how they're dressed, they're floated to other units without any respect for their expertise, they have limited time off. They have to be there until 3:15 and then punch out. If they punch out at 3:13 they'll be called on the carpet despite the fact that they might have just spent the busiest 8 hours of their professional life.

An example of the difficulty in communication between intensive care nurses and nursing supervisors was given by Mary Roberts, a nurse who worked in a community intensive care unit. The anecdote shows the staff nurses' feelings that nursing supervisors not only expect them to work an unrealistically high intensity but in addition they fail to acknowledge that ICU nurses, as nurses on other units, do in fact have very strong feelings for the patients with whom they work.

The patient arrested and died and the nurse was upset. He had been there for a while and it bothered her when he died. I called to tell the supervisor he had died and her response was, "Great. Send that nurse down to relieve on medicine in half an hour."
   "Half an hour?" I said. "She has to pull all the tubes, stop the bleeding, clean him up, wrap him, deal with the family, clean the room, get him onto the stretcher, and into the morgue—he's really overweight—and she's upset to boot. How do you expect her to be down there in half an hour—an hour maybe she could be there." But no, the answer was, "I want her in half an hour to relieve for supper on medicine."
   Before that patient died, the nurse wasn't going to have to relieve, but all of a sudden he's dead and the supervisor wants to pull her. What are you supposed to do with your feelings in this kind of a situation?

Nurses in specialty areas derive a fair amount of pleasure out of being able to diagnose and understand the illnesses with which they're working and they can be fairly critical of coordinators who do not have the same ability to diagnose. They are particularly critical when the coordinator cannot diagnose but will attempt to criticize for something that the nurses consider to be a non-issue but which is something that the coordinator can usually understand. "You're with a patient with 'V tach' and the supervisor is looking at the monitor and doesn't know what's happening. She complains about beds in the hallway and you feeling like saying, 'Can't you see what's happening—what are your priorities?' Staff nurses were also not above testing their supervisors competence by doing such things as taking apart a monitor and asking the head nurse to put it back together. These tests seemed to be designed to test "how much would I get from you if I really needed your help."

There were also several complaints about supervisors not understanding the violence with which caregivers were confronted. "Our administration became upset because we kept calling in the police to restrain aggressive patients. They gave us self-defence lessons and told us to stop calling the police, but eventually they got us security guards" And:

A patient walked in with a rifle and pointed it at one of the nurses. A report was filled in but the coordinator wanted to know why no incident report was made out before one of the nurse's colleagues called the police. This was while somebody is pointing a gun at one of her colleagues.

The final significant problem with administration concerned the possibility of closing emergency rooms when the nurses on duty felt that they had more patients than they could handle.

We asked the supervisor to call the ambulances and advise them not to come to our hospital because all the beds in the hospital were full and all of the emergency stretchers were full. Instead of calling the ambulances, the supervisor sent the orderly for more stretchers from the operating room.

They have a lot of difficulty closing the emergency room because our board of governors are good citizens who don't want their names to be spread across the newspapers as being associated with emergency rooms which have no beds. We find stretchers if there are no beds any place because we're afraid of what the coroner might say or what the Minister of Health might say.

In these situations, however, nurses who were feeling misunderstood by coordinators said that they gave the patients who were complaining about the lack of service they were getting, the names of hospital administrators and ministry officials, and told them to please call and complain because they felt if enough complaints were received, then staffing and financial resources would be improved. They worried though, because, "Patients are afraid to get the nurse in trouble so they won't complain when they get such poor service, but we wish they would complain, so things could improve around here."

POORLY DEFINED AUTHORITY AND RESPONSIBILITY (6%)

This problem has been noted in the work of Schmalenberg and Kramer (15) and Rosenthal, Marshall, MacPherson, and French (16). This section will use only one anecdote to illustrate a fairly typical example of this problem.

Norma Diamond, a nurse on a surgical unit said that in the teaching hospital where she worked it was often difficult to interact with the house staff covering on nights.

They don't know how to glove or catheterize or do blood gases. I have to babysit because they don't know what's going on. I tried one night to get the intern to give chemotherapy on evenings, and his response was, "I'm not going to chart that I gave chemo—chemo kills people" He didn't want to do it and tried to leave the floor. Sometimes I feel like I'm a guard dog, but if I don't do it, who will? I feel that if the 12 hours on a shift I'm responsible for a patient, I want others to be too. That's what I mean by accountability.

POOR ORIENTATION AND EDUCATION (5%)

Caregivers often felt that their educational programs did not prepare them for what they would face as professionals. Dr. John Smart spoke of the difficulty he had in his medical training.

One major factor in medical school is the disillusionment—the tremendous amount of ego battering you take. For some students it provides a motivation to improve yourself, but often leaves the student with little sense of self-esteem. We're left in despair. It's education by intimidation. We had one surgeon teaching us who used to yell and scream at everyone who would take it. He was glad when they didn't take it and when they spoke back. Medical school is full of people like that. Those who are different stand out like stars. Recently my chief said to me, "Nothing you do will be perfectly acceptable to me. I know what you're capable of and I'll push you." There's the feeling that to learn and to be best it has to be painful.

McCue (17) states that physicians are often not taught the type of skills that they will need in practice. Never having learned these skills and having poor role models, physicians find it difficult to perform the kind of tasks and functions expected of them in practice. Other professional groups also mentioned this lack of practical education as well as the absence of a supportive milieu in which to learn. A chaplain noted: "The clergy here have only been trained to deal with death issues intellectually. They're not in touch with their feelings at all. The university has built up a lively little system that covers everything and keeps personal involvement out of it."

Nurses mentioned the lack of preparation for the types of roles they were expected to perform, and a lack of proper evaluation of their performance within these roles. A study by Dr. Derek Doyle (18) examined some of the information deficiencies experienced by nurses working with dying patients. It was found that only 52% of nurses had had specific training in the assessment and control of pain in dying patients, that only 36% knew about the distresses experienced by palliative care patients, that only 44% were aware of the special emotional problems of the patients, and that only 35% had had specialized training in dealing with families in bereavement prediction and counseling.

Social workers also complained of a lack of orientation and education, particularly when working within a medical environment where other staff familiar with the language discussed medical procedures. A social worker commented: "I feel inadequate lots of times because I can't do anything physical to help people. I don't understand lots of stuff that the staff talks about. I go to rounds and read, but that isn't quite enough."

A lack of adequate education may preceed beginning work on a specialty unit and then a lack of an adequate or ongoing orientation program may well complicate the issue.

> A resident recently said to me, "I'm so scared, what am I going to do? I have to take care of this man on a balloon pump. I'll have to get a book to know how to take care of this man" At least he had the guts to have the book there, others don't. I've seen medical students or interns try seven times in order to be able to get a catheter into a patient. They won't go to the staff man to admit their lack of knowledge and the patient winds up with seven holes in his legs.

Orienting new staff members to the technical aspects of an intensive care unit is clearly quite crucial, but in addition, caregivers also need to have some understanding of the emotional aspects of the unit. Randy Little, a nurse clinician on a CCU said that:

> Here there's lots of orientation for the new nurses but no orientation to how they're apt to feel about this place. I think we should have orientation to how you're going to feel with what you're going to be doing. The new nurses are afraid to talk with the head nurse about the feelings they have because they're afraid that she'll sense that they're not coping. Perhaps some kind of nonthreatening group situation would be helpful—some place where they could discuss what it feels like to be working for the first time.

Nurses who had been actively working in a number of different settings sometimes mentioned that they felt that they should have more ongoing education, and yet frequently when units attempt to offer this, staff members do not feel that they have the time to attend. Some nurse clinicians and head nurses have suggested that nurses in this type of situation should have an obligation to do at least some of their educational preparation on their own time. When, however, units are beginning to bring in new technology, then it behooves them to provide adequate training and preparation for the caregivers to use this equipment. Despite the fact this seems quite logical, it was interesting to note how often staff complained that it was not done.

REFERENCES

1. Vreeland, R., & Ellis, G. L. (1969). Stresses on the nurse in an intensive care unit. *Journal of the American Medical Association, 208,* 332-334.

2. Gentry, W. D., Foster, S. B., & Froehling, S. (1972). Psychologic response to situational stress in intensive and nonintensive nursing. *Heart and Lung, 1,* 793-796.

3. Huckaby, L., & Jagla, B. (1979). Nurses' stress factors in the intensive care unit. *Journal of Nursing Administration, 9*(2) 21-26.

4. Anderson, C. A., & Basteyns, M. (1981). Stress and the critical care nurse reaffirmed. *Journal of Nursing Administration, 11*(1) 31-34.

5. Nichols, K. A., Springford, V., & Searle, J. (1981). An investigation of distress and discontent in various types of nursing. *Journal of Advanced Nursing, 6,* 311-318.

6. Steffen, S. M. (1980). Perceptions of stress: 1800 nurses tell their stories. In K. E. Claus & J. T. Bailey (Eds.), *Living with stress and promoting well-being: A handbook for nurses.* (pp. 38-58). St. Louis: C. V. Mosby.

7. Yancik, R. (1984). Sources of work stress for hospice staff. *Journal of Psychosocial Oncology, 2,* 21-31.

8. White, W. L. (1978). *Incest in the organizational family: The unspoken issue in staff and program burnout.* Rockville, MD: H.C.S., Inc.

9. Campbell, D. W. (1980). Death anxiety on a coronary care unit. *Psychosomatics, 21*(2) 127.

10. Lowry, F. (1982, June 15). Opening abortion clinics. *The Medical Post,* p. 15.

11. Segers, M. C. (1982). Can congress settle the abortion issue. *The Hastings Center Report,* 12(3) 20-28.

12. Bourne, J. P. (1972). Abortion: Influences on health professionals' attitudes. *Hospitals, 46,* 80-83.

13. Gentry, W. D., & Parkes, K. R. (1982). Psychologic stress in intensive care unit and non-intensive care unit nursing: A review of the past decade. *Heart and Lung, 11,* 43-47.

14. Marshall, R. E., & Kasman, C. (1980). Burnout in the neonatal intensive care unit. *Pediatrics, 65,* 1161-1165.

15. Schmalenberg, C., & Kramer, M. (1979). *Coping with reality shock: The voices of experience.* Wakefield, MA: Nursing Resources.

16. Rosenthal, C. J., Marshall, V. W., MacPherson, A. S., & French, S. E. (1980). *Nurses, patients and families.* New York: Springer.

17. McCue, J. D. (1982). The effects of stress on physicians and their medical practice. *The New England Journal of Medicine, 306,* 458-463.

18. Doyle, D. (1982). Nursing education in terminal care. *Nurse Education Today, 2*(4) 4-6.

5

Life as a Professional

Role Stressors

Not only did professionals experience stress within their work environments, they also found certain aspects of their professional roles to be difficult. Variables related to stressors in ones' work environment accounted for 26% of the occupational stressors mentioned ($N = 808$ anecdotes). Physicians were somewhat more apt to report role-related stressors than were other professionals. This was perhaps due to the fact that their more independent role left them somewhat less vulnerable to environmental stressors, while at the same time their role presented its own particular and unique stressors, as will be seen throughout this chapter.

The occupational role stressors that we will discuss are derived from two different sources: (1) the professional role that one occupies, and (2) various aspects of our professional roles. For example, there are different role stressors inherent in the role of physician and nurse or clergy and social worker, yet each professional group, while experiencing some unique professional stressors, also has other stressors such as role overload, or role conflict in common. This chapter will therefore discuss both the stressors unique to each professional group as well as those they share in common, albeit perhaps in somewhat different ways.

OCCUPATIONAL STRESSORS AND PROFESSIONAL ROLES

Table 5 in the Appendix shows that in response to the demands of their professional roles, each of the three major professional groups surveyed experienced different stressors. From this table it can be seen that nurses most often reported difficulty with team communication problems, dealing with patients and families who have personality problems or difficulty in coping with their illness, factors relating to the type of unit on which they work, and inadequate resources or staffing. Their stressors can be seen to reflect their perceived role as coordinator of patient care; their close proximity to patients and families when problems are acute; and the fact that they are the team members most often assigned to a particular unit, without the freedom to "escape" to other activities such as going to other wards, teaching, attending rounds, etc. This close proximity to the unit's stressors makes them particularly vulnerable to experiencing stress because of constant exposure to dying patients and their families, high technology, inappropriate bed utilization, a "fish-bowl" environment—or other stressors in the unit. In addition, their role makes them particularly aware of inadequate resources— a lack of supplies and outdated equipment, or a lack of qualified staff to carry out basic patient care.

The stressors reported by physicians differed from those mentioned by other caregivers. Their greatest stressor was difficulty in communicating with others in the organization, usually other physicians, but sometimes with other departments. This was nowhere near as great a problem for other caregivers whose roles tended to isolate them somewhat more from others in the environment outside of their unit and may have thus caused them to focus on team communication problems. This difference may also of course reflect the fact that physicians might not have seen themselves as being members of an interdisciplinary team. Hence, they might have seen problems with other team members as being communication problems with "others." The two other stressors that were major problems for physicians also presented much less difficulty for other caregivers. These were role overload and role strain, which usually involved difficulty in decision-making. The stressors reported by physicians can be seen to reflect some of the lack of understanding or the rivalry they experience with their colleagues when they are trying to develop new programs, secure the type of care they want for the people they are treating, obtain recognition for their work, or when fighting political battles. They were more apt to report role overload because their professional role was most likely to encompass multiple roles—teaching, research, patient care, administration, etc. Those caregivers reporting multiple roles related that their greatest role stressor was role overload. Physicians were more likely than other groups to report difficulty with decision-making because theirs is the professional group with the major legal responsibility for decision-making in patient care. The difficulty and stress sometimes experienced in making these decisions will become clear later in this chapter.

The counselor group included social workers, psychologists, and clergy. Their greatest stressors came from role ambiguity, patient/family personality or coping problems, and communication problems with administration and other team members. It is interesting that the group of caregivers whose major role is communication report that their greatest stressors are related to communication problems.

OCCUPATIONAL ROLE STRESSORS

Research has shown that the profile of a "good job" for many people would be:

> ... one in which the work is interesting, I have a chance to develop my own special abilities, and I can see the results of my work. It is a job where I have enough information, enough help and equipment, and enough authority to get the job done. It is a job where the supervisor is competent and my responsibilities are clearly defined. The people I work with are friendly and helpful; the pay is good and so is the job security (1, p. 48).

It was clear in Chapter 4 and will become more clear in Chapter 5 that these factors are not always characteristic of the positions held by our respondents.

Coburn reported that men who found their work interesting and challenging tended to be satisfied with their jobs but to experience a good deal of stress. Comparing those who were satisfied with their work with those who weren't however, he found the stress levels to be quite similar. The two most important factors that affected feelings of stress were the number of deadlines experienced and the degree to which the job was seen as interfering with one's family life (2).

Somewhat similar findings emerged from a study by Hawk (3) of family practice residents where it was found that the more hours a week the residents worked, the greater were both their feelings of personal accomplishment and the stress they reported in being a resident. However, the frequency with which the residents felt a sense of accomplishment seemed to decrease with the increase in the problems they experienced in trying to combine their personal and professional lives. Female residents reported significantly higher levels of symptoms of stress as well as stress in response to trying to combine personal and professional lives.

Similar findings were also reported by entry-level nurses. In a study conducted by Schmalenberg and Kramer (4), the competition between nonwork interests and activities and the job caused these neophyte nurses to feel that they were being consumed or swallowed up by the work of nursing.

Fry, Lech, and Rubin have stated that group members need to develop ways of achieving goals. They have found that in any group there are questions concerning: "a) the extent to which such expectations are clearly defined and communicated (role ambiguity); b) the extent to which such expectations are compatible or in conflict (role conflict); and c) the extent to which any individual is capable of meeting the multiple expectations (role overload)" (5, p. 35). Similar findings were found with the caregivers surveyed for this book in that three out of the four top stressors cited were role ambiguity, role conflict, and role overload.

ROLE AMBIGUITY (20%)

Kahn et al. have stated that "Each member of an organization must have certain kinds of information at his disposal if he is to perform his job adequately" (1, p. p. 22). To adequately perform in one's role, an individual must understand the expectations that others have of the role. One must understand the rights, duties, and responsibilities of the office, what activities on the individual's part will fulfill these responsibilities, and how these activities can best be performed. When there is a lack of clear, consistent information about what is expected of a person in a role, or when an individual does not understand what others expect of someone in that role, then role ambiguity exists. In general, the more ambiguity one experiences in one's role, the more tension and anxiety are felt. Furthermore most people want less role ambiguity than they have (6).

In the present study, role ambiguity was greatest amongst the social workers and clergy and was the major role stressor in palliative care, pediatric chronic care and intensive care units. Social workers frequently felt that nurses were defining their role in such a way as to overlap with the role that social workers felt belonged to them. This was particularly a problem between social workers and either clinical nurse specialists or primary care nurses.

Some social workers mentioned that part of the difficulty with role ambiguity was that their profession itself was frequently unclear on what it should be doing and this lack of clarity then extended to the institutions in which social workers were employed. Theresa Little, an oncology social worker, stated:

> There are lots of problems in the social worker role which haven't been sorted out yet. We can't decide whether we really should be focusing on doing placement of patients, or on doing psychotherapy. There don't seem to be any long-term goals in the profession. As a group we have a lot of ambivalence about both ourselves and our role. We still feel that being assertive is being aggressive. From my perspective you have to like what you do and sell it. This is the only way we're going to get credibility, but social workers don't work to establish credibility. We also have great difficulty banding together to help the profession. I ask myself why, when the job of social workers is processing through relationships, they have so much difficulty processing through their own career.

The clergy also experienced considerable role ambiguity. Wood (7) has noted the uncertainty that is often present with regard to the role of the clergy in that ministers are frequently uncertain about proper procedures, what expectations are held relative to their behavior, and what the consequences of any given action might be.

Reverend Dave Tracy is a chaplain who moved from a large teaching center to a small community hospital. In the university hospital he was used to attending rounds, reading patients' charts, and being a member of the health team. When he undertook his role as pastoral care coordinator in the community hospital, he found it difficult to define his role where no previous pattern existed.

> You go to the desk and introduce yourself to the nurses and doctors and say that you're the new pastoral care coordinator and you'd like to be involved on the team. They look at you like you're crazy and say, "Why would we need you? We're the nurses and doctors—we're the professionals. We don't need any help." But then they call you after the death has happened—after the vase has been shattered on the floor, and you're supposed to talk about how God needed another angel so he reached down and plucked Margaret to be an angel with him in heaven. It doesn't work. They don't acknowledge all the training we've had in psychology, theology, counseling, grief. We can be a lot of help if they'll let us in.

Another aspect of institutionalized role ambiguity arises from the fact that what nurses are expected to do during the busy day shift when all the other members of the health care team are present may be very different from what they are expected to do on evenings and nights when other staff are at home. A nurse in a community hospital labor room said: "On days when the doctors are around we 'yes them' to death. Then on evenings and nights we have to handle it all and only call them when it's time for them to be there. Your head is on the chopping block if there's a problem or you don't call on time, but likewise you're also on the chopping block if you call too early."

Those working in palliative care also reported significant stress that often evolved from the fact that their role was not clearly defined. Similar findings were reported by Mount and Voyer in their most impressive descriptive analysis of the stressors at the Royal Victoria Hospital Palliative Care Service (8). As we saw in Chapter 4 hospice or palliative care programs or teams were often started without having worked through the resistance of the other professionals in the hospital or community. Frequently the hospice team was accorded a token role but did not really have the power to influence the care that the patient received.

Such an example was given by a palliative care coordinator in a community who said: "Recently one of our most resistant physicians stopped me to chat on the stairs and to ask us to see one of his patients about symptom control. It was really nice of him to ask but he turned out to be like so many others, they feel like they've done their 'bit' by giving us the consult but they won't do anything we suggest."

Part of the reason for this unwillingness to follow through with the suggestions of the consult team derives from the fact that other staff members may either not want suggestions about improving their care, as it implies certain deficiencies in their competence, or else they may want someone else to "do something, rather than just making suggestions." When the role of a hospice or palliative care team is ambiguously defined then stress responses may be seen both on the team and with other staff members. A palliative care consultation team spoke of the difficulties they had in their setting:

> Originally the plan was for a hospice unit but the hospital finally settled on the concept of a symptom control team. It wasn't clear, however, what each team member would do and where. They hadn't really looked at issues like leadership, decisions, referral systems. Ours is a hospital rich in resources with a clinical specialist, clergy, and social worker on each floor. The environment just wasn't prepared for what they considered to be the "intrusion" of consultants. We've now learned that lots of times when staff are 'swamped' they want someone to pitch in and help, and not just someone who wants to "just talk about feelings." Now we sometimes do primary care and with 'heavy cases' we may share the load with the staff.

The role ambiguity in hospice work is further exacerbated by the presence of volunteers as integral members of the team, yet members whose role is often quite ambiguously defined. Rita O'Neil, a hospice volunteer coordinator described the advantages and disadvantages of role ambiguity for volunteers when she said:

> The role of a volunteer here is fairly open, because to be effective there cannot be too many rigid guidelines. That means, however, that the multitude of options which are open to volunteers may cause them to feel stress. Because their role is not clearly defined, they may also tend to overdo and become 'little green gods'. So maybe their role should be more clearly defined—but its beauty is in not being too over-structured.

Not suprisingly this role ambiguity leads to comments like that made by a nursing director. "One of the nurses' major problems is the volunteer who needs constant nurturing. The nurse knows she is doing a good job because she knows what good nursing is. ... the volunteer has more trouble because (she or he) doesn't know what good volunteering is."

Staff working with chronically ill children also reported difficulty with role ambiguity. Since all staff members were endeavoring to do a good job in taking care of chronically ill and dying children, and were usually willing to "go the extra mile", it was not surprising that the roles caregivers were expected to assume were not always clearly defined. This lack of clear-cut definition caused significant difficulty for many caregivers. One of the major difficulties in defining roles came in the interaction between social workers and nurses. In a pediatric oncology unit the arrival of a new social worker led to difficulty with role ambiguity when nurses who had previously counseled patients were told this was now to be the social worker's role and they were to call her 24 hours a day if family counseling needed to be done. "There's no question there's resistance from both sides. We've been burned before when social workers got too involved with patients and decided that they couldn't handle things and walked out. The message this gives off to staff is, 'This is too much to cope with'—we're the ones who know that we have to be able to stay there and hang in."

Intensive care units also experienced difficulties with role ambiguity. Rosini, Howell, Todres, & Dorman (9) state that the required teamwork and the emergency crisis orientation of an ICU means that doctors and nurses often perform tasks not normally their responsibility. In these situations there are frequently a lack of clearly understood role expectations and task definitions that can lead to role ambiguity, confusion, and strife. When mistakes occur there can be accusations of blame and feelings of guilt.

With the issue of decision-making surrounding the cessation of treatment, role ambiguity can provide considerable stress. Nurses spoke of the fact that in this situation the physician clearly has the legal right to make these decisions. Yet he or she may be hesitant to put this decision in writing. The nurse is then put in the uncomfortable position of a decision being made but no order being written. Nevertheless, she is generally expected by physicians to follow this unwritten order while she questions herself about what her legal responsibility is in this situation. "No one writes the order, but a ventilator gets either turned off or turned down sometimes. The nurse has to figure out what to put in the chart. We have to figure out what to say in the chart to explain why it looks like a child was under active treatment and then dead with nothing in between."

Physicians are often hesitant to write any orders about turning off or turning down ventilators for fear of the legal problems that may ensue. Nurses frequently get caught in this situation as they are aware that the physician has turned down the ventilator but feel that there is little that they can do to clarify their own role in this situation. Nurses who clarify their roles and develop clearly defined roles and areas of expertise run the risk of being negatively labeled.

The nurses on one unit were left with unresolved feelings when an anesthetist, completing a month's rotation on the unit left with the parting comment, "You're the most castrating bunch of females I've ever met." The comment hurt, although they knew it was partly a tribute to their competence, a reflection of his feelings of inadequacy, and a comment on the role ambiguity that existed on the unit.

ROLE CONFLICT (19%)

Kahn has found that "persons subjected to high role conflict report greater job-related tensions, lower job satisfaction, less confidence in the organization itself, and more intense experience of conflict" (10, p. 5). In addition, role conflict is associated with poor interpersonal relationships in that those who experience high role conflict are more apt to report that they have less trust in members of their role set, respect them less, like them less, and communicate with them less. These findings of course explain many of the problems with team communication discussed in Chapter 4. Yet not everyone responds to role conflict in the same way. People who tend to be anxiety prone experience more intense conflict and react with more tension than do people who are not anxiety prone. Similarly, introverts react more negatively to role conflict than do extroverts in that the former suffer more tension and report more deterioration in their interpersonal relationships as a result of role conflict. Kahn also reported that the more frequent the communication between role senders and the individual, the more the individual is dependent on others in his role set; and the greater the power of the role set, the more signs of strain they show when role conflict occurred. Finally, in this study Kahn found that almost half of his respondents reported being "caught in the middle" between two conflicting persons or factions, more or less frequently (10).

In view of these data, it is not surprising to find that role conflict was the major stressor for nurses, and the second greatest role stressor for social workers. Both of these professional groups frequently find themselves in a variety of the role conflict situations to which we have already alluded. It is perhaps also not surprising to find that with regard to specialty areas, those in obstetrics had the most difficulty with role conflict. Much of this difficulty was in direct response to the stress experienced with the issues surrounding abortion.

Schmalenberg and Kramer (4) have identified four types of role conflict, derived from the earlier work of Kahn et al. (1):

(a) interrole or role-role conflict
(b) intrasender conflict
(c) intrarole conflict, and
(d) "self-role conflict"

"Interrole or role-role conflict results when a person holds two or more roles simultaneously and the expectations of one role conflict with the expectations of the other" (4, p. 205).

Dr. Ed Travers, a family practitioner, reflected on the interrole conflict of a physician and a family member, and the job-home interaction conflict that could ensue:

> I look around the office and think to myself that I'll be finished by 5:30 and by 6:30 I'll be home and ready to take the family to the cottage for the weekend, as I've been promising them. Then at 4:30 p.m. Mr. Jones calls to say that his wife is on the floor and can't move. I take a careful history to know if I have to go there to do a house call or whether to call an ambulance. I then have to call the ambulance myself because if he called, they'd just take her to the nearest hospital instead of the hospital where her records are. Then I call the hospital to prepare the resident for her arrival. When all that's done it's 5:30 and the office is still full.
>
> I'm late leaving and on the way home in the car the stress begins to build up. I know the family expects me to be there already and they're going to be mad when I get home. They don't care that Mrs. Jones is on the floor—they want to go to the cottage. There have been too many Mrs. Jones over the years.

Interrole conflict may also be experienced by people who have two or more professional roles that may be in conflict. A physician who worked temporarily as a researcher stated that the most difficult year of his professional career was the year that he did a study on the issue of abortion.

> I was constantly listening to opposing people, many of whom were entirely too biased one way or the other. From 6:00 a.m. to 10:00 p.m. every day I thought, wrote, and talked abortion. Then there were crank phone calls in the middle of the night of babies crying.
>
> I wound up being very ambivalent about the whole abortion issue. Then my first day back in the clinical setting the whole issue was resolved. With individual patients with specific problems it's a fairly straightforward issue. Many people can resolve the

issue on a one-to-one basis but it is much more difficult to decide the abortion issue for community or society.

Another anecdote regarding interrole conflict came from a nurse who experienced conflict between her own concept of her role as a professional nurse and her role as an employee of an institution accountable to a supervisor within an authority structure.

> I was working nights and a woman who had a prostaglandin injection aborted a live fetus. It was at least 24 weeks and wouldn't die. I didn't know what to do or what my responsibilities were. I called the night coordinator who said, "Package it away and have a cup of tea." It lived for 45 minutes. When I first handled it, it started moving. I said, "Hey, this isn't a fetus, it's a baby." It changed its status. I didn't tell the mother.
>
> I felt lost. What do you do? Usually prostins come out burned, not alive. I was angry towards management. They don't know what we're going through. When I couldn't get help from the coordinator I weighed the baby and decided that if it was over 500 grams then I would consider it viable. It was under 500 grams.

Interrole conflict in obstetrics was most often experienced by caregivers who had to work simultaneously with abortion and obstetrical patients. A chaplain said:

> It's a crazy world; in my last job I was part of the staff of the abortion unit but would be called up to the neonatal unit to baptize babies just slightly older than the ones being aborted.
>
> One day I followed a woman through the whole abortion procedure. I felt that I had to observe the reality of what happened so that I knew I wasn't playing games with myself. That afternoon I was called to the neonatal ICU to baptize a baby just 2 weeks older than the one aborted.
>
> It really served to focus my own ambivalence in this area and to make me aware of how fuzzy the lines of life and death are as technology pushes us to the outer limits. No one could give me a clear ethical guideline to fit both situations. . . .

Intrasender conflict occurs when the person sending out messages is giving double or contradictory messages. An obstetrical nurse said, "I really have trouble when I'm rushing around caring for ten patients—five new C-sections and five postpartums, and the head nurse who gave me the assignment stops me to tell me to clean up the utility room. How I'm supposed to do all these things at once is beyond me."

Intrarole conflict results because caregivers operate in roles in which there is more than one group of people who have expectations of how they should perform. A pharmacist complained that he could not tell the people in his drugstore about the interaction of the multiple drugs they were taking without causing their physicians to become angry. He felt conflicted because he felt his responsibility lay with the patients, yet he feared professional censure from the physicians in his community who threatened to boycott his store.

Miss Barbara Thompson, a nurse-coordinator in obstetrics and gynecology described a staff nurse's intrarole conflict:

> When the doctor "gets it all" with cancer surgery, they are so proud of themselves and spend lots of time with the patient who feel that they're like a god. When he can't get it all though he gets out of the room as soon as possible and the nurse is left holding the bag. She knows that the patient hasn't been told what's really going

on, and she feels torn between loyalty to the doctor and feeling that the patient should know.

Schmalenberg and Kramer found that new nurses whom they studied eventually decided which role pressures from which members of their role set would take precedence. "Depending upon which role relationship is more important to her—the physician's or the patient's—and consequently which role pressure is more effective—the physician's or the patient's—she makes a choice. The tension generated by the conflict is reduced with the choice and by concentrating future involvement with those members of the role set whom the nurse has decided are more important to her" (4, p. 224). Unfortunately the caregivers in this study did not seem to have quite the same smooth adjustment to such a decision. Caregivers frequently tended to feel torn over extended periods of time.

Multiple sources of role conflict sometimes interacted simultaneously. This was particularly well illustrated by a social worker from the midwest whose physician colleague resolved his role conflicts in a manner that in turn created role conflicts for her. She said:

> The chief of my service feels that all the professionals on staff should do more than just work with cystic fibrosis children, but that the CF kids must always come first. He feels that he should always be able to have his secretary call and tell you to be there on a weekend or whenever he wants you to be there. It's not at all unusual for me to get a message from his secretary saying that a certain patient is coming in at noon on Saturday and Dr. Jones want you there. My husband gets mad at me. Furthermore, Dr. Jones never shows up himself. He's now at the stage of life where he takes a lot of time to be with his own kids, but he doesn't allow us as staff members the same option. It really became clear to me when one of his private patients was dying and I found myself completely alone with this patient for long hours with no physician, nurse, or anyone else. I went to him and told him that I felt really abandoned in this situation. Things weren't the same between us for the next 2 months. He really seems to expect us to sacrifice everything because his patients are dying. I have to ask myself what kind of message we're giving parents when we overextend ourselves like this. Do we give them the message that they too should be constantly overextending?

Self-role conflict occurs when the expectations of the role are in opposition to one's personality characteristics or needs. For example, a 22-year-old nurse said:

> I've always believed that abortions were okay, but I never had to work with abortion patients. One day I was floated to labor and delivery. A saline abortion patient was yelling in pain. I went to get her medication and returned to find that she had aborted. She passed the membranes—that's the grossest part. I refused to go back in. I just couldn't.
> I wouldn't have expected this reaction from myself. I was shocked that I was repulsed. I thought it would be a challenge. I've been okay on obstetrical units when a woman had a spontaneous abortion in bed—that didn't bother me at all. But this did. I suppose I made a value judgement on the girl and the grotesqueness of the situation got to me. I thought to myself, "I'm relieving, I don't have to cope with this. I'll go start IVs."

Similar findings were noted by McCue (11) who wrote of the difficulty that physicians face when they discover they have psychological discomfort with fundamental professional activities, or when they find that there are conflicts between their long held expectations and the reality of medical practice.

Winnifred Hummell, a birth control counselor in her early thirties who had worked in the area for several years reflected on the self-role conflicts she still experienced, how she had resolved them, and how she might resolve these conflicts differently in another role.

> I have to constantly ask myself, "What's my involvement? What's my complicity in abortions?" Usually I can separate them. I know though that if I were a physician I'd be more discriminating about who I'd work with. There are certain reasons that I just wouldn't accept like, "I just bought a house and it's not the right time."
> As a nurse I am there to support the woman in her decision. It took me time to realize that it's not my decision—it's hers. I'd feel differently if I were a doctor though because then it would be partly my responsibility and I would be more selective.

Role conflict in neonatal intensive care units is evidenced in the literature in articles by Kachoris (12) and Marshall and Kasman (13) but the concepts they describe can equally be applied to other settings, especially in pediatrics. They suggest that the staff members in a neonatal intensive care unit, in addition to their professional roles often, at a symbolic level, become surrogate parents to the children. This may result in self-role conflict. Kachoris suggests that the physician often unconsciously plays out the paternal role while the nurse plays out the maternal role. The physician assumes the role of protector and provider and undertakes the responsibility to help the infant survive by combatting the factors that could lead to death. In the paternal role the physician has enormous authority and control because he is seen as having a fund of knowledge and experience. He can order, prescribe, and control interventions that lead to feelings of omnipotence, grandiosity, and an elevation in his feelings of self-esteem and worth. The nurse, as the maternal surrogate often assumes the role of provider of care, love, and nurturing. She administers medications and treatments, she feeds, cleans, bathes, changes, holds, cradles, rocks, and sings to the baby. She comforts and soothes the baby, learns its pattern of behavior and gradually becomes more and more sensitive to the nuances of this behavior. NICU nurses often speak of "my baby" and "your baby" and compare the babies' progress and chances for survival. The nurse spends long hours at a baby's side and frequently smiles, coos, and speaks to the infant for some kind of acknowledgement.

When it becomes clear that the child will die the nurse may then be caught between continuing to provide ministrations to the baby or withholding them because of impending death. This process creates ambivalence in the nurse about the quantity of attachment she has available to offer, and yet she may still desire to do so (12). Marshall and Kasman (13) and Fulton (14) suggest that the nurse who becomes a surrogate parent then feels a personal and deep grief with each baby or child's relapse or death.

In this current study, nurses and pediatricians at one children's hospital experienced considerable role conflict because both groups wanted to perform the warm, maternal functions for the children, particularly for those who were dying. The staff physicians often felt that nurses were usurping part of their role when they became increasingly involved with dying patients and their families.

In another situation, a volunteer observed that her flexible role created role conflict for nurses because she had the time to do the special things for children with cancer that the nurses would have liked to do personally if they were not already burdened with multiple role demands.

Mrs. O'Hara became a volunteer in a cancer treatment center because her own child had died of cancer. She spoke of her role and the insight she had developed into how it caused conflict for nurses:

> When kids are sick they need to have somebody spend time with them, talking to them, helping them to take a bath, being considerate in caring for that person. The nurses have a calling to do this kind of work, but very often they get taken away from being able to do it by technology. They may become angry when along comes the volunteer with hours to spend with the patient doing the sorts of things that the nurses would love to be able to do. Imagine what happens when I then develop the type of relationship with the children that they used to have. Initially it was pretty hard, but now we've been able to work it out.

The issue of pain relief was also a source of role conflict in many settings. One nurse said: "We want to be able to give the kids enough medication for pain without killing them. We all want to be able to give a shot to cope with the pain, but not the 'last shot', so we find we get into bargaining with regard to who'll give the 'last shot'."

LACK OF CONTROL (12%)

According to Kahn et al. (1), job control is associated with autonomy and generally refers to the control a worker has over his or her own time and activity. A lack of control over one's job, especially in relation to the pace of work and working methods has also been associated with increased job stress (15), especially if one has an internal locus of control and wishes to be able to have control over the work environment. Dr. Sam Toomey, a resident, spoke of the lack of control he had over his own time and activity. "I have absolutely no control over the environment. Lots of times, I vow that today will be different. I'll run like hell and get out on time. I run like hell and get so exhausted that I have trouble when an emergency crops up. I'm at the beck and call of everyone—staff doctors, nurses, the admitting office, switchboard."

In the health care system a lack of control is also related to issues of authority. Within the present study nurses reported somewhat more difficulty with a perceived lack of authority than did other professional groups. Rosenthal, Marshall, MacPherson, and French (16) point out that within the health care system, nurses have power and authority over patients but are themselves subject to the power and authority of physicians, administrators, and in some respects the law. They note that with the exception of patients, no group within the health care system more keenly feels the effect of physicians' superordinate status, even sometimes with regard to nonmedical activities. The impact of physician control over nursing decisions may, of course, vary with particular settings and may be reflective of the role of nursing and medicine within a particular setting. For example, a nurse who had previously worked in a university teaching hospital and was now working in a community hospital, commented, "When I was at the University Hospital we adopted nursing process and it was of no concern to the physicians. Here it has to go through medical committees and we almost weren't allowed to do it. They really object to our doing nursing histories and asking about such issues as sexuality."

Caregivers in obstetrics and emergency rooms were most likely to report difficulty with a lack of control. This was often related to the fact that they felt they were exposed to stressors, which were inherently potentially stressful to begin with but then elicited a greater stress response because of the perception that caregivers had a complete lack of control over the situation. For example, nurses in obstetrics who worked with women having abortions often felt that they had little control over the situation and felt that they were "dumped" into the role of working with these women. They had often come into obstetrics wanting to work in a "happy" setting, caring for newborns, and instead found themselves caring for abortion parents.

But nurses can sometimes exert control. Neubardt and Schulman (17) reported that in their clinical setting when staff complained about their distress in aborting fetuses beyond 19-20 weeks of gestation, their setting refused to do them beyond that point except on medical grounds. Other professional groups also developed mechanisms of control as a coping mechanism that served to decrease the stress they felt. Dr. Ed Hines said:

> Even though intellectually aborting a particular pregnancy makes sense, I can't think of even one of our physicians who doesn't have doubts, especially in the second trimester.
> Part of the way they get around it is like dropping atomic bombs on Hiroshima—they aren't around to see the result of their actions when the patient expells the fetus in bed. Or, when he sees it after a saline abortion it's macerated—a darker color because of the blue dye we use, and very lifeless.

While the physician gains control by "not being around to see the result of their actions when the patient expels the fetus in the bed" the same option is not open to nurses who have to handle the fetus. They often feel abandoned by the physicians who performed the procedure. Thus it becomes obvious that one professional group's attempt to gain control over a particular stressor may lead to another professional group's increased stress. Several of the nurses interviewed were exerting their own form of control. They had worked in the area for several years and were planning to gain control by leaving their jobs. None of the other professional groups interviewed planned to leave, but they exercised control in a variety of other ways. Dr. Deborah Devine said that she managed to continue to work in the abortion field by no longer doing saline abortions.

> I did them day in and day out for 6 years. They were so time consuming. Often there were complications such as the placenta sticking. I didn't have to be there to see the fetus but I still had to be around in case of problems.
> They took a lot of time and a lot of hospital visits. You never knew when they'd abort—anywhere from a few hours to 2-3 days. They took a lot of time and there were a lot of complications.
> I decided that I'd prefer to spend that time doing my research.

Not all physicians have the power to exert control over their clinical practice. For some, their position in the status hierarchy is such that they may feel obligated to perform procedures even when they feel they should not. A psychologist related that a young staff physician who seemed to love the challenge of doing radical surgery such as pelvic exenteration and vulvectomies called "in hysterics" one day. He had been told by his Chief of Staff that he had to do an abortion on a woman 4-5 months pregnant. "They're alive then. The infant is alive at that point and they want me to murder it. I can't say 'no' to my chief. I have to scream at you because I have to let it out."

Other caregivers described how junior medical staff were treated as "low men on the totem pole"—being in the powerless position of having to perform more abortions than they might want to. This situation can be compounded by their age and stage of life as they are in the process of starting up a new practice and, perhaps starting a family themselves. They felt pressured to take all the work referred to them by their colleagues while at the same time they resented their position and lack of control. They tended to take out this resentment in a variety of ways. One nurse described the actions of one doctor:

> Most of the doctors around here don't talk much to the nurses about how they feel about abortions, but one used to talk to the head nurse because she was a friend. He would get angry once in a while and would say "these sluts." He hated doing abortions but had to because he had a new practice without much gynecology.
>
> Part of the problem was that he was religious and had feelings about the morality of abortions. Now his practice is going and he's much more caring with his own patients—maybe even with the abortion patients.

Other low status groups reacted in a different way in order to gain a sense of control. The chief of a large teaching hospital's Department of Obstetrics and Gynecology mentioned that the residents in that institution were increasingly more resistant to performing abortions, feeling that they were not learning experiences but rather repetitions, unpleasant technical acts. (See also 18). Gradually the number of residents choosing to do their residency in this particular hospital decreased. As a result, staff physicians decided to limit the number of abortions residents would be expected to perform. This shift in role expectations may be to the patient's advantage as well, for studies have shown that inexperienced residents can cause considerable distress to patients. Brachen (19) found that patients aborted by less skilled operators were up to four times more likely to report continued anxiety after the procedure than were women aborted by more skilled operators.

Often physicians resolve the issue of doing abortions and gain some sense of control by having one or two physicians in a particular institution or community perform most of the abortions. Hall (20) suggests that these people are often held in fairly low regard by their colleagues. Often they are willing to accept this hostility because they see their role as having an important social function. The physicians interviewed who did a large number of abortions had developed a sense of meaning in what they were doing but found it important to integrate their abortion work with other types of professional work. This use of multiple roles served to decrease potential job stress and increase personal job satisfaction. Dr. Norm Herron serves as a good illustration: "I get lots of referrals for teenage abortions because I'll take them even if they don't have money. So I say okay. I'll do four abortions every morning then I'll go and try to fix up tubes because the real stress of my job is working with the women who constitute 99% of my practice who are infertile."

Sometimes the lack of control that caregivers feel may not be so much a reality as one's perception of the situation. Doctor Norman Thomas, a psychiatrist, suggested that the lack of control and powerlessness felt by nurses in an emergency room might be in part a reflection of the interaction between their own personality and the environment in which they work. He mentioned a psychiatric resident who was choked in an interview room by a patient. As soon as this occurred, the hospital set about improving the interview rooms for patients in order to minimize the possibility of this happening. It was recognized that the interview rooms were very small and windowless, which might well increase certain patients' paranoia and no protection was offered for anyone interviewing patients in this situation.

> The head nurse said to me, "You doctors can always get things done. No one bothers when we're getting assaulted." I realize that it wouldn't have mattered to hospital administrators who was assaulted in this situation. They would certainly have taken the necessary precautions to keep it from happening again. I could also see that this nurse had a hell of a lot more power than she recognized that she had. I said to her, "This is how to do it if you want to get something done" but she didn't want to know that she had power. The feeling of emergency room nurses that they have no power and clout has to do with their fear of injury. In the emergency care situation a patient is rendered helpless and gives himself over to the caregiver. The fact that this really competent lady was saying that I have more power than she does reflected the fact that nurses have a need to rescue those rendered helpless, but in part this contributes to their own feeling of helplessness.
>
> Our need to rescue helpless victims is often a reflection of our personal feelings of helplessness. One has to question whether in fact this is a long-standing personality trait of helplessness or whether it's a response to the environment in which these caregivers function.
>
> In any event this way of seeing helplessness in the patient rather than in one's self makes it a patient problem and one doesn't have to recognize one's own sense of impotence and lack of control; but in reality, that's where the difficulty is.

ROLE OVERLOAD (10%)

Role overload or the feeling that there is too much to do in one's role was the greatest stressor in oncology and the second greatest role stressor in emergency. With regard to professional groups, this was the single biggest role stressor for physicians, as already noted. Quantitative work overload has been associated with job stress but usually this is related to a heavy workload imposed by external forces (15). This might be the case for nurses but the physicians who mentioned role overload acknowledged that much of this was self-induced. Dr. Patrick Nelson, an oncologist, said: "Lots of us feeling overloaded and overworked create it ourselves. We start dancing to a tune that you're called to play by yourself."

Dr. Eric Towne, another oncologist, commented:

> You work all the time—not that you want to do it, it's just what happens. People keep giving you things to do and you can't say no, because you figure "I may need something from this person later." You can't afford to say no to someone who'll have some control over your academic future, grants, etc. You have to satisfy the fellow higher up in the pecking order. In the pecking order, all anyone wants to do is succeed—papers, presentations, peer reviews, accolades.
>
> But if you keep saying yes, you jeopardize some of what you're doing. If I'm doing research I have to keep asking myself if I'm really keeping up clinically, so you take on more patients. The system is a series of paradoxes. If you do A you can't do B, but if you don't do B you can't do A. You wind up working harder and harder. It seems to me now that the way out isn't to say yes and work harder—clearly the thing to do is to botch it up. Be a poor administrator, misspell, be late with everything you do.

Another oncologist commented,

> I could cope a whole lot better without so much on my plate constantly. Overload comes at different levels for different people. Some can cope with only a small amount

of stress, but each of us needs to know what our overload point is. Things are particularly difficult here because overload is not only with individuals but with the physical
plant as well. There are the problems in dealing with the patients' illness, then there are
no rooms to see patients in. The appointment desk is overloaded and they start hassling
me. Then there are the radiotherapy machines which may be treating up to 80 patients
a day. . . The patient wants to talk, you're trying to schedule all the patients, talk to the
people who need it, and keep your colleagues happy. This all serves to increase the
normal stress you feel.

Oncologists were not the only group to experience difficulty with role overload;
physicians in a variety of other specialties did so also. Dr. Ed Travers, a middle-aged
general practitioner said:

Little sources build up and they start niggling at you. I vow I'll say "no" more often
or I'll delegate more, but it doesn't always work out. It's the problem of saying "Yes,
I'll deal with your problems" when you know deep down you won't have the time.
It happens with counseling, information-giving, and some of the other softer things.
Then when an emergency occurs or a baby is about to be born, everything else gets
dropped.

It has been noted that persons attracted to the caregiving role are those who
feel a strong need to help other people and are frequently willing to listen to others
when they are outside the work situation. This can lead to role overload and
eventually become emotionally draining as a person may come to feel that she is
never "off duty". Mrs. Lois Meier, who runs a bereavement program commented:

Sometimes I get the feeling that everybody is sucking on me and it's give, give, give
all the time. At a social function, if I identify the kind of work I do, then I identify
myself as a certain type of person and people begin to tell me their whole life story.
This week I went to my child's nursery school, and even her teacher started telling
me about her whole life. I hardly even got a chance to talk with her about how my child
was doing. It seems sometimes like everyone is making demands and there's little control
over it. I tell the volunteers in the program not to advertise their role when they're
out socially, because otherwise people are going to take everything they have to give,
and pretty soon they're going to wind up having nothing left.

PROXIMITY TO STRESSORS (9%)

Some caregivers, because of the role they occupy, are in the position of being
constantly confronted by stressors. Dr. Patrick Nelson said: "I think it's much
harder to be a nurse than to be a physician. The nurse is there on a minute-to-
minute basis whereas the doctor doesn't have to be as involved, he can get out.
The nurse is often younger, she doesn't have the same kind of control that the
doctor has, and she's expected to be there with the patient."
For the NICU and ICU nurses in particular, one of the major role stressors
experienced was the close proximity to a variety of stressors. The physician role
often allowed for the flexibility to leave the unit to perform a variety of other
recognized functions. He or she can leave to go on rounds, fulfill academic or
teaching responsibilities, or carry out some other work. Nurses are often confined
to the environment and often must stay at the bedside for hours at a time. Marshall
and Kasman describe the NICU environment which may be a frenetic atmosphere
where nurses must be on their feet much of the day. There is always the "intense
awareness that at any moment a crisis may occur: a baby's condition may suddenly

deteriorate; transport of a patient may be required; an unexpected birth or death or a grief-stricken family may intrude at any time. One must remain on edge, and that is exhausting" (21, p. 1163).

Learning to deal with a high technology role can be a significant stressor on the ICU, especially as technology continues to change. Both physicians and nurses have talked about the types of difficulties they encounter as they familiarize themselves with new machines. Many of the young nurses interviewed said that they had come into the ICU setting because they liked the technical challenge and enjoyed functioning under a high degree of stress. They found their early months on the unit both frustrating and challenging, and were able to say that much of that time was spent learning "how to nurse the machines." Particularly in pediatric ICUs, as they became more comfortable with the machines, they seemed to almost abruptly realize that these machines were attached to children and that these children had families. Some of these young nurses said that this realization suddenly exposed them to a whole new set of stressors for which they were ill-prepared.

For the caregiver whose personality is such that he or she feels uncomfortable with technology, dealing with these machines can be exceptionally difficult and may give rise to a feeling of constant inadequacy.

Caregivers on an intensive care unit not only have to deal with critically ill and dying people, but they may have to face several people dying at the same time. Multiple role demands, stemming from the kind of illness situation, difficult trajectories, the caregiver's relationship with the family, the caregiver's role, and the environment in which he or she functions often combine to lead to a very stressful situation. A group of nurses on a pediatric intensive care unit described the particularly difficult nightshift they had the previous night:

A baby came in as a crib death, but she hadn't yet really stopped breathing. The parents were told that the child was essentially dead, and they elected not to stay to watch her final death, although they kept calling us on the phone every few minutes and asking why she hadn't died yet. We were really short staffed and there wasn't enough staff to take care of this child who was to be left to die.

At the same time a 6-year-old came in with his spinal cord severed at a place so high as to be incompatible with life, but he was not yet brain-dead. He and his mother were in an accident and his mother was killed.

His father said, "Please don't try to save him. If he's going to die, let him die and be buried with his mother."

The young resident said to the father, "I understand how you feel." But then he turned to us and said, "How can anyone say this about his own child?" We understood. We'd seen this sort of situation before.

The tension on the ward was very high, and I was the nurse assigned to take care of both of these children. When I came on duty I was told that the infant was "dead" so I shouldn't try to do anything. Yet I knew the boy was also "dead" and it was a real stress interacting with his father and trying to know what to say to this man whose wife had just died and who was now watching his son die. In addition, I felt torn between the father's feelings and those of the resident.

Things were really hectic and so the charge nurse carried the baby with her all night as she went around helping the rest of us. Everyone was upset by seeing this child and hearing her gasping, but we just couldn't stand to put her into an isolette and let her die alone, and we couldn't stay with her because things were so hectic.

Obviously, such situations have no quick and easy solutions, but one must really question the staffing on a unit like this, and examine the conflicting role demands occasioned by this close proximity to stressors as caregivers are expected to simultaneously treat one child and ignore another when both lack the real possibility of living. Despite the fact that the nurses agreed that this had been a horrendous night, they also agreed that they managed to cope and survive because of the strong sense of team camaraderie. While they didn't want to see the charge nurse carrying the baby around, reminding them that they could do nothing to save it, at the same time they understood her compassion and all felt they would have done the same thing in a similar situation. This shared value system of people who have worked together, who are willing to help one another in stressful times and then openly share their experiences, and who praise one another for "helping out" in difficult times goes a long way to decrease stress in this type of situation. If as sometimes happens staff members disagree about how such a situation should be handled, then tension really mounts.

Part of the difficulty with constant proximity to stressors had to do with multiple deaths. As one staff member said, "We need some light days once in a while to recuperate. You need some time to fool around and laugh. We haven't had it in a long time and we're really feeling it. There are too many sick, sick kids and too many deaths."

The close proximity to people who were living and dying with life threatening illnesses over an extended period of time also presented problems to caregivers in oncology. In the process of getting to know patients, caregivers were always aware that they were running the risk of being hurt. A nurse commented that she became tired of having one patient after another die of cancer. "I got so that I wanted to go up to each new parent with their set of hopes and dreams and say, 'Forget it, your child is going to die the same as all the others.' I could work with the ones who were dying because I had a long relationship with them, but I was not about to get involved with one more new patient."

Another group whose constant exposure to bereaved relatives served as a role stressor were funeral directors. They commented on the stressors inherent in their role with their constant proximity to death. Ed Green, an experienced funeral director in a large urban setting made this comment:

> It's always a death. People are always upset. Every time you pick up the phone it's another death, it rings your bell a little bit. If everyone's in their seventies, it's okay, but in one community I worked in the average age of death was 33 and the known suicide rate was 13%, although we all felt it was really much higher. This proximity to death is a strong element. Even if there's not lots of tragedy and young people dying, it's still trouble, and you're constantly dealing with grieving people.
>
> The more you do, the more tuned in you get to grief. Even with those I wouldn't have become involved with before, some of the older people in their seventies, I still feel involved. It gets to the stage where you're always thinking, "It could have been me, I'm that age—Or, what if it were my mother left?—That could have been my kid." I'm always asking, "How do I help? What can I do?" And it's especially hard when it's kids who've died.

ROLE STRAIN (7%)

Role strain or having difficulty performing various aspects of one's professional role for the most part, involved difficulty in decision-making and was the most common role stressor in the area of chronic care and in intensive care. Of all professional groups, physicians mentioned it most often, and next to role overload it was their greatest role stressor. Nancy Nichols, a head nurse in an intensive care unit described the pressures of role strain inherent in her position:

> With all the pressure in the head nurse role I find I'm getting more tense and miserable. I never feel happy or relaxed the way I used to as a staff nurse. Then, if I had a really bad day I'd think, well, tomorrow might be better and I'd come in happy the next day — at least I could point to something positive in those days.
>
> Now, whenever something goes wrong it comes to me and it seems like nothing's ever right. I was supposed to go on holiday last week and we were supposed to leave on Saturday morning. I had worked 7 days in a row and couldn't move. I actually couldn't go away. It's ridiculous that I got so exhaused that I couldn't even go away on my holiday.

Whereas the difficulty that nurses had with decision-making was often reflective of problems within the team situation, physician difficulty or role strain with decision-making had to do rather more with the comparative isolation of their position in making these decisions and with the fact that "the buck stopped here." Dr. Bob Tracey commented that, "Decision-making, which is not properly defined, is a real source of stress on the ICU." Dr. Elaine Harding, who works in both oncology and cardiology in a large medical center said that, "You can always code a heart patient because they're never really defined as terminal. Cancer patients become terminal and they are no code, but things are a lot less clear in cardiology which can make it more difficult." While Dr. Chuck Cartwright said, "The stress in ICU evolves from what you're comfortable with as a physician. During my early time in ICU I was uncomfortable making decisions. The big difference between then and now is the effort I used to have to put in just to make sure I wasn't making mistakes. With maturity I'm pretty sure of my judgement and that makes a big difference."

Reverend Ruth Nevens commented that the situations in which caregivers found themselves where they had to decide whether or not to "pull the plug" often caused them difficulty.

> The terminology frequently gets in the way of us and the family. These decisions often happen in lots of forms and shapes and it's not always that we've had a patient here for 3 days, he or she has no brain activity, we pull the plug and they're dead in 5 minutes. Often there are surprises—there are times when initially we felt quite sure of which way it was going to go and it didn't. Last week we had a patient here who had apparent brain stem damage following a caesarian section. We were all set for her die and then she didn't.
>
> You have to realize that whenever you make the decision to discontinue aggressive treatment, whether it's with a cancer patient or a palliative care patient or with a patient on the intensive care unit, it's always done not knowing for sure whether or not that decision should be made; but that's the world we live in. We need to be able to take responsibility for decisions when we make them. In addition we need to be able to structure in as much attention as possible to what these decisions mean for the patient and the family, but it's hard for us to live with this. We would like clear-cut procedures but we have to realize that what I'd be willing to live with in this situation might be very different from what someone else would be willing to live with. In these sorts of situations we need time and support to wrestle through these issues.

The problems of role strain that evolve in chronic care settings are different in that staff members have often come to know patients over an extended period of time and may have warm personal friendships with them. Dr. Cathy Young, a physician in a chronic care hospital commented that in her setting staff members often had difficulty in making the decision to avoid aggressive life-prolonging treatment with patients with multiple sclerosis. "Once they're on the unit even 2 or 3 months, the staff become attached to them and there may be difficulty around making the decision whether or not to treat them aggressively. I feel that my decision is often questioned by the junior staff—maybe it's my own guilt."

Needless to say, when these decisions are taking place at a time when there are conflicting values or team communication problems are a major stressor in the unit, then decision-making and the carrying out of these decisions can come to be a stressor for all concerned.

Role strain may occur not only during one's official professional job but may also result from the fact that professionals are often expected to continue to perform in their role when they are outside the clinical setting.

One family physician observed:

It's the sudden stress of having to deal with an unexpected demand—like a cardiac arrest in the cafeteria when you're relaxing, or like someone fracturing his skull while you're at the cottage. When you're fatigued and physically exhausted and you have an intellectual problem like this and you're asked to make a snap decision, it's stressful. It's the stress of being expected to know things all the time whether you're on duty or off duty.

CAREER PATH CONCERNS (7%)

Career path problems or concerns about where one would be able to go with one's career were primarily mentioned by nurses, who made comments such as:

You're given no respect in nursing, there has to be a job better than this. You see how staff are treated in this hospital. They blame nurses for problems when they're not really their fault, they get fired, you have to fight to get a day off to get married—things that would normally be given in a job outside. There's no future in this hospital. In 20 years I'd still be doing the same thing."

You move from being a staff nurse to a team leader or a teaching position, but where do we go from here? Most of us aren't happy with what we're doing or with the return from the job, but the question is, what do you do about it?

SHIFT WORK OR TIME SCHEDULE (5%)

Despite the fact that shift work is a problem often associated with the caregiving professions, it was mentioned less often than one might expect as a stressor. This may in part be because many of the caregivers surveyed were in positions where they had at least some control over their work schedule but it may also have reflected the fact that the caregivers surveyed did not see shift rotation as a problem that affected their care of critically ill or dying persons.

None the less, it is worth mentioning that there have been a number of recent well-done literature reviews concerning the effects of shift work on persons working in a variety of professional disciplines. It has been found that workers who are forced to rotate shifts have more difficulties than those who work fixed shifts (15). Sleep and digestive problems are major concerns. Social problems and problems of health and well-being often occur in the same people. Those on permanent night shifts have a better biological adaptation than do those on rotating shifts, regardless of the length of exposure to rotating.

Often studies found an increased consumption of caffeine, cigarettes and alcohol, decreased performance with an increased length of rotation of night work, and higher turnover in organizations with rotating shifts (22). In addition rotating nurses tended to take slightly more sick days than all workers assigned permanently to a shift, regardless of what the shift happened to be, they reported disruption of sleep patterns and interference with domestic life, particularly with respect to sexual activities and child-rearing responsibilities (23).

The nurses in the present study made the following comments relative to the stress they suffered as a result of shift work:

An Australian nurse—"Working back-to-back shifts over the years is really depleting."

A nurse in a U. S. community hospital—"One of the problems with nursing is the working hours and the rotating shifts. The whole time schedule in general—you work weekends and holidays and begin to feel that you're the only one working."

Physicians also experienced stress as a result of their work schedule. Several studies on the effect of sleep deprivation on residents have been done. Increased depression was noted in residents who were on services where there was an increased number of work hours per week (24). A decreased ability to recognize arrhythmias on electrocardiograms was noted as well as transient mood changes and the fear that they would lose control during long periods without sleep (25).

One of the interns in the present study said: "For this year I have time for only two out of the three important things in my life—family, climbing, and medicine. I've given up climbing. I just keep telling myself it's temporary for me. . . The only way a nurse can get out of her routine, however, is by stopping being a nurse."

While interns expressed sympathy for nurses, the reverse was often also true. An ICU nurse commented:

It's disgusting the way the hospital makes interns and residents work, especially if they're medical residents. They're on call one night out of three or one night out of two if someone's sick. They're expected to do so many things—not just making decisions. With the number of hours that they're on, I don't know how they can function, let alone think. Then if they try to go home early to get caught up on sleep they get almighty shit. The senior staff say, "we had to do it when we were interns and residents, you can too." But you can bet your life that when the senior staff did it, it hurt as much as it does with these guys now.

REFERENCES

1. Kahn, R. L., Wolfe, D. M., Quinn, R. P., & Snoek, J. D. (1964/1981). *Organizational stress: Studies in role conflict and ambiguity.* New York: Wiley (reprint ed.). Malabar, FL: Krieger.

2. Coburn, D. (1978). Work and general psychological and physical well-being. *International Journal of Health Services, 8,* 415–435.

3. Hawk, J. (1982, October). *Sources and levels of stress in family practice residents: A descriptive study.* Berkeley, CA: Unpublished doctoral dissertation, The California School of Professional Psychology.

4. Schmalenberg, C., & Kramer, M. (1979). *Coping with reality shock: The voices of experience.* Wakefield, MA: Nursing Resources Inc.

5. Fry, R. E., Lech, B. A., & Rubin, I. (1974). Working with the primary care team: The first intervention. In H. Wise, R. Beckhard, I. Rubin, & A. L. Kyte (Eds.), *Making health care teams work.* (pp. 27–59). Cambridge, MA: Ballinger.

6. French, J. R. P. (1973). Person role fit. *Occupational Mental Health, 3,* 15-20.

7. Wood, J. (1976). The structure of concern: The ministry in death related situations. In L. H. Lofland (Ed.). *Toward a sociology of death and dying* (pp. 135-149). Beverly Hills: Sage.

8. Mount, B., & Voyer, J. (1980). Staff stress in palliative/hospice care. In I. Ajemian & B. Mount (Eds.), *The R. V. H. manual on palliative/hospice care.* (pp. 457-488). New York: ARNO Press.

9. Rosini, L. A., Howell, M. C., Todres, I. D., & Dorman, J. (1974). Group meetings in a pediatric intensive care unit. *Pediatrics, 53,* 371-374.

10. Kahn, R. L. (1973). Conflict, ambiguity and overload: Three elements in job stress. *Occupational Mental Health, 3,* 2-9.

11. McCue, J. D. (1982). The effects of stress on physicians and their medical practice. *The New England Journal of Medicine, 306,* 458-463.

12. Kachoris, P. (1977). Psychodynamic considerations in the neonatal I.C.U. *Critical Care Medicine, 5,* 62-65.

13. Marshall, R. E., & Kasman, C. (1982). Burnout. In R. E. Marshall, C. Kasman, & L. S. Cape (Eds.), *Coping with caring for sick newborns* (pp. 5-15). Philadelphia: Saunders.

14. Fulton, R. (1979). Anticipatory grief, stress and the surrogate griever. In J. Tache, H. Selye, & S. B. Day (Eds.), *Cancer, stress and death.* (pp. 87-93). New York: Plenum Medical Book Co.

15. Elliott, G. R., & Eisdorfer, C. (Eds.). (1982). *Stress and human health: Analysis and implications of research.* New York: Springer.

16. Rosenthal, C. J., Marshall, V. W., MacPherson, A. S., & French, S. E. (1980). *Nurses, patients and families.* New York: Springer.

17. Neubardt, S., & Schulman, H. (1977). *Techniques of abortion* (2nd Ed.). Boston: Little, Brown.

18. Bourne, J. P. (1972). Abortion: Influences on health professionals' attitudes. *Hospitals, 46,* 80-83.

19. Brachen, M. B. (1977). Psychosomatic aspects of abortion: Implications for counseling. *The Journal of Reproductive Medicine, 19,* 265-272.

20. Hall, R. E. (1971). Abortion: Physician and hospital attitudes. *American Journal of Public Health, 61,* 517-519.

21. Marshall, R. E., & C. Kasman. (1980). Burnout in the neonatal intensive care unit. *Pediatrics, 65,* 1161-1165.

22. Vander Doelen, J. (1982). Problems and approaches to shift work. *Occupational Health in Ontario, 3,* 37-47.

23. Tasto, D. L. (1977). The health consequences of shift work. Conference on Occupational Stress (pp. 37-41). Los Angeles, CA.

24. Valko, R. J., & Clayton, P. J. (1975). Depression in the internship. *Diseases of the Nervous System, 36,* 26-29.

25. Small G. W. (1981). House officer stress syndrome. *Psychosomatics, 22,* 860-869.

6

Patients and Families

Living, Dying, and Grieving

While patients and families were not as much of a stressor for caregivers as one might have expected, that is not to say that they presented no problem at all. As we have already seen much of the stress that caregivers experienced in response to the environmental and role stressors to which they were exposed derived from the fact that they were trying to deal with these issues while simultaneously attempting to care for seriously ill and dying patients. Thus, it may be that their tolerance for dealing with occupational stressors was decreased as the stress responses these stressors elicited interfered with the ability of caregivers to perform the way they felt they should with dying people and their families. Likewise, when dealing with dying persons one's tolerance for occupational stressors may also be decreased.

It is also of course possible that at least some of the stress caregivers reported in response to environmental and role-related stressors was a displacement of the stress they experienced in response to caring for particular dying patients or else to their exposure to large numbers of dying people and their families.

This chapter will focus on the specific stressors caregivers reported as they dealt with the people involved in life and death situations. The reader will quickly become aware that even if all of the environmental and role-related stressors we have thus far discussed could be alleviated tomorrow, caregivers would probably still experience some stress in response to their exposure to the difficult clinical situations they will soon describe. Nonetheless, their ability to cope with these clinical stressors might well be improved through alleviating some of the environmental stressors to which they are exposed.

Stressors related to patient and family variables accounted for 22% of the occupational stressors mentioned. Patients and families who acted in a way that was unexpected, those with whom caregivers could most readily identify, and those with whom caregivers had difficulty communicating caused the most stress. The noted nurse researcher Dr. Jeanne Quint Benoliel noted similar findings as early as 1967 (1). She observed that nurses had difficulty in providing care to dying patients when: (a) the patient was assigned a high social value in that many people would be affected by the death, (b) the family behaved in a manner that disturbed the staff or ward milieu, or, (c) the patient behaved in an upsetting way by being aggressive or moody or highly emotional—perhaps by talking in a way that bothered the nurse.

Patient-family stressors were most common in pediatric chronic care settings and oncology. In both of these settings caregivers usually had long-term relationships with clients and their families, thus they were more likely to identify with the suffering patients and families experienced, and have difficulty in their interactions if there were personality or coping problems or when there were communication problems about treatment. Patient-family stressors were also problematic in obstetrics in that there were often value conflicts between caregivers and consumers with regard to the issue of abortion. In addition staff members in obstetrics readily identified with the suffering of clients and family members when confronted with congenital anomalies, stillborns and most difficult, with unexpected maternal death.

PERSONALITY OR COPING PROBLEMS (27%)

This largest category of patient and family stressors consisted of interacting with people who were seen to either have preexisting personality problems or else to be responding to their illness or dying process in a way that differed from the norm. Patients or families who became extremely depressed, angry, withdrawn or psychotic; those who completely denied what was happening; those who acted out by drinking or taking drugs; and those who engaged in avoidance behavior constituted this group. Personality or coping problems presented somewhat more difficulty for nurses and social workers than for physicians, perhaps because the role of the former groups required more direct contact with patients and families who had personality or coping problems, whereas the physician role allowed for more limited contact with problem patients and families.

The sources of difficulties with patients and families with personality or coping problems varied across clinical settings depending on whether the caregiver's relationship with the client was long or short term; whether one was dealing primarily with the client or the family; whether this was a response to an acute crisis or a chronic stressor; and the meaning of the particular event for the client, the family, and the caregiver.

Caregivers working in gynecology for example, generally defined abortion patients as having problems coping with their situation if they had delayed seeking an abortion or if they were having repeat abortions. Studies have shown that women who delay seeking abortions have a greater background of psychopathology, denial, are ambivalent towards the pregnancy, have difficulty with decision-making, have lower social support and chronic difficulty with contraception. They are apt to be younger adolescents or older married women ambivalent about another child, primigravidas, and less well educated (2-4).

Approximately 31% of women who have one abortion later go on to have one or more additional abortions (5). Research has shown that these women were no different from women having first abortions in their preabortion scores on depression and anxiety. After abortion, however, the repeat aborters were found to have significantly higher emotional distress scores in dimensions relating to interpersonal relationships (6). Often these women have not been practicing contraception at the time of conception, or have used methods that have inherent imperfections. Some studies have classified them as impulsive, lacking reflectiveness, unable to foresee consequences, having a reduced capacity to plan ahead, having a low sense of self-esteem, more depressive tendencies, and feelings of inadequacy (4).

> We don't have much trouble with a woman who had an abortion at age 17 in 1971, has been using an IUD and is now pregnant again. The ones we really have trouble with are the young girls who have sex once or twice, get pregnant and have an abortion. Often they feel so badly that they say they won't use birth control because they're never going to have sex again. Then she comes back with the same story, again she feels terrible, and again she refuses to use anything.

Sometimes repeat abortions are also reflective of unresolved grief as was the case with a single mother in Australia who had a child die. She could not afford another child as she had two others and very little money, but she repeatedly got pregnant to prove that she could still conceive, lest another of her children died. A teenage patient treated by two of the caregivers interviewed had a very strong grief reaction following her abortion and insisted on having a funeral and full Christian burial for the products of conception. She continued to return on many occasions, thinking she was pregnant again. When she actually became pregnant for the second time she insisted on another abortion. Caregivers involved in such situations often understand that they are dealing with a complicated grief reaction but are uncertain how to handle it.

Caregivers in obstetrics also have difficulty when family members do not grieve in a manner that they have come to consider to be appropriate. Consider, for example, nurses working in a situation described by Mrs. Fran Shields, a nurse clinician. Mrs. Shields was working with a woman with a threatened miscarriage. It gradually became evident that the woman was going to lose this baby, and the woman began to talk about the importance that the baby had for her. She was a single woman who had conceived the child in the midst of an affair that then ended. She had not really grieved the end of her affair, and felt it was going to be essential to her to see the baby in order to grieve not only for the baby, but for the death of the relationship as well. Once the baby was born at 23 weeks gestation, the nurses were willing to show the baby to the mother, but then they began to feel a fair amount of distress when the woman kept wanting to see it again and again.

> By midnight she had finally reached the stage where she wanted to see the baby for one last time, and became quite stable. I shudder to think what would have happened had the nurses not allowed her to see the baby. As it was, she did just fine, but I think it would have been a disaster for her had she not been allowed to see the baby. My problem as the nurse-clinician was in reassuring the staff that they really were doing a good job in allowing her to have contact with the baby. They wondered if they were really helping the woman or if this was a really "sick" situation.

Parents may also have considerable difficulty when babies are born with congenital anomalies. Karen Irish, a nurse in her early twenties described a day with a new mother who was just thrilled with her baby. She was convinced that the child was the most beautiful baby ever born. The nurses realized that the baby was a Down's Syndrome child, but the parents didn't. When the pediatrician told the parents, the mother completely rejected the baby. She refused to allow anyone to come in to see her unless it was absolutely necessary. Karen tried to reach out to her while respecting the woman's privacy and put a note under the door saying, "Please call me if you want to talk." Neither the patient nor her husband ever discussed the issue. They left the hospital unexpectedly, going down the back stairs and leaving the baby behind.

In the neonatal intensive care unit caregivers are often confronted with family members with personality characteristics that may not be dissimilar to those that their colleagues confront in working with women having abortions. Studies have found for example, that the parents on the neonatal intensive care unit may have suffered previous stressors causing them to be more at risk during this current life situation. Neustatter (7) reports that babies born to mothers in lower socio-economic groups are more likely to need intensive care units. Marshall and Kasman (8) also suggest that families who have high-risk babies may be high-risk families with lifestyles different from those of the professionals. This difference in lifestyle may be reflected in families reacting differently from what the caregivers may expect. For example, some families may not visit the child at all, while other families may express their frustrations in verbal abuse of staff members. Other studies have shown that women delivering preterm babies have experienced other recent stressful life events. This may mean that these women must also resolve some of those problems while coming to terms with the unexpected outcome of their pregnancies. If caregivers do not understand the difficulties these women are experiencing they may misinterpret their behavior and then experience stress in caring for them.

Even without other stressors, parents in an ICU may have difficulty coping with their child in this environment. For example, a social worker interviewed about NICUs found that the parents in the unit on which he worked often focused on the technology that was sustaining the life of their child, but separated themselves emotionally from the child. He observed that parents on the NICU were often unable to relate emotionally to their children as they did not yet have a clearly developed relationship with them. He felt that it was as though these parents whose children were on the NICU often "put their relationship with their child on hold" until the child was transferred to a more normal environment. If caregivers do not see this as a normal response to this crisis, they may tend to label the parents as uncaring or inadequate. The social worker mentioned came to see his role as being to facilitate relationships between parents and their newborn infants; this was in contrast to his work in oncology where the relationship between parent and child was already developed. Caregivers may have particular difficulty in dealing with grieving parents in that they may often be angry and irritable right after the death of their baby. Hildebrand and Schreiner (9) suggest that this anger may be directed towards the physician, the nurse, the hospital, family, and friends. Rather than labeling such behavior as problems in coping with stress, caregivers should see it as a normal response to grief. The death of a child may create particular difficulty for parents in that it may recapitulate an earlier sense of helplessness and failure and "the possible re-emergence of a sense of self that is inadequate to cope with circumstances, accompanied by the emergence of a strong sense of guilt for reasons that are not overtly rational. The patient may unconsciously feel that she "caused" the loss" (10, p. 503). This may cause her to act in a way that may cause distress to the caregiver.

While mothers are often discussed in the literature, the problems of fathers are frequently pushed into the background. The caregivers interviewed reported finding it particularly difficult to deal with grieving fathers as they were unused to seeing men cry, or had difficulty with the grieving patterns that the fathers exhibited. If caregivers do not have the time to sit with families and listen for clues as to the sources of their behavior, they may tend to label such parents and distance from them. This also keeps caregivers from acknowledging the fact that witnessing the grief of these family members may deeply threaten their own sense of competence and self-esteem.

In other settings it has been found that children living with chronic illness not infrequently develop personality or coping problems secondary to their diseases. Such difficulties have been documented in cystic fibrosis patients (11), cancer patients (12), and in pediatric chronic illness in general (13). Pfefferbaum and Lucas (14) describe the conflict that may develop when a child's perception of his illness is significantly different from that of those around him. They suggest that in these situations, children may become depressed, withdrawn, or conversely, begin to act out. In such situations it is possible that their attitude may hasten their death.

A nurse who has worked with over 300 patients with cystic fibrosis felt that abut 75% of female patients in their late adolescence to early thirties tried to find some meaning in their deaths. This searching frequently involved a period of great suffering for the patients, and for the caregivers as well, but the resolution of their search often led to a new sense of calmness. For many, the search for meaning led them to God and the sense that their life here was temporary and that there was something better waiting, particularly if they handled this final period well. According to this nurse, this new sense of meaning seemed to help these young women die more peacefully. Other caregivers observed that the behavior of female patients perhaps reflected the fairly typical socialization pattern of females who were taught that they should accept their lot in life. Male patients did not seem to have this same need to find a meaning in their lives. Perhaps in a "typical male fashion" their methods of coping were to engage in risk-taking behavior, defy death by smoking, not taking their treatments, etc. They seemed somewhat more apt to deny the reality of impending death, but as it became obvious that death was inevitable, they sometimes simply died with little struggle. A good example was the young man who said to the nurse: "If I take these treatments this time can I be guaranteed a few months at home with my family, without having to be back and forth to the hospital with all the disruption that leavetaking involves?" When told there were no guarantees, he said: "Thanks for telling me; I won't bother then." He died peacefully the next day.

Caregivers from other settings working with children and young adults having cystic fibrosis also mentioned coping problems they had experienced. A nutritionist described the difficulty she experienced as adolescent girls with the disease became anorexic. Frequently their mothers insisted that they take their medication, even when the children wanted to stop; but when the girls wanted to show their independence they refused to eat, or if forced to eat would vomit. While the nutritionist understood this behavior as an indication of their need to separate themselves from their parents, she also found it very difficult to cope with this situation. When children die of malnutrition, nutritionists can often feel they are somehow inadequate and to blame for not having been able to resolve the problem.

Schowalter (15) suggested that patients who are complaining, demanding, or abusive, and who cause nurses to try and avoid being assigned to them, are often people who elicit an angry response from both physicians and nurses. While this emotion may not always be fully conscious, the staff may become at least somewhat aware of a feeling of dislike. Caregivers, however, can seldom experience pure dislike because they are under social and professional pressure to care for their patients. Schowalter notes that when this type of troublesome patient dies, there is often an inordinate amount of grief among the staff, in part because of the guilt they feel at not having been able to do better.

The personality and coping problems experienced by parents of children with chronic illness have also been well documented. Pakes (16) studied families of children with cancer, finding that 90% of them blamed the original physician in some way for the child's illness. He found that this scapegoating phenomenon left the parents angry at the physician, who then experienced the stress of feeling helpless to intervene because a specialist took over his patient.

In the early phases of adapting to the diagnosis of a chronic illness in a child, denial is often the paramount emotion. Easson (17) says that parents may maintain this denial for a long time, sometimes until the child's death, but usually denial is dropped and reality is confronted. As family members begin to confront the reality of impending death, they may begin to experience anticipatory grieving. This may include feelings of sadness and anger, and the reinvestment in other family members. Easson states that clinicians need to be aware of the ways in which mourning behavior can be understood and to realize that mourning families always feel anger. This feeling of anger may well be projected onto nursing staff and sometimes to medical staff. Goodell (18) suggests that nurses must realize that the anger that parents direct to them during hospitalization is often a stress response to a crisis situation. She suggests that nurses are often recipients of hostility and anger because they happen to be closest to the situation causing stress when it occurs. Readers who are particularly interested in parental coping in chronic illness are referred to Easson (17), Lewis and Armstrong (19), Bywater (20), and Holroyd and Guthrie (21).

Perhaps the area of chronic illness in which parents had the most difficulty in coping was in adjusting to the fact that their children had muscular dystrophy and were going to continue to deteriorate and eventually die. One caregiver spoke of parents from two families who talked openly about wanting to kill their children to spare both themselves and the children the future suffering involved in the disease. In both of these instances the child's illness very much represented the death of a dream. Fathers in particular, seemed to have great difficulty in accepting the fact that their sons were never going to be able to play baseball with them. In some of these situations where fathers had difficulty in adjusting to the reality of their child's chronic illness, they began to proposition the nurses with not so subtle hints that they have a sexual relationship in the belief that somehow the healthy nurse working in conjunction with the father could "make a healthy kid—not like this dying one" (22).

Staff members on intensive care units could also get upset with long-term patients who did not seem to be working to get better. Mrs. Patricia Philpot is an intensive care unit nurse in her early sixties. She stated:

Work doesn't get to me anymore but recently I had worked for 5 months with a woman who I just knew wasn't going to get any better. It really bothered me when I saw that she wouldn't work to get better. I think she was so sick that she had no heart left by the time she finally died. Her heart muscle had gone but they resuscitated her twice. She finally died but what was so hard was that while she didn't want to die, she didn't really want to get to work at getting any better. I found it particularly difficult to deal with her 84-year-old mother who wouldn't look at her and refused to acknowledge the fact that her daughter might die. When I got the doctor to tell the mother that the daughter was going to die, she just wouldn't see it.

There were far more problems reported with personality and coping problems with family members on ICUs than with patients. Sometimes this had to do with the difficulties that the family had in accepting the patient's illness and the possibility of impending death; other times it had to do with families' responses after someone had died; and sometimes it had to do with preexisting problems.

Sometimes when the patients are kept alive on ventilators, their condition begins to deteriorate so much that family members find it difficult to continue to visit. Diane Young spoke of such a situation:

The ones that really cause stress are the ones you end up nursing for weeks but know they won't make it out of the unit. Some of these are patients who have gone for surgery and then one thing after another goes wrong until they wind up with multisystem failure. They live with a dopamine drip at 4 times the normal strength, they're ventilated, dialyzed, and eventually their skin starts rotting off. It's really rough. I can remember just going in and standing at the bedside of one such patient. When I walked away the front of my uniform was soaking and oozing serous fluid. His skin was just coming off in layers. The skin gets glassy and edematous and looks like if you touch it, it will break and indeed it does. This is because there's no oxygen or nitrogen getting to their cells so when you touch their skin it rips and tears. The patient has lots of sores and just doesn't look the way he originally did. You can see that there's a face there but would never recognize it as being that person.

With one such man, his wife finally stopped coming in and we understood. She called in and brought in a photograph album of the last few years that they'd had together. This was helpful to us because we almost didn't recognize this man as a person with all these machines going 12 hours a day. She put up pictures around his room to show this was a person and we were able to separate "this was, what was" from "this is, what is now." When a person gets to this point and you know they'll never come back to any sort of life, and there's no way they'll ever get off machines, sometimes it's easier for us to see pictures to know what the family is grieving over. That also helps us to understand why the family has such difficulty in coming in to see the patient and we're not apt to be as critical.

Sometimes though, in that sort of situation, the family projects their anger onto the staff afterwards and we get letters like the one that recently came to a doctor saying, "Thank you so much for what you did for my husband, but how could you have let him get so big with fluid in your hospital? I had to pay for a double coffin to find one that would fit him." We all have nightmares when this sort of thing happens.

Caregivers in oncology reported difficulty in dealing with patient and family problems that arose both from preexisting personality problems as well as in response to the disease. An oncologist and nurse who worked together in a breast cancer clinic commented that breast cancer patients seemed to be the most "twitchy" patients in their setting. Indeed, studies have shown that breast cancer patients are referred for psychiatric consultation at twice the expected rate (23). "We suppose that it's the combination of endocrine problems, mutilating surgery, possible sexual problems, and the psychosocial stressors which accompany these. Often there isn't support forthcoming from family and friends and the woman is somehow expected to cope at a somewhat higher level than other cancer patients."

The nurse went on to observe that she spent about one third of her time ". . . on the phone talking to patients and families who are not coping at home either because they are deteriorating physically, not doing well or having problems coping. Often the husband can't cope. The wife has been the stronger person and the message from the husband is, "if she can't cope, how can I?" Even the women who are now separated or divorced were usually the stronger ones in the relationship."

Speaking of cancer patients in general, Dr. Walter French noted that:

> Cancer itself isn't stressful. What is stressful is some patients and their reactions to stressful situations when you perceive them as being unrealistic. There seems to be an increase in patients with cancer expecting that they can and should be cured. They used to assume cancer was synonymous with death. Perhaps the publicity on cancer drugs such as interferon led patients to assume that the physician can and will erradicate their disease. It's then stressful when expectations don't live up to reality and you feel impotent.
>
> Recently I had a young man with cancer of the testes who had a football size mass which had shrunk down to a miniscule amount of tumor. I gave him his final treatment and he developed drug toxicity, got pneumonia, and died. It was my error in judgement that led to his fatal toxicity. His father feels that I murdered his son and calls my office to ask my secretary, "Are you still working for that murderer; I'm going to come and kill him." That's stress for you—especially since I know that he has a gun.

IDENTIFICATION WITH PATIENTS AND FAMILIES
(22%)

Caregivers may particularly identify with certain patients or their families. In psychiatry the term "counter-transference" is used to describe this phenomenon in which "the conscious or unconscious emotional reaction of the therapist to the patient may interfere with psychotherapy (24, p. 372). This counter-transference may be either positive or negative and is often based on variables from one's personal life.

As a result of factors in their own lives, caregivers may be more likely to identify with particular patients, and to invest their emotional energy in their patients and thus they may be more at risk of developing stress responses when these "special" patients begin to deteriorate or die. Certain patients are most apt to evoke these responses: "socially valued patients" such as children, young people, or those who will be leaving young families; intelligent and cooperative patients; those who are similar in age, social class, or lifestyle to the caregiver; those with prominent positions in the community; those who have responded well to treatment over an extended period of time; and/or those who for a variety of reasons have managed to work their way into the hearts of caregivers. Certain caregivers will identify with particular patients who are similar to them in personality or who remind them of one of their significant others, or who have a disease that the caregiver suspects he or she may some day develop. Not only individual caregivers are at risk of identifying with patients, sometimes the total group will identify with particular patients and then have great difficulty when the person either begins to deteriorate or die.

Reflecting on how her stage of life influenced her identifying with a patient, a female surgical resident commented: "The first cancer patient I saw had advanced breast cancer. . . . she was 24 and had a new baby. I was 24 and had to give her poisons. I wondered about why we were each in the position we were." A male medical intern said, "I got quite close with one woman with leukemia who reminded me of what my wife would be like 15 years from now. She died with her chemotherapy running—we just never managed to pull her back. It's hard to be critical of the staff men though. Maybe chemo could have pulled her back but I sure didn't like to see her die the way she did."

Dr. John Nielson is an oncologist who worked with the intern just quoted. Dr. Nielson spoke of what this identification is like for caregivers who may work with patients over periods of many years.

Sometimes it hurts lots more when certain patients die. You've become attached to them. I can't single out what type of person I get attached to. I don't know why I'm a little closer to one than to someone else. I'm used as a crutch by some and that's okay... A lot of closeness probably comes from the fact that in dealing with leukemia patients we see them so often and follow them so closely. It's endogenous to the disease. They require this close contact. It's the medical "name of the game" that you need to learn more about the individual and the family. The advantage of the longevity of close contact is that it lets you know about patient and family development... It's more than a business-like approach. They're more like your next door neighbor—you know them better... But then it hurts...

An oncology nurse reflected somewhat similar sentiments when she said, "The worst case is when we have people for whom we care and we can't do anything, for example, to keep their pain under control. At those times I feel so awful. I get a pain in my stomach when I go into the patient's room. We all feel extremely helpless in these situations and keep asking ourselves, 'when is something going to work?' "

Caregivers in oncology are not the only ones who have known patients over an extended period of time, identify with their distress, and then experience their own stress in response. This may happen as well to family physicians. Dr. Ken Hertzberg, a general practitioner in his early sixties said: "People think that it's easy for me to make housecalls on those who are dying. I do it in an easy, sort of low-key way, but it takes a lot more out of me than anyone will ever know. Those people are my friends. I've cared for them over the years and I love them."

Dr. David Travers, another middle-aged family practitioner described the difficulty experienced by his colleagues when caring for people they had known for much of their lives. "There are real problems when you lose a patient that you delivered. Recently, an adolescent girl I had delivered came to me and I diagnosed her as having an adenocarcinoma. She was the third person that I had known closely that I diagnosed as having cancer within a particular one week period. This is really stressful."

Staff members in community hospitals may also have the experience of having to deal with tragic issues involving friends or patients they have come to know over many years. When problems develop there may be a very strong identification with the patient's plight. Sally Morrow, a single, middle-aged nurse in a community hospital spoke of her patient, Mrs. Smith who had already had seven babies born at this particular hospital.

She was really a remarkable woman and had a very strong faith. She had gone through a routine seventh pregnancy and then suddenly, just shortly before her due date, the baby died in utero. She came in knowing that the baby was dead. I wasn't sure what to do with her or what to say to her, so finally I went up to her and said, "I'm very sorry about what's happening here." Patients like to be touched so I held her hand and then said, "Now we have to get on with what needs to be done." She was even able to bring some humor into the situation and tearfully said to me that as she was going to the hospital to have this baby her other children, who had already been told that the baby was dead asked "Couldn't we turn in Jackie, our 'bratty' brother for this new baby?"

I must say that working with her gave me an incredible lift; it really convinced me that there's something to be said for faith. She was going home to another beautiful child who was only about a year and a half, but she pointed out to me that no baby really could replace this one who had just died.

When the situation of identifying with a client is complicated by questionable treatment, significant stress may result. Another nurse in a community hospital was on duty in the nursery when a colleague's baby was admitted. This baby had appeared to be fairly normal, but within a short period of time the nurse saw the baby having seizures. She called the physician, but said that since he had not himself seen the baby have a seizure, he did not believe that this had happened. The nurse had a lot of difficulty in finally convincing the physician that the baby was having problems, because other people thought she was overreacting to her friend's child. The child was eventually diagnosed as being severely retarded, and the nurse then had to deal with her own feelings and those of her friend, both of whom were concerned about whether the situation had been properly handled.

Children with deformities who are born to nurses or doctors with whom caregivers can identify can also cause difficulty for many staff members. One nurse said, "I find it ironic and much harder to deal with when it's a child of a doctor or nurse, and I ask, 'Why did it have to happen to them?' With other nice couples, I just feel sad for them, but when it happens to a doctor or nurse I always think to myself, 'It's only supposed to happen to someone else.' "

Similar problems were found when caregivers in oncology or hospice work developed cancer. Jean Cameron, a social worker who formerly worked on a palliative care unit wrote of the rejection she felt from her former colleagues when she became a patient on the unit (25). A recent article by Deborah Welch-McCaffrey also documents the problems of oncology nurses who then develop cancer (26).

In obstetrics, caregivers could often identify with women who had fertility problems. Caregivers stated that the death of an infant when the woman was reaching the end of her fertile years, or when she had a series of miscarriages proved to be difficult and stressful for them to deal with.

Even more difficult for caregivers in obstetrics, however, was dealing with women whose own lives were at risk because of carrying on with the pregnancy. They could identify with the woman's dilemma even though they did not always agree with how it was handled. In this anecdote the reader can see how it was difficult for staff to support a woman who made a decision that was contrary to their beliefs. This is a form of negative counter-transference that then interfered with the care they were able to give this woman.

We had a woman admitted from out of town. She had three children at home, the youngest of whom was 7. When she was 3 months pregnant she discovered that she had cancer of the ovary. The gynecologist-oncologist said that if she went to term she had a 50% chance of survival. If she was delivered a month early she had a 70% chance of survival. Her gynecologist, who never does second trimester abortions, advised a saline abortion.

She was a very religious Catholic woman whose husband said that he'd go along with whatever decision she made. She grappled with the issue and consulted a priest who told her to go ahead and have the baby. She returned at 8 months to have a C-section and to have the tumor removed. She was thrilled with the baby and never seemed to regret her decision. That's why I respected her so much in the beginning—because she followed her own value system.

But then 2 months later she was admitted with widespread metastasis. We all had trouble then. She didn't stay with us very long because she was transferred to another hospital where I heard she wound up in ICU. I guess she's dead now.

There are four kids and a father but no mother to bring them up. It doesn't seem right.

I felt angry about it. I agree with abortions for those who make mistakes, or for genetic, or therapeutic reasons. I felt that she should have been content with her three kids and should have had the abortion. If she aborted, had surgery, and treatment she had a 70–90% chance of survival. I was angry at her and at her priest but realized that with her religious beliefs she felt that she'd be killing the baby and she couldn't do this. I felt she had really made her decision. The doctor, the nurses, and the head nurse all talked to her. She was adamant she knew the risks and was willing to take them. I was angry at the doctor who tends to say "you *should* do this." He was more concerned with her health than the baby. He was angry because someone said that she didn't want his help at this time.

Caregivers are not always conscious of identifying with patients. They are often unaware of how their personal experiences may sometimes lead them to have unexpected difficulty when some of their own unresolved conflicts unexpectedly emerge and they overreact to a situation because of a counter-transference that they do not understand. Reverend Deborah Jones, a chaplain in a large teaching hospital said:

The head nurse called me to see a young nurse saying, "She's having problems after a death; could you just pop by incidentally and see her." The young nurse had become really upset with a man who died after neurosurgery. She had coped very well with him before his surgery and couldn't understand why she became so upset when he died. As she started talking she realized that he reminded her of her divorced husband. She was still really upset regarding the divorce and the circumstances surrounding it. She hadn't realized that she was involved in a counter-transference relationship. She had become very upset when she started to cry in the room when the patient died and had no understanding of where this emotion was coming from.

A similarly unexpected complicated response to a child's death was mentioned by a nurse clinician. She was called in because the staff physicians were having problems dealing with one of the residents who had just had a patient die.

Dr. Paul had come from a third world country where he had previously seen a lot of death. There, children died from GI problems, or in wars. There were lots of really tragic deaths, and he never had the opportunity to become involved with dying kids back home. When he moved to the United States he became very involved with children, in part because he was technically very competent, and the kids would ask for him to do their IVs. He liked this and began to get close to them.

One of the children that he had been very close to died at home. The staff man called me and asked me to come in to help Dr. Paul because he had begun to fall apart. He began to question why he had risked caring for kids and why he was a doctor. The other doctors had trouble coping with this and left me with him because they were afraid of what might happen to him, and didn't want to stick around. I had a colleague with me and we held him and let him talk, but drew him back to other situations where he had felt incompetent. He spoke of the problems he had in his relationship with this young girl, and about what he had been able to do and not do. We helped him to see that he hadn't been isolated in caring for her, that others too had helped, and we were able to draw from him that this child had a good time because of the treatment he had been able to give her. It involved several hours of working with him and letting him talk.

  This was the first time I'd seen a doctor fall apart like this and it made me question what was going on in the team that this could happen. I could see why he got involved with this girl, but why weren't his medical colleagues around to help him?

In an attempt to provide improved care for chronically ill children, many hospitals and clinics have developed a staffing system that allows for a particular physician or nurse to be a primary care provider for the child. This often provides very good care for the child and family, and can offer a great role satisfaction for the professional. Closeness between the child and the care provider may however, cause the caregiver to identify with the patient and to grieve when the child begins to deteriorate. Articles by Brunnquell and Hall (27), Schowalter (15), and Fulton (28) note that nurses involved in long-term relationships with children can experience severe grief when these children die. Schowalter states that the longer a nurse has known a child prior to his death, the more depressed she tends to be following that death. In addition, he found that the closer the contact the nurse had with the child, the less eager she was to agree to protracted attempts to prolong the child's life, once it was clear that such efforts would not be curative.

In NICUs caregivers often develop "special baby relationships." One physician suggested that it was easy to say that the more one is involved with a particular baby the better one can relate; he pointed out that on his unit, however, there were often problems when staff members became strongly attached to certain babies and then something went wrong. In such cases the staff had to deal not only with the family, but also as happened with Dr. Paul, with their overinvolved colleague who would have to be helped to cope with the crisis. Nurses in NICUs often develop special relationships with the babies under their care and they may give them amusing or pet nicknames. The babies may become like their own, sometimes to the exclusion of parents who may be seen as intruders into the nurses' territory. Parents in turn may feel that staff members are holding their babies hostage in a totally alien environment. Nurses can come to resent the presence of parents on the unit and may be upset at discharging "their babies" to the care of parents whom they feel are not really "deserving" of the child.

This problem is complicated by the fact that there is some evidence to suggest that parents of premature babies, whether because of preexisting problems or because of the stress imposed by the birth and the isolation from their baby, are at greater risk of neglecting or abusing their children in later years (29). The caregivers who have developed strong relationships with these babies may come to feel that these parents are "not deserving of their children," fearing that they may be abusive to the children caregivers have worked so hard to save.

A different type of relationship may develop between caregivers, patients, and families on the pediatric ICU. Here caregivers sometimes become emotionally involved with the long-term patients and with their parents as well. This involvement sometimes extends to a very strong identification with the parents to the point of adopting them and spending off-duty time providing support, entertainment, and by showing them around the city. This can be a source of stress for caregivers for parents may come to expect increasing amounts of time and support from staff members who may find themselves withdrawing in response. When caregivers become very involved, either with parents or with a child, it is not uncommon to find them withdrawing when the patient begins to take a turn for the worse, or when he or she dies. In other instances, caregivers may become very involved at this point and may find themselves incapacitated by grief over the loss they have experienced. Some caregivers make a point of not allowing themselves to become close to either patients or family members. Sometimes, however, the system interferes with caregivers' desire to distance. For example, on many intensive care units there are photographs of children before their traumas. One nurse said:

> While it's good to have the pictures here, sometimes it's hard as I'm not sure I really want to know what the child was like before. I can get involved in dealing with this child as long as he's fairly anonymous, but when I come to know more about him I find it much harder to deal with him. The parents are often difficult though, because you can put yourself in their position. They have one shock after another. They're completely distraught and are trying to deal with the machinery, an ICU environment, and their critically ill child.

Long-term involvement with patients and families from the time of diagnosis, through phases of hope, relapse, deterioration, death, and possibly beyond often involves identification with patient and family and this may be stressful. That does not of course mean it should therefore be avoided. Miss Frances Haynes, a head nurse on a pediatric oncology unit said:

> You become attached to them. They creep into different corners of your heart. The problems come when it becomes evident that they're going to die, particularly if it goes on too long. You struggle to care for them through pain and wondering how much they really know. They make comments like, "Why do you bother, I'm going to die anyway," or "I'm sorry I'm dying because I know you wanted me to get better," or "I know things are bad because I hear the doctor's voice outside my door. She won't come in because she doesn't know what to say."

Caregivers may have difficulty with these close long-term relationships, especially if the children are very open about their impending death. A physiotherapist working with children with cystic fibrosis said: "The kids whose deaths are especially hard are the ones who have come to terms with it themselves and are so open about what's happening. They seem more able to accept what's going on than we are."

COMMUNICATION PROBLEMS (22%)

This category includes patients and families who came from different social or cultural backgrounds and/or those whose value systems were in conflict with those of the caregivers. Some of the examples given by caregivers involved a fairly straightforward cultural discrepancy. For example, an Australian nurse commented: "When the nurse is Mrs. Middleclass Australia, she has very little to say to the aborigine dying in the hospital who previously would have been left under a tree to die. In addition, she may have very little patience with Indian people sleeping under the beds of their dying family members, or on the floor."

Dr. Mark Parr, a Canadian oncologist said that he often wondered about the rights of families especially when he was dealing with immigrant groups with a different value system. This case he mentioned is the opposite of the frequent problem of the family not wanting the patient to be told his diagnosis or prognosis and involved the patient not wanting the family to know.

> As an intern I had a patient with acute leukemia who was dying. He had no will and refused to let me tell his wife he was dying. She was going to be left in dire straits. I've always been struck with the patient's right to know he's dying but I think the family also has rights. . . . Especially if it's the breadwinner who is dying, he's always kept his wife fully dependent on him and she has had no preparation for his death. Now I tell the patient his diagnosis and tell him that I think his family should know about his diagnosis because I think it's ridiculous to say I can't talk with them.

Learning the cultural patterns of various groups proved to be a stressor for caregivers in a variety of settings in that they were often not sure what should or should not be accepted within the culture of their hospital. Staff in a pediatric hospital, for example, were horrified when an Italian family started dressing in black when told their son had leukemia.

In another setting, a palliative care team in Western Canada reported that they found it a challenge to deal with the variety of ethnic groups that congregated in their city.

> Some tend to be more reserved while others tear up and down the hall yelling. One man slept under his father's bed because as a child his father had slept under his hammock and saved his life with his spirit as he hovered near death.
>
> Usually we can work with their beliefs as happened with the woman who didn't want her husband's body to leave the hospital alone. We got the funeral director to come to the front door of the hospital and she accompanied her husband's body to the funeral home.
>
> Another time an Indian family was weeping, moaning, wanted incense and sitar music. We weren't sure what to do so we called an Indian nurse who told them to stop this behavior, this was Canada. They seemed to accept this from one of their own but we would never have done this and don't really know what should have been done.

Often caregivers have found it helpful to use translators from other departments in the hospital to communicate with those of different cultural backgrounds. The palliative care team just mentioned had a relationship with the head of house-keeping for example in which housekeeping staff could be called upon to serve as translators for up to 3 hours. As already noted in Chapter 2, this may of course be difficult for the translator. A Chinese dietician for example, spoke of being called in when a patient refused treatment.

> I was asked to come in because the doctor felt that the patient hadn't really grasped how bad things were with her and she was refusing chemotherapy. I was asked to tell her that if she didn't have a "bag" of chemotherapy she would be dying by the next week.
>
> I sided with the patient and identified strongly with her and asked the doctor why he didn't get her husband to translate. This was my way of escaping having to confront dealing with this patient about her death. Prior to this time I knew the patient and saw her losing her hair, getting fed up and then she said, "no more treatment." I tried very hard to convince her to go ahead and have chemo. I didn't feel obliged to the physician just to the patient and her survival. . . . From then on everything was taken care of. We only talked about food. We never talked about death and dying or her disease again.

Families of different cultural backgrounds may also wish to use alternative forms of therapy that may cause difficulty for the caregivers. Carol Myles, an oncology nurse clinician reported:

> I have difficulty when families take as many worldly goods as they possess and give them to the church in order to get prayers said for the cure of the child. I have trouble if I think this child's care or the future of his siblings are going to be compromised by giving away all of the family resources.
>
> As staff members, we accept the fact that families have a right to do whatever they feel they can to save the child, and yet we do get very anxious in the hope that these parents are not going to be caught by charlatans. We also make it a point to ask the parents to please let us know about the alternative treatment that they're using so we can take it into consideration in planning the treatment program.
>
> One recent situation that we had caused a lot of us difficulty. A religious group came and prayed over the child and performed a laying on of hands. The family was told that the child was healed and that treatment should be stopped. We reached the stage where we wondered if we were going to have to go to court to continue treatment. You hate to have to get confronted with that sort of situation.

Obviously it is not only patients from a different cultural background who choose to opt out of traditional therapy. A nurse and an oncologist at the same cancer clinic were interviewed at different times. The nurse said, "A young woman was offered adriamycin. We all knew it wouldn't help but the doctor wanted to do it anyway. The patient asked to be able to go home and make her decision and we all agreed. She came back and said she didn't want any treatment. To the doctor it felt like a professional failure. He kept saying, 'Did I present it right?' "

From his perspective, the physician said, "One of the real problems I have is when patients insist on using alternative forms of therapy at a point when I think that some of the current therapies would be of real help. Too often they then come back wanting to do what you suggested in the first place when it's too late for therapy to do any good."

Communication problems may also evolve when family members are of different cultural backgrounds. Their discrepant value systems may surface, particularly at times of crisis and may require intervention by caregivers. Reverend Ian Hardy, a chaplain in a large pediatric hospital mentioned such an incident.

> A child had a cardiac arrest but hadn't actually died. Clearly he was going to die but remained unconscious in the ICU for a few days. The mother's main concern was with the surviving child. She knew this one was going to die, but she wanted to be sure that the other one survived. Her husband was from a different cultural background and felt that he shouldn't show his feelings in front of the healthy child. Therefore he kept joking with the healthy son as though the other child weren't dying. The mother felt a need to talk to her little boy and to be natural with her feelings of anxiety about her dying child. She asked me to please talk with her husband and to help him to understand what she was going through. We met as a family and it really went very well. It was a very positive experience. He agreed that he wasn't the cold, callous person that his wife saw, but admitted to her that he was covering up his feelings. With some help from both of us he was able to work through some of these feelings that he had previously kept hidden.

Family value systems may also sometimes involve setting different priorities than caregivers might expect. Dr. Ed Travers, a family practitioner reported:

> I had a 56-year-old man who had had a stroke. He couldn't speak, was dysarthric, and

his lungs were quite congested. He was doing okay, although he still had some pulmonary effusion. He was up and about so I decided to let him go home for the weekend to sort himself out. From what I can piece together after the fact, he apparently had chest pain on the weekend and figured "I've had it." He apparently took an overdose of Valium.

There had never been a hint of depression in this man, but apparently with the chest pain he figured, "The hell with it." He wrote a note saying goodbye to his family. The son found him and brought him in to the hospital, and didn't tell us anything about the note. We assumed that he had had a brain stem infarction and weren't too sure how aggressively we should be treating this, given his previous stroke.

Two days later, his son came to me and said, "Can sleeping pills do this? If he took something, could that be responsible for the way he is now?" This was 2 days after the man had been admitted. The mother hadn't seen the note; I immediately knew we had to change our treatment and realized that the wife had to be notified. The son refused to let me speak to her, saying "I won't let her be upset. I'd rather he died."

This family gave a really bad time to the clinical clerk. I told her, "Remember, they killed the bearer of bad tidings in ancient times." She kept putting herself out for this family, and yet got crapped on. You get to feeling that you do everything in your power to help a family, and they turn and spit and claw at you, particularly on the person who's turned herself inside out.

It didn't really bother me, other than a temporary upset when I realized that they hadn't let us know the real story, but the internist, when he found out, said, "I can't deal with this family, I'm giving them back to you." As a family doctor, I'm not set up to practice in-hospital medicine, and I couldn't handle him. Trying to get someone else to cover was a real problem. No one wanted to take responsibility at that point. The doctors became really uptight because other physicians in the hospital are up on legal charges at this point for the way that another situation was handled. I had to really hunt around to find someone to cover for this patient.

Legal problems were another aspect of communication problems that came up several times with various caregivers. A surgeon said:

What stresses me most is a family that threatens you with a suit when you've done the best you could, and some son of a bitch starts tinkering with reality. That gets me really mad. It's a problem for a patient when there's bad communication between the patient and the doctor and there's the threat of a suit, and these problems usually come up when there is a lack of communication. It's a shattering experience when it happens to you and you know you're being sued. Society has to have a public way of dealing with complaints, but it's hard for the doctor who knows he's done his best. As far as the insurance company is concerned, it's almost not whether you're right or wrong, but how much money you're going to pay people. They seem to have the feeling, "It's not worth it to fight. Give these people 5 thousand dollars.

Such legal action sometimes results from a failure to accurately communicate with patients and families. Some caregivers sometimes feel they are doing their best by telling patients about "appropriate" treatment while neglecting to mention problems which may result that seem of little import to the caregiver, but may be significantly associated with the patient's life values. Cathy Eagan, an enterostomal therapist worked with surgical oncologists who did not feel that male patients about to have a cystectomy or illeal conduit should be told that there was a very strong probability that they would be impotent postsurgery. "If the patient brings it up pre-op I'll answer but the doctor gets very angry and says, 'Hey, that's no consideration when we're talking about my saving his life.' "

Patients who wish to have second opinions or consultations with other physicians, especially those who practice less than completely orthodox medicine, may find themselves in communication problems with physicians. A patient who mentioned to his oncologist that he planned on going to a physician who used alternative methods reported that his oncologist said, "... 'You're going to see that voodoo doctor? What can he give you that I can't? What you need is a concerned doctor and you've got one in me.' He then showed up at my door at 8:30 p.m. that night saying, 'I knew you were upset and wanted to let you know that I knew.' "

Communication problems were a major source of stress in obstetrics where they often reflected value clashes between clients and caregivers in the area of abortion. Caregivers frequently found it difficult to cope with a woman's reason for wanting an abortion, her attitude towards caregivers involved in the procedure, and her response to abortion. If a woman wanted an abortion for "legitimate" reasons—that is reasons that were congruent with the caregiver's value system—the decision for an abortion was generally regarded as justified. A first pregnancy in an adolescent, a failure of birth control methods, and the presence of genetic anomalies were generally seen as "acceptable" reasons to abort.

Dr. Nina Ryan noted that the staff members she worked with in a birth control clinic could be sympathetic to the teenager who became pregnant with first intercourse, or to the pregnant single mother, but they had less patience with women whose reason for aborting was that pregnancy was not convenient at that particular time.

The attitude that patients had towards their abortion also made a difference to whether or not caregivers were comfortable with their decision:

> It is okay with me if the experience has some meaning for the woman—if she has some feeling of what she is going through and just isn't looking on the light side. She doesn't have to be guilty or uncomfortable about it but she has to acknowledge it. I have trouble with women who have no doubt about having an abortion, don't feel guilty but just look on the pregnancy as an inconvenient thing that happened that they want to eliminate.

Caregivers also reported feeling distressed by patients who did not communicate verbally but were withdrawn, as they wondered if they should be doing more for them. "Often the TAs are not talkative. They're quiet and ashamed and don't want to deal with a nurse who may be passing judgement. There's more to discuss with gynecology surgery patients with whom you identify and have something in common."

Other obstetrical patients also caused caregivers difficulty when their values conflicted. For example, although caregivers are gradually becoming accustomed to offering to show mothers their children who have died, they may feel uncomfortable if the parents disagree about whether the child should be seen. Some caregivers spoke of the conflict they felt when fathers wanted to be with their dead children, and mothers refused to see them. Other caregivers have found that fathers, wanting to protect their wives, will frequently refuse to allow the wife to see the dead baby, and the caregivers are then not at all certain about how they should handle the situation.

Nurses also had trouble communicating with parents who had children with congenital anomalies. Helen Edwards recalled one mother who would reject every overture when the nurses tried to speak with her, and yet they would hear her complaining on the phone to her friends that no one would come near her to talk. She would give the nurses signals that she wanted to talk, and then reject them. Ms. Edwards said, "You know she's grieving, but you just don't know what to do about it."

Communication problems may also result when caregivers do not understand the normal family responses to a diagnosis of life-threatening illness. Heller and Schneider (30) referred to the communication problems that arose between parents and physicians when parents were afraid that their behavior might offend the doctors, and that they in turn would not work to save the child. These authors have suggested that such parents come to feel that the hospital was not a safe place to express their true feelings, for fear that their distress might alienate hospital personnel and their anger might cause the physicians to withdraw from dealing with their children.

There may also be difficulty in dealing with educated consumers whose awareness of medical treatment and corresponding demands may threaten the caregivers' sense of competence. One oncologist described his feelings when confronted with a father who had done a computerized literature search on the treatment approaches for his son's cancer. The father wanted an accounting from the physician of whether or not he had considered the data contained in each of the articles. "It was 9:00 p.m. now. My own kids were waiting for me to come home to say goodnight, and he caught me in the hall with this." When families expect to be treated as partners in decision-making and challenge the authority of the caregivers involved, and when they insist upon knowing exactly what is going on with the patient, caregivers who themselves have a strong need for control may experience considerable stress.

Caregivers obviously do not always have difficulty dealing with patients who come from a different cultural background, or with those who have different value systems. One chaplain spoke of being asked by a Hindu patient who believed in reincarnation to be present as a "holy man." The patient believed that the presence of a holy man at his death would enable him to return later at a higher level. The chaplain said:

> What struck me about the death was the complete passivity to death. He simply lay down and died. For me it was a big question on the whole palliative care movement and on getting people to talk about their death. I watched a woman, whose husband had just left her, simply lie down and die. From these people, I've learned to be quite comfortable with those who want to lie down and die without talking out their feelings.

Allowing people to die in their own way rather than in the way caregivers believe to be the best is extremely important in alleviating some of the communication problems we have. Nurses in a palliative care unit said, "The hardest part to accept is the person who wants to die alone. There's a real place for growth for us to allow patients that kind of freedom." An experienced oncologist spoke of a conflict he had with a young intern.

> We admitted an older woman who had recently had 2 MIs, an aortic aneurysm repair 2 months ago, and now she had leukemia. I told her about her disease, its poor prognosis, and the expected treatment. She responded, "I'd like something for pain and a tranquilizer at bedtime." The intern said, "Call the psychiatrist. This is completely unrealistic. She isn't getting appropriately upset." I told him that this was her way of handling it and her daughter agreed. She said, "Mother has had three or four life-threatening illnesses in the last couple of years. She may seem unrealistic to you but she knows what's going on and that she could die at any time.

YOUNG PATIENTS (9%)

Dealing with illness and death in young people was a specific stressor for certain caregivers. This was not necessarily because they identified with patients so much as they found it difficult to watch the suffering these young people endured. Caregivers were often led to question the meaning of life and why young people had to become ill, suffer, and die.

Much of the stress in pediatrics comes from the fact that illness and death seem to be particularly unfair in this age group. Caregivers made such comments as:

> Death is different with children. There's a different intensity of feeling. The staff feel the agony of the parents' loss which is untimely and unacceptable. There's grim despair.
>
> When a baby dies there is a raw grief, particularly in men. The woman seem to be most devastated by the "motherly" things that are denied them, especially if they have older children and know what they're missing.
>
> With prolonged illness there's a tremendous void and a colossal loss. Death is a release for the children but a tremendous sorrow for the parents, even though there might have been very little quality of life for a long time.

In adult intensive care units, caregivers often have considerable difficulty in dealing with younger people, especially those who will die. Rita Pearson, an ICU nurse in a large teaching hospital, spoke of a situation that was particularly difficult for her.

> The older isolated patients and younger patients really get to me. I can remember one young woman of 27 who was brought up from the emergency room with a ruptured brain aneurysm. She had been on a round-the-world trip when her aneurysm ruptured. She'd had rheumatic heart disease as a child and had had a variety of medical problems. A few weeks ago she'd had an abortion and had become septic while on her trip, and then her aneurysm ruptured.
>
> I looked after her from the time she came in until she was taken off the ventilator 4 days later. It was just awful. I knew realistically that there was no way that she could get better because her brain was shot. Yet I kept doing things for her and didn't want her to be alone. The physicians would come out of the room and say, "You can't do anything for her, she has brain death." But I found that hard to accept. I became very emotionally upset when they said "that's the end" and they pulled the plug. I was very angry with them. At that time the physicians and residents we had on the unit were very good and I expressed anger to them and to my fellow workers. I became miserable at home following her death and cried during my days off which followed her death. I talked to my friends as well. When I came back there were more patients and I had to take care of them. You tend to push back what's happened when you have new patients to care for. Nonetheless, that incident happened 8 years ago and she's still very clear in my mind.

SOCIAL AND FAMILY PROBLEMS (7%)

This category included people with preexisting social and family problems that caregivers could do little to resolve. These may have included multiple marriages, marital breakdown, poverty, and long histories of drug and alcohol abuse. An example of such problems was given by Kathleen Tower, a public health nurse who said:

> We had one situation where a daughter kept putting her mother into the nursing home until her welfare checks would stop, and then she'd take the mother back home. The mother was consistently admitted with malnutrition. She would eat very well in the

hospital and obviously wasn't being fed at home. The social worker said that she was not going to allow the woman to go home again. The daughter said that if the social worker tried to keep her mother in, she'd sue her. The hospital says "back off." This made us very frustrated and gave us a high level of stress.

When patients come from homes that have a number of family and social problems, there is sometimes a tendency for caregivers to become even more involved with them and to assume the role of surrogate family. A nurse from Arizona described the involvement she had with a young boy who was dying of cystic fibrosis.

Johnny was 5 years old and his mother had lived with five different men over his lifetime. I didn't know who his father was nor, I suspect, did he. He would be in for 2 weeks out of every four. She'd bring him in and wouldn't visit until it was time to take him home, but she'd send him lots of expensive gifts. I became quite close to him—almost a surrogate mother.

When he was dying I kept calling his mother to get her to come in, but she kept saying, "No he won't die, he's been like this before." I told her she'd better come in for her own sake because she'd feel really guilty after he died if she didn't. I admit that I laid it on a bit thick. She was there when he died and broke down once saying, "God, why are you making me suffer like this?" When he died she kept saying, "I'm not guilty. I did everything I could. Look at all those toys I brought him."

I was in the corner boo-hooing. I'm never sure what to do standing in the room of someone who's dead. Nothing is being said. She was being comforted by her boyfriend who came over to comfort me saying, "He's out of his suffering now."

My teammates and I went to the funeral. I couldn't be much help to the mother because I stood in the back and boo-hooed while she was stoic. I came to feel I was doing her crying for her, but I was glad that I was there. The only people were the mother, her boyfriend, and an uncle—there were no friends.

I felt like I was "doing justice" to him. He was a neat little boy and he deserved someone to cry over his death.

OLDER PATIENTS (6%)

Older patients served as a stressor for some caregivers. Sometimes this was because the caregivers empathized with their plight, especially their loneliness. They made such comments as: "I feel most upset with people who have been together for years. As a spouse is dying, they'll say to me, 'Oh my dear, how will I survive? We've been married 45 years; we have no children—all I have is my little dog.' I want to do more, and I'm apt to get emotionally involved with this type of person." On longer term units caregivers often felt particular sympathy for the older person who was dying alone, having outlived all relatives.

In other cases, stress was experienced by caregivers because they questioned the ethics of performing heroics on older patients, particularly in intensive care units or oncology units; while other caregivers disliked caring for older patients, for whatever reasons, or became angry because of a number of older patients "filling up active hospital beds." In a study of head nurses, Leatt and Schneck found that they noted the care of elderly patients as being more stressful than any other group with which they were dealing (31).

In intensive care units caregivers often experienced considerable stress and staff dissention when they were dealing with elderly dying patients. Rosemary Young, a head nurse in an intensive care unit said that on her unit the nurses had particular difficulty

... with an old person about 80 with tubes, and a ventilator doing all sorts of things. The patient is dying but we don't let them die. The nurses ask me, "Why are the doctors treating this poor soul" and when I ask them they'll say, "He's salvageable." In my mind if you put an 80-year-old in bed he'll never go back to the way he was before, but the doctors will often say, "He's salvageable, he was walking before he came in here." In these situations I ask the resident, "If this were your mother or father, would you do it?" They'll often respond, "It's the staff man's decision, not mine." But often I know that it's the referring staff man who doesn't come to visit the patient on the ICU but insists that he be treated and resuscitated. Whether these doctors are under pressure from the family, I don't know. But we're there all the time and under constant pressure as a result of these decisions.

PATIENT OR FAMILY CULPABILITY (4%)

Caregivers experienced stress when dealing with patients seen as responsible for their plight. Caregivers in obstetrics were the only group that cited patient culpability as one of their major stressors. Here, not unexpectedly, the difficulty again involved abortion patients, primarily those women using abortion as a form of birth control. Karen Ginsburg, a birth control counselor working with adolescents said:

I don't think that I could work in an adult setting. It's different with an adolescent, essentially I see them as a child who made a mistake. Somehow I expect an adult to be more responsible.

During some of my training I sat in on interviews with women coming in for their second or third abortion. They were using it as a form of birth control. There was no question that they expected that they should be able to get an abortion on demand.

With adolescents I feel that they've made a mistake. They are not yet mature so I have a sense that they can still change. They worry, "Will I be passed by the committee?"—as opposed to the adult women who assume "of course I'll be passed."

For some women the issue of abortion on demand is a political one, and that can cause a caregiver stress. Dr. Norm Herron found that he experienced the greatest degree of stress dealing with "the women's libber who doesn't want to put any chemical into her body and feels she has the right to abort. These are the same women who won't go to their own gynecologist but come to see me because they know I do abortions. They aren't really dealing with it at all."

Caregivers also sometimes had difficulty with people who had developed medical problems as an outgrowth of their life styles; e.g., lung cancer in smokers, or heart problems in the obese, or AIDS in homosexuals, but perhaps the most difficulty with culpability came from issues of wife and child abuse.

Nurses in a community hospital emergency room spoke of the difficulty they had in dealing with adults who were abused and who showed up in the emergency room. They spoke of numerous women who had been abused by their husbands and yet returned home to live with them.

Husband-wife abuse is so difficult. The wife knows that she can't exist within the environment but she's afraid that if she reports it, something will happen to her husband, and he's the only one who has any positive feelings for her at all. So they'll come in and say she fell down the stairs. You'll talk to them and threaten that if they don't report their husband, this violence is going to continue. You see them almost in tears with suffering and yet they'll go out arm-in-arm with the same man. One woman we kept for four days after her husband beat her and threw hot water all over her, burning her quite badly. Some of us were physically sick when we saw the damage that he had done to her, and yet she left the hospital with him and dropped the charges that she had initially laid against him. There just aren't enough police to guard women like this against the violence to which they're exposed. The police think she eggs him on and yet that's not what we think.

Probably the most difficult anecdote involving family culpability was that of an 8-year-old girl who was brought into a southwestern hospital. She had been murdered and her body was mutilated. The nurse said:

> I realized that her body had to be identified but there was nothing left of her head. Her mother was so bereaved that she couldn't come in and I said to the doctor, "There's no way I can have the parents look at this child, you'll have to have them identify her by her clothes." I suppose I should have twigged when the mother looked at the paper bag and said, 'Is that her teeth?' How would anyone else have known that those were her teeth? The mother was so sedate that she carried on with her grieving. They seemed to be such a decent family that my heart went out to her and I thought, "This is her baby, it must be so difficult for her." I had heard that the same couple had had a baby die a crib death just 9 months before and I said to myself, "how much can one family take?" Then I found out that she had killed not only this child, but the child that we had thought had died a crib death. We were all horrified.
>
> This situation was made so much worse by the fact that since we're a community hospital, the relatives who came to realize that this woman had killed both of her kids, kept coming to emergency dealing with their grief over the next several weeks so we had to keep reliving the situation over and over again.

REFERENCES

1. Quint, J. C. (1967). When patients die: Some nursing problems. *Canadian Nurse, 63,* 33–36.

2. Kaltreider, N. B., Goldsmith, S., & Margolis, A. J. (1979). The impact of midtrimester abortion techniques on patients and staff. *American Journal of Obstetrics and Gynecology, 135,* 235–238.

3. Kaltreider, N. B. (1973). Psychological factors in mid-trimester abortion. *Psychiatry in Medicine, 4,* 129–134.

4. Brachen, M. B. (1977). Psychosomatic aspects of abortion: Implications for counseling. *The Journal of Reproductive Medicine, 19,* 265–272.

5. Center for Disease Control. (1983, May). *Abortion surveillance 1979–80.* Atlanta, GA: U. S. Dept. of Health and Human Services.

6. Freeman, E. W., Rickels, K., Huggins, G. R., Garcia, C., & Polin, J. (1980). Emotional distress patterns among women having first or repeat abortions. *Obstetrics and Gynecology, 55,* 630–636.

7. Neustatter, P. (1981, September 22). Neonatal care is a minefield of woes. *The Medical Post,* p. 53.

8. Marshall, R. E., & Kasman, C. (1980). Burnout in the neonatal intensive care unit. *Pediatrics, 65,* 1161–1165.

9. Hildebrand, W. R., & Schreiner, R. L. (1980). Helping parents cope with perinatal death. *American Family Physician, 22,* 121–125.

10. Turco, R. (1981). The treatment of unresolved grief following loss of an infant. *American Journal of Obstetrics and Gynecology, 141,* 503–507.

11. Strauss, G. D., & Wellisch, D. K. (1980–1981). Psychological assessment of adults with cystic fibrosis. *International Journal of Psychiatry in Medicine, 10,* 265–272.

12. O'Malley, J. E., Koocher, G., Foster, D., & Slavin, L. (1979). Psychiatric sequelae of surviving childhood cancer. *American Journal of Orthopsychiatry, 49,* 608–616.

13. Geist, R. (1979). Onset of chronic illness in children and adolescents: Psychotherapeutic and consultative intervention. *American Journal of Orthopsychiatry, 49,* 4–23.

14. Pfefferbaum, B., & Lucas, R. H. (1979). Management of acute psychologic problems in pediatric oncology. *General Hospital Psychiatry, 1,* 214–219.

15. Schowalter, J. E. (1974). Pediatric nurses dream of death. *Journal of Thanatology, 3,* 223-231.

16. Pakes, E. H. (1979). Physicians' response to the diagnosis of cancer in his child patient. (Mimeo).

17. Easson, W. M. (1980). A child's death and the family. *International Journal of Family Psychiatry, 1,* 401-412.

18. Goodell, A. (1980). Responses of nurses to the stresses of caring for pediatric oncology patients. *Issues in Comprehensive Pediatric Nursing, 4,* 2-6.

19. Lewis, S., & Armstrong, S. H. (1977-1978). Children with terminal illness: A selected review. *International Journal of Psychiatry in Medicine, 8,* 73-82.

20. Bywater, E. M. (1981). Adolescents with cystic fibrosis: Psychological adjustment. *Archives of Diseases of Children, 56,* 538-543.

21. Holroyd, J., & Guthrie, D. (1979). Stress in families of children with neuromuscular disease. *Journal of Clinical Psychology, 35,* 734-739.

22. Vachon, M. L. S., & Pakes, E. H. (1984). Staff stress in the care of the critically ill and dying child. In. H. Wass & C. A. Corr (Eds.), *Childhood and death* (pp. 151-182). New York: Hemisphere.

23. Silberfarb, P. M. (1984). Psychiatric problems in breast cancer. *Cancer, 53,* 820-824.

24. Osol, A. (1972). (Chairman of Editorial Board). *Blakiston's Gould Medical Dictionary.* Third Edition. New York: McGraw-Hill.

25. Cameron, J. (1982). *For all that has been.* New York: MacMillan.

26. Welch-McCaffrey, D. (1984. Oncology nurses as cancer patients: An investigative questionnaire. *Oncology Nursing Forum, 11,* 48-50.

27. Brunnquell, D., & Hall, M. D. (1982). Issues in the psychological care of pediatric oncology patients. *American Journal of Orthopsychiatry, 52,* 32-44.

28. Fulton, R. (1979). Anticipatory grief, stress and the surrogate griever. In J. Tache, H. Selye, & S. B. Day (Eds.), *Cancer, stress and death.* (pp. 87-93). New York: Plenum.

29. Jeffcoats, J. A., Humphrey, M. E., & Lloyd, J. K. (1979). Role perception and response to stress in fathers and mothers following pre-term delivery. *Social Science and Medicine, 13a,* 139-145.

30. Heller, D. B., & Schneider, C. D. (1977-1978). Interpersonal methods for coping with stress: Helping families of dying children. *Omega, 8,* 319-331.

31. Leatt, P., & Schneck, R. (1980). Differences in stress perceived by head nurses across nursing specialties in hospitals. *Journal of Advanced Nursing, 5,* 31-46.

7

Patient Illness as a Stressor

Having discussed patient/family variables in Chapter 6 we will now turn to a discussion of the accidents and illnesses with which these people were so involved. Illness variables can be divided into two major categories: type of illness, and trajectory, or course, of illness. A category labeled "illness variables" may appear to ignore the fact that illnesses occur in individuals and cannot be legitimately separated from these persons. Nevertheless, this section is meant to show that there are some illnesses that in and of themselves are particularly difficult for some, if not all caregivers. The fact that these illnesses occur in people with whom caregivers may identify, like, dislike, or feel neutral towards, may serve to increase, decrease, or neutralize the stress the caregivers experience. Similarly the fact that these illnesses or accidents occur in people who may or may not have personality problems or difficulty in coping with their illness, social or family problems or communication difficulty with caregivers, may also affect the caregivers' response to the illness situation and those involved with it. For the most part illness stressors will be seen as being most problematic in settings wherein the caregivers do not have close and prolonged contact with clients and their families. Longer term contact of course often serves to cause caregivers to see the problem somewhat more in terms of the people involved, rather than the illness per se.

The only specialty area where the major source of stress involved illness-related variables was in the pediatric and neonatal intensive care group, where unexpected illnesses or accidents resulting in a short illness trajectory leading to death served as a major stressor.

Variables related to illness type accounted for only 10% ($N = 305$ anecdotes) of the occupational stressors mentioned.

TYPE OF ILLNESS

Unexpected Illness (34%)

This category included illnesses of sudden onset such as heart attacks with no previous history, accidents resulting in severe injury or death, tragic illness such as the discovery of advanced cancer in a pregnant woman, suicide, homicide, etc.

Dealing with unexpected or tragic illness was the second greatest stressor for caregivers in the emergency room. When patients come in and are dead on arrival from a particularly tragic accident, or when family members come running in and have to be informed that someone has just died, the fact that the physical setting allows for no privacy, that one may be having difficulty with a colleague, and that one may feel that one is expected to function far beyond the role for which he felt prepared, may lead caregivers to experience considerable stress.

A group of nurses in a large urban community hospital emergency room reflected on the deaths that gave them particular difficulty.

> The worst ones are the deaths of children or young people. The first crib death of anyone really bothers them. They fall apart. Particularly if they're married, they identify with the thought of losing a baby and we all get really upset.
>
> If it is a severe accident it can really destroy morale for the rest of the shift. I remember one day around Christmas which was really dead with nothing going on and the next minute there was a house fire and five kids came in who had died together. They were so charred and we all felt like it was one of our own kids. They looked liked steak and we just couldn't get over this. I can deal with burns but not with burns like this. A situation like this you keep bringing up constantly for 2 to 3 days after the event and it continues to resurface over time as we "remember when."
>
> A paramedic in a similar situation recalled having to be the person to go into a Multi-Patient Unit (ambulance bus) to confirm that six children from another family were in fact all dead.

Other caregivers spoke of the stress involved with cardiac arrests and the fear that they were not going to be able to perform in an adequate way. A group of nurses in another community hospital emergency room said:

> I don't think there comes a time in any nurse's life when it becomes natural and comfortable to deal with a cardiac arrest situation. There's real nervousness when these patients arrive and you never really get used to dealing with them because everything happens so quickly. After it's over and you've lost the patient, the next thing is to deal with the family which is another whole stress. I can't deal with it. . . I just go and cry. Even after 6 or 7 years in emergency I still can't face the family of someone who's died. I find that I can function in the code situation and do everything to save a life, but the reality when it's over with and the person is actually dead, I find so hard to deal with. When I have to confront a woman who has just lost her husband after 50 years of marriage, I find it hard to talk to her because I feel so bad.

Probably the most difficult of all deaths for most of these caregivers were the deaths of children. Numerous tragic situations were given and just a few examples will be related to give the reader some sense of the types of stressors to which these caregivers are exposed.

A large group of emergency room nurses attended a conference in western Canada. They compared anecdotes about the most stressful situations that they experienced and many of these revolved around the deaths of children. They made the following observations.

Relating to the death of a child is different before and after you have your own children. If you have your own, then you relate to them realizing "there but for the grace of God go I." You also come to realize that for the real horror stories to happen, the seconds have to be perfect. You see parents thinking, "If I got up instead of drinking that cup of coffee, my child would have been fine." Or, the fire that started when a parent left to go to the store for a few minutes and got back to find her child dead. Or the baby who was crying for an hour and then the father notices that the baby's not crying and goes for a shower and then returns to find that the baby has died of crib death. This situation was particularly difficult because they were told by the doctor to let the child cry himself to sleep and not spoil it. The first time they decided to do this, the child died a crib death.

Caregivers in pediatric ICUs also found it difficult to deal with unexpected illness and death and the effect this had on families.

One hour the child is fine, the next hour he's critically ill or dying with tubes coming out of all orifices. It's one shock on top of another for parents who are already distraught. They must deal with the impact of the accident, all the machinery and the intensive care unit environment. . .

Norman Carr, a social worker who worked in both oncology and ICU reflected on the particular problems involved in dealing with parents who must confront a sudden or unexpected illness or accident:

The critical care cases are the most difficult. The kids whose chances of dying by tomorrow are great, and they were healthy yesterday. These families are in an intense state of shock and death is imminent. In such situations I can't hand them a book to read, but I have to try to do some instrumental facilitative things, and perhaps facilitate the system for them. I find it really hard though because I feel my hands are tied with these kids in terms of giving hope. With the children with cancer that I've worked with I can often provide hope, or at least I have time to work with the family if the child is going to die. On the trauma unit so often it's a situation of just getting in there and coping and doing something as quickly as you can.

The issue of perinatal mortality was crucial in the area of obstetrics. As one obstetrician pointed out, as short a time ago as 1964 in the province of Ontario (where he works) there was a 2.4% perinatal mortality rate. That is to say, 24 out of 1,000 infants died. Today only one women in 100 who makes it past the 20-week abortion stage will lose her infant. This physician suggested that both women and caregivers have become used to having 99% of babies delivered alive, so when a baby dies this is seen as really being quite unusual.

Most of the caregivers interviewed very quickly recalled some of their stillbirth experiences, indicating perhaps the way in which they stay with them. One obstetrician said:

Last week I delivered a woman who had a smooth pregnancy. There was a cord entanglement with the cord over the baby's shoulder, and the baby died. It couldn't have been predicted. It didn't upset me as much as it would have 15 to 20 years ago, but it really upset the nurse who was there.

I said to her, "You're really going to have to somehow manage this in your own mind. This woman's Braxton-Hicks contractions forced the baby against the uterine wall and it got tangled in the cord. You musn't let it ruin your day or your week. There was nothing we could have done differently."

It really bothered her; she really helped the woman, but was quite short with us. She felt that we were delaying delivering the woman, but she knew that we knew the baby was dead. She kept trying to hurry us into doing the delivery, and was urging the anesthetist to top up the epidural. I was trying to do the delivery with as few stitches as possible, but she was primarily interested in getting the baby out.

The nurse visited the woman on the gynecology floor and was really very good with her, but seemed to blame me for the fact that the baby died. She was sulky and wouldn't talk to me whenever she saw me in the coffee room for a few days after the delivery. She's a friend and I want to help her with this; she's an excellent nurse, and I want to keep her doing this work. She wants to go into medicine so that she can have more of a part to play in things in the future.

When a stillborn is reasonably straightforward, as was the case in this situation, experienced caregivers usually realize that in fact they had very little responsibility for what happened to the baby. When caregivers question whether an infant has died because of their own management of the situation, the feelings that they experience become much more problematic.

Dr. Walters said:

The stress involved with a problem patient in labor can really be quite intense. It used to be even more so before the days of fetal monitoring. There you are, flying by the seat of your pants trying to rely on your training and experience to tell you what to do, but you're not always right. I can remember back to my early days of practicing obstetrics and can recall two or three patients whose babies died. The thing that really stands out is that they felt terribly sorry for me. They had a sense that there was a certain inevitability of some deaths, and they were willing to accept that this had happened to them.

They would wind up feeling sorry for me. They were university graduates, the kind of people I could relate to. They would ask, "Why did it happen?" and I'd say, "I don't know why, maybe I made a mistake. I'm awfully sorry." What else can I say?

A neonatologist had some interesting observations on the relationship that develops between an obstetrician and his or her patient. He suggested that there is often an unwritten contract between a woman and her obstetrician in which the nonverbalized message is that if the mother does certain things, everything will be okay:

There's an unwritten deal that if she does as she's told all will be fine, then if something happens the reaction of the obstetrician often is, "Look, I can't cope with this right now; give the mother a heavy sedative and we'll cope with it later on." The real message of the obstetrician is that he needs a sedative to cope. As the neonatologist, I'm often put in the position of being asked to intervene in this situation because I'm not emotionally involved. I can take charge as an outsider or as an interested observer coming in cold, and can use that as an opportunity to provide the kind of support that the mother needs in this situation, and which the physician is unable to provide.

Another source of stress in obstetrics and gynecology and probably the most problematic for most caregivers arose from situations where a mother was either diagnosed as having a potentially life-threatening illness during pregnancy, or else died during childbirth, or in the immediate puerperium. Although maternal death is a very rare phenomenon, a few of the caregivers interviewed had experienced this crisis.

In three out of five situations where caregivers discussed maternal death, they had known the patient previously. This caused more intense grief at the time of the woman's death. One group of nurses spoke of a patient who had been on their unit for a few months in an attempt to maintain her second pregnancy and to deliver a live baby. The previous year she had had a stillborn. The woman had chronic cardiac disease and had been told from childhood that she would never be able to have a baby because she was too sick. When she married, she was told by her cardiologist that she wouldn't live long enough to carry a baby. She decided to get pregnant anyway, and after her first stillborn had a second pregnancy. She was admitted to the hospital in an attempt to maintain this pregnancy. The nurses interviewed were quite upset by the fact that the woman's cardiologist had not come to see her during this pregnancy, a fact that seemed to indicate he was angry that the patient had gone against his better judgement. One of the nurses spoke of having developed a very close relationship with the patient, and just a couple of weeks before delivery she had spoken with her about the possibility of impending death.

I asked her how she felt about herself dying, and she said, "I'm not really that sick. I do gymnastics, and I really think I'm okay."

I said to her that as far as her heart problems went, she had about the worst problems that one could have, but she listened and said, "I'll be okay." I asked her if her husband was willing to take care of the baby should she die, and she said he was. I was hesitant to discuss this any more since she was so firm in feeling that she had made the right decision. I thought, "Who am I to try to force her to go through all the stages of looking at what might possibly happen."

I asked her obstetrician what he thought was going to happen, and he told me, "Well, it'll be okay, but it'll be tense." I knew that statistically, there was a 60% chance that the baby would die. But none of us really thought that it would happen. She didn't die during delivery but died soon after, and she actually didn't die of her heart disease, but of another disease which no one realized she had. She bled to death, and we all had the feeling that it shouldn't have happened here at a big teaching hospital.

When I heard that she had died, I became very angry. First of all I became angry at her because she'd gotten pregnant. I felt sorry for myself but then I quickly began to feel badly that I should feel sorry for myself when I thought about her parents and her husband. I felt guilty that I should have talked more to her towards the end but we were both always so busy. I was angry that she, of all people, had to die; she had so much love and gave so much to other people. She went through so much and I kept asking myself why someone else hadn't died instead of her.

When I went to work the next day I became completely hysterical and had to leave report twice. When I started work I completely blew a catheterization on one patient, and gave a mean Fleet enema to another. I was really upset that I didn't handle her death better. I felt that I had specialized in gynecological oncology and this shouldn't have upset me. I wanted to develop some kind of strategy to help the family. I kept feeling I didn't do as much as I might have. I guess it just completely threw me.

I can still see her happy, smiling face. I can still see the afghan that she was knitting. I can still remember sitting with her and picking out the baby's name. I don't think I'll ever forget her.

A clergyman also spoke of the difficulty that he had when one of his parishioners died in childbirth.

I work very well with dying patients, but the two things that I can't deal with are dying kids and maternity problems. Last week in maternity, a girl that I had known for years died of preeclampsia. I got terribly angry at the futility of her death. I got angry with God about the fact that it had happened, and got really uptight and threw my anger around in all the wrong places. When this sort of thing happens I throw my anger in all directions. It gets directed at external issues or gets completely misplaced on to parish issues. I bend over backwards not to give any of this anger to the family and that just increases its intensity. I find that when something like this happens, it just leaves me completely empty. I have no solution to that kind of problem. I cope by taking up some kind of cause and working at it very hard until the grief finally passes.

The final example of maternal death was particularly difficult for staff members involved because the woman, whom they knew well, predicted her own death. This is not an uncommon phenomenon where sudden death is concerned, and often leaves the bereaved survivors as well as the caregivers involved feeling quite stunned. The reader who is interested in this phenomenon would do well to read the paper by Doctors Weisman and Hackett (1) who describe patients who predict their own death. They stress that when a person calmly predicts that he or she will die, caregivers must take special precautions.

A nurse in a community hospital gave an example of such a predilection to death:

> We had a gravida 13, para 12 whom we'd had in and out lots of times. The day before she had her 13th baby she was admitted to the hospital and took off her wedding rings and all of her jewelry, giving it to us and saying, "I don't think I'll need these anymore. I don't think I'll get to see this baby."
>   We didn't know what to make of this and said to her, "Of course you'll see the baby. Don't say things like that." The next day she delivered. Then her uterus ruptured, she hemorrhaged and died. We could do nothing to save her. It's the first time that I've seen a husband left totally alone. No one could go near him for half an hour. We were all completely stunned.

Unexpected or sudden illness served as a major stressor for personnel in intensive care units in part because each unexpected or sudden illness caused them to question their own competence in dealing with this type of situation, and secondly, in part because of their identification with the fact that this type of illness could happen to them as well.

Dr. Bob Tracey spoke of the difficulty that caregivers on his unit experienced when people that they thought were getting better died suddenly. He said,

> You become upset and wonder what you missed. You wonder what went wrong. Was it the equipment, did the support system fail? You question the whole system that was involved with the patient, not just the machines. One of the stressors of dealing on an intensive care unit is dealing with people that you know are dying and the failure of the system that cannot keep them alive. You identify with them as visions of our own mortality and somehow on an ICU there's the feeling that something went wrong with us when a death occurs.

The unexpected suicide was a stressor for many caregivers, especially those in the community who were left to deal with the bereaved relatives. A chaplain commented that when he was first ordained he was sent to the outback of Australia to work in a small deprived community.

> I had seven suicides in my parish in a year and a half. One boy killed himself the day before marrying his pregnant girlfriend. Another hung himself in a tree, one cut his throat, another shot himself. I developed a job-induced depression and started driving my car at 110–120 miles an hour in a suicidal way.

Another chaplain spoke of the role conflict he experienced in dealing with an unexpected suicide. He was called off the golf course to deal with a nurse who had been attacked by her estranged husband.

He cut off her finger and thumb, stabbed her in the eye, halved her clavicles. She was in fear and trembling of his coming into the hospital and finishing her off and was under a police guard. The next thing we knew he and I had to tell her of her husband's death.

He was found dead at the end of the garden. One part of me said she'd be relieved; another part said she'd be upset. We sat in silence for 45 minutes then she said to me, "You'll have to do the funeral." I was dealing with someone I really hated and had wanted to kill him before he did it himself but she said to me, "If you can accept him and his death the others in the hospital will too."

Disfiguring or Difficult Illness (21%)

Radical neck dissections, hemipelvectomies, or radical vulvectomies were among the stressors categorized as difficult or disfiguring illnesses. This was especially true if the caregivers questioned whether the surgery would actually prolong life or offer good survival time. One caregiver commented that, "Heroic surgery may demand a hero to go on living afterwards." Caregivers had particular difficulty dealing with open, gaping wounds discharging considerable purulent material, as the close physical contact and extensive nursing and medical care created a situation which was difficult for patients and caregivers alike. Frequently, but by no means always, these illnesses involved disturbances related to the patient's sexuality, such as radical vulvectomies, or to elimination functions (e.g., colostomies). Problems with radical surgery were more common in teaching hospitals than in community hospitals.

Caregivers were sometimes able to see beyond disfiguring illnesses to sense the personhood of the individual undergoing the experience. In such a case, the illness experience often was no longer perceived as a stressor, except when patients were seen to suffer in a way that caregivers could not alleviate. A particularly poignant insight, albeit one unlike that most caregivers will experience, was given by Father Edward Connors:

I worked in a lepersarium which gave me an understanding of a specially chosen God-people. When one of them died the others had a peculiar whine—more like a dirge than a moan. It communicates their special closeness to God. It was like a religious experience to me—it communicates peace to me and I ended up with positive feelings about the deaths of lepers.

They are isolated and have worked out their own life style. They don't want to be back into other communities. They have a closeness to nature working out of a small colony as self-supporting as they can be without fingers. They have great self-respect and a real mutual support system. Their tremendous sense of acceptance and peace with their lot in life is communicated to you.

Dr. Elaine Harding commented that nurses working in an ENT unit had trouble dealing with patients with head and neck cancers that can involve, "foul and offensive tumors and drainage." Initially it was difficult for the staff. "But then it became the 'fat girl in kindergarten syndrome'—you'd point to the girl as fat until you got to be friends, then she was Mary-Jane and you didn't see the fat. The same thing happened when they came to know the people with head and neck cancers."

In obstetrics, particular difficulty was experienced with women having second trimester abortions.

Dr. Devine, a physician who had elected not to do second trimester abortions described the stress she experienced when a patient had not been appropriately assessed as to the stage of pregnancy, resulting in an unexpectedly difficult abortion. As will be obvious, this type of situation can be particularly stressful when one has developed certain techniques and rituals to gain control over one's work situation.

> We do 16–18 suction abortions 5 days a week. I think of myself as having a primarily technical role. I think of the schedule, being careful, on time. I concentrate on my technical performance and on doing a good job—maximizing safety and minimizing complications. I think of an abortion as simply a technical procedure. I don't think of the contents as being anything other than the contents of the uterus. I don't see any fetal parts, the products of conception go down the tube and I don't think of it as anything. There's no stress. The fastest and easiest part is doing the operation. The patient is put onto the stretcher, gets anesthetized, has the procedure done, and is back to recovery in 17 minutes. Occasionally however, one slips by at about 15 weeks. I recognize limbs, parts and think to myself, "this shouldn't be a suction abortion. Who assessed the size of this woman's uterus. Whatever ding-dong did it doesn't know the size of a uterus."
> It becomes unsightly. There are fetal parts on the floor. I have to break up the pieces. I have to probe to make sure it's not incomplete so that the patient doesn't wind up expelling recognizable parts at home. I'm also concerned for the patient because of the risk of hemorrhage or infection and because the fetus is so big.
> I'm also concerned for the nurses and the anesthetist because the operative time is prolonged.
> It's bad. Everyone in the room sees tiny legs on the drapes because they haven't gone down the suction tube. They are there and visible. If there is someone observing like a student nurse or someone new, I apologize and say, "It's not always like this."
> I try to clean up so the floor cleaner doesn't have to experience this. After a delivery I wouldn't think of cleaning up if a placenta fell on the floor, but with this type of abortion I always do.

Finally, a nurse described how difficult it was for herself and her colleagues to cope with malformed infants. She said that the ones that were particularly painful to deal with were those whose deformity made them appear really ugly. She said that their physical appearance disturbed the nurses, and ways of coping varied between becoming very involved with such babies, or avoiding them as much as possible. She stated:

> If you have some unresolved need within yourself, and then get a malformed baby, you're apt to put yourself in that position and give the baby lots of love. Some nurses just refuse to be assigned to these kids, while others are quite willing. There's a real problem if the nurse doesn't want to care for the child, but is forced to.

Ethical Problems (12%)

This category involved caregivers confronted with such issues as abortion, and the prolongation of life with life support systems. One caregiver referred to this as making "judgements in uncharted territories."

Many nurses spoke of questioning whether in fact older people should be resuscitated in emergency or whether they should be allowed to die. Mary O'Hare, a psychiatric nurse-clinician who provides consultation to emergency room nurses spoke of the difficulty that some of them were having with the admission of burn patients to the emergency room. In this situation the physicians were now speaking to patients before their trachea started to swell and they went into electrolyte imbalance and explaining the problems of survival and what the final injury would be like.

We're really surprised at how alert they are and with what good judgement they approach things. The doctor says, "If you survive you'll have artificial limbs but we really expect that you'll die of infection." So far we've had two people who have opted to allow themselves to die in this situation. They both had burns over 95% of their body with 50% of these being deep burns. But then again, we have a 60-year-old, 275 pound alcoholic man with 60% burned and everything against him, but he's doing very well. We don't make a lot of serious irreversible mistakes, but we probably make some.

Even when there are guidelines, decision-making in situations where ethical issues arise is never easy. Caregivers must be open to changing many strongly held ideas. This was well illustrated by Cindy Robbins, a 25-year-old nurse who reflected on her early days in an NICU:

I was assigned to care for a 21-week-old fetus with tubes coming out of all its orifices—umbilical IVs, ventilator, he arrested twice and was resuscitated. It made me really confront my values and what I thought we were doing. I began to think that it was morally wrong for me to be working there and participating in all of this. Then a mother came to visit, holding the hand of a 2-year old toddler. This was the earliest survivor the hospital had—22 weeks gestation. Suddenly I looked at this baby just one week younger in a totally different way. If that one could survive, maybe this one could too. What I was doing suddenly was justified.

Iatrogenic Illness or the Presence of a Threat of Lawsuit (11%)

Problems arose when caregivers either suspected or knew that an illness was unintentionally induced by a physician or other caregiver. Sometimes these errors occurred at the caregiver's hospital; in other cases patients were transferred to tertiary referral centers following the mishap. This type of illness was most prevalent on intensive care units and was of greater concern to physicians. It was more commonly mentioned by caregivers in teaching hospitals.

The situation with multiple physicians on a unit becomes particularly difficult when there is a possibility of iatrogenic problems. One nurse spoke of a young boy who arrested in the out-patient recovery room within minutes of being discharged. It appeared that the surgeon had ligated his carotid artery on one side by mistake. She said:

The other physicians tended to ignore the problem. The nurses not looking after the boy were openly hostile to the surgeon, while the nurse looking after him had as little to do with the doctor as possible. In this situation nurses talk in terms of reporting the physician, but never actually do. I have talked with the chief of medicine about people I think are bad. He knows what goes on but says, "Ya, ya, ya." Who knows what goes on between chiefs. I'm sure these sorts of situations must be discussed but they don't come back and tell the nurses. When it really comes down to it, a doctor is a doctor and a nurse is a nurse and we don't share our problems together.

Dr. Chuck Cartwright, an anesthetist who directs an intensive care unit said:

On our ICU I haven't seen any iatrogenic problems in a long time. The problem that nurses don't always understand is that you can have a routine procedure like an ulcer and by mistake cut the common bile duct and it becomes a problem. In terms of decision-making for the physician you do all that's possible. The stress for the doctor isn't in terms of decision-making but in terms of handling the family. We stress that in this situation we do all that we can do and we do everything that can be done. We do, however avoid talking regarding what happened in the operating room. If the nurse is uncomfortable communicating with physicians then she may find that she gets lots of different stories about what went on. In these situations the family often also gets lots of different information and they begin to have a real distrust of the system.

We've found in our system that if we have a resident there who is the one person who talks to the family all the time and gets to know who's the spokesman for the family, then we manage to decrease a lot of the stress that we would otherwise get into with these iatrogenic problems.

Illness with a Poor Prognosis (9%)

Some illnesses, by their very nature carry a negative prognosis. Some caregivers found it particularly difficult to work with illnesses where the prognosis is certain death, where they feel there is little they can do. This might be especially difficult if the disease will progress quite rapidly, as in some forms of cancer, or if the progress of the disease will be a constant downhill course, as often occurs in Duchenne Muscular Dystrophy. A psychologist observed:

> The deterioration is harder than death. There's a relief with death even though I miss them. Watching a child gradually deteriorate from a healthy 2- or 3-year-old through to be a severely distorted, shriveled adolescent who has only enough energy to move the "joy stick" on an electric wheelchair is hard. When the diagnosis is made we as staff tend to telescope things. We're not just looking at this 7-year-old child, we're projecting what he'll be like at 17.
>
> The staff in the Outpatient Department who work with children with a variety of problems say that the Muscular Dystrophy Clinic is the hardest to work in. It goes on and on and never gets any better. For 12-16 years you see the same child continually getting worse" (2, p. 165)

Other illness types that evoked caregiver stress were *illnesses that resulted in personality changes (4%)* such as may often accompany brain tumors, AIDS, chronic illnesses, or the aging process. This was a particular problem to caregivers in palliative care and chronic care settings, perhaps because they have had a long-term involvement with patients and find these changes difficult to reconcile with their previous picture of the person.

"Unnecessary" or Self-Inflicted Illnesses (2%) such as lung cancer or chronic obstructive lung disease in heavy smokers; diseases related to obesity; and suicide attempts cause difficulty for a small number of caregivers in oncology, critical care units, and emergency. Recently, AIDS has become a major issue.

TRAJECTORY OF ILLNESS

In their important book *Time for Dying* Glaser and Strauss (3) wrote that illness and death are temporal processes, that is they take place "over time." "In hospitals where death is a common occurrence, the staff's work is organized in accordance with the expectation that dying will take a longer or shorter time. Sometimes the organization of hospital work fits an individual patient's course of dying—'his dying trajectory'—but at other times the work pattern is, at least in some respects, out of step with the dying process" (3, p. 1). Not only are hospitals organized with certain expectations for a given patient's illness or dying trajectory, so too are caregivers' mindsets organized with particular expectations in mind.

When the patient's illness or dying trajectory differs from what caregivers expect, caregiver stress may result—this may be true if a patient dies unexpectedly, especially in a specialty such as obstetrics where death is a rarity, if a patient who is expected to die dies sooner than anticipated, or if a patient takes "too long" to die.

The differences observed between the unexpected death and the one that takes "too long" often reflect the differences between acute and chronic stressors in caregivers—that is the sudden unexpected death results in a sudden surge of adrenaline calling for a crisis response. Caregivers respond quickly. If the patient dies, caregivers may be very upset, the group mood may become one of anger, guilt, depression, conflict, but this is usually relatively short-lived. If a patient is taking "too long" to die, however, particularly if the dying trajectory is quite difficult or if the patient is either very much liked or disliked by caregivers, a group chronic stress response may result. Group morale is low, depression is obvious, staff conflict arises, tempers flare, caregivers may avoid or become over-involved with the dying person, absenteeism increases. Likewise if the illness does not proceed as expected, caregivers may also experience stress. Reverend Deborah Jones compared the emotions surrounding death trajectories in different hospital units: "In Emergency, it's a panicky thing. In ICU/CCU/Cardiology, everyone's alert—there's a tension of being aware of everything happening. In oncology with the terminal case it's a matter of waiting, not knowing when, dealing with the family and the staff's personal involvement with the patient and the family."

Variables related to illness trajectory constituted only 5% of the occupational stressors (N = 168 anecdotes).

Trajectory Too Short or Unexpected Death (26%)

This category, which Glaser and Strauss call the "unexpected quick trajectory," was a stressor primarily in intensive care units which, while set up to deal with death, may not be prepared for the death of a particular patient at a particular time. Glaser and Strauss (3) assert that the crucial structural condition in a hospital staff's handling of an unexpected quick trajectory is whether the "surprise" comes as an emergency or as a crisis. According to these authors, an "emergency situation" usually implies that the facilities to initiate prompt action are readily at hand. In a "crisis situation" adequate preparation for mobilizing action is lacking, so the need to act immediately may tend to immobilize the staff. Glaser and Strauss found that the resources available within the hospital environment were determining factors as to whether a particular dying trajectory was an emergency or a crisis (e.g., in an ICU or emergency room the impending death is an emergency, while on a unit not as prepared to deal with death, it is a crisis). However, the caregivers interviewed spoke more in terms of their own psychological preparedness for a death rather than the unit's preparedness. Rita Pearson, a 30-year-old nurse on a busy intensive care unit expressed the problems with the unexpected trajectory in the following: "If a patient was expected to die and he died, the nurse looking after him would come out and say, 'he's dying'—either an arrest would or wouldn't be called. It had been worked out ahead of time and wasn't a big problem. If the death isn't expected, especially with a young person, then the tone of the unit is much quieter. People express their feelings. It's really awful."

A different type of unexpected death which could be termed a "crisis" was reported by Mrs. Kathleen Tower, an experienced public health nurse:

> I went out to do a routine home visit and found the woman dead. She was a 75-year-old alcoholic woman who had hemorrhaged to death and looked just awful. The landlady who had let me in just stood there and screamed. I looked after the landlady for 20 minutes before being able to look after the woman who had died. The landlady said, "Her eyes are open. She's looking at me." I tried to decrease her guilt by telling her a bit of the woman's history and explained that this was the outcome of this type of drinking pattern.
>
>   I didn't mourn because I felt this woman had caused lots of problems to her family. I felt that her death was predictable. . . I just hadn't expected to come upon it like that.

Sudden unexpected trajectories presented stress for caregivers who worked with people with chronic illness. These caregivers came to expect that they would be able to anticipate and thus prepare for death. If staff in any way feel responsible for the unexpected death then of course their stress is increased. For example, particular stress was experienced by the staff of a muscular dystrophy clinic where two adolescents suicided in order to avoid the stages of the disease that they knew were yet to come.

Another staff member described a death on the oncology unit where she worked.

> One of the worse deaths was that of a young girl who died in the operating room during a routine staging procedure. No one knew what to do, so they brought her back to the ward. We gave her family a private room and let them spend time with her. What was hardest on us was watching her father brush her hair—tears streaming down his face.
>
>   We all gathered around them and tried to do what we could. We cried with them because we all felt so bad even though we didn't really know the family. . . The doctor even drove them home because we feared for their safety driving and wanted to do something for them.

In the same oncology unit where both nurses and physicians frequently became very involved and invested with their patients, another stressor arises when children begin to die of infection as a side effect of the chemotherapy they receive. Frequently, the physician has not prepared the family for death and finds it extremely difficult to confront the fact that this child might die. Rather than allowing the child to die on the unit with the parents and the caregivers who have taken care of the child for so long, physicians sometimes transfer such children to the intensive care unit. There, the intensive care unit staff often have great difficulty:

> The leukemic kids within hours of dying are brought down and put on ventilators and pavulonized. We asked the doctor, "Why are you doing this to them?" The doctor said, "She has only one-tenth of one percent chance of making it but I'll give her that chance." The nurses on the hematology service come down with the patient and the family and we say to them, "Why is this happening?" They don't know either, and they too question why the children are being separated from their family at the time when death is happening. Are we justified in doing this or is this simply the physician unable to accept the failure implied by death?

Adams (4) also refers to the fact that death may be more difficult when children die suddenly and without warning from infections when on an oncology unit.

He suggests that this is because the parting process is severed and parents and siblings do not have the time to resolve their own feelings and say their farewells, but one might also suggest that the same holds true of the caregivers working with the child or with any person who dies unexpectedly of a chronic illness.

Even in Palliative Care Units death trajectories may be unexpectedly brief and thus cause caregiver stress. Dr. Nina Thompson commented:

> Last Wednesday we had a difficult death. He was 31, quite well, and married only 1½ years. He had been at the Halloween party on Friday dressed as Sir Galahad. His death was sudden from a pulmonary embolism. We could all say, "He would have wanted it this way."
>
> His death was good for him but bad for his wife, son, and us. We would have liked to have had him with us for a longer time, to get to know him better.

Unpredictable Illness Trajectories (16%)

These occurred in those situations where caregivers really did not know what to expect with a given illness trajectory, or when things did not progress as expected. This could occur, for example, when a patient on life-support systems who is expected to die, suddenly regains consciousness. Physicians found this a somewhat more difficult trajectory than did nurses. This is probably a reflection of the fact that the physician sees it as being his/her role to predict; whereas the nurses' role in prediction is much less clearly defined (which certainly does not deny that it exists, as nurses are constantly being asked by patients and families to make predictions, yet their prediction often carries less official sanction).

An experienced ICU nurse commented:

> I can't answer if I'm asked if someone will live or die. I saw a person with three flat EEGs–clinically dead, come back. I saw him start to trigger the ventilator and was told I was crazy. I said, "I don't think he's dead," but no one would listen to me.
>
> His face was huge and swollen and his eyes were wide open. A doctor came in and took pictures and his sister sat there crying. He woke up on Christmas Eve and said he dreamed that he saw Mary and Joseph on the way to Bethlehem. He talked to them and they told him to come back.
>
> His coming back sure scared lots of people. People were really guilty about what they had said. The doctor and sister denied that they had taken the picture and cried. People denied all the horrible things that were said and the fact that everyone came in and had a gawk.

Illness Trajectory "Too Long" (14%)

Illnesses that linger much longer than either caregivers or family members expect may begin to lead to stress responses. The message almost seems to be, "Would you either get better or die, but don't just hang on." Two visiting nurses described patients having this type of illness trajectory as ". . . the people you see three or four times a week, 52 weeks a year for 5 to 6 years." ". . . those who go on forever but don't die." A private duty nurse described working with a woman who lived much longer than expected.

> When I went to work with Mrs. M. she was expected to live for 3 months, then they thought maybe 6 months, but she lived a year. She kept coming close to death. She'd go into a coma. We'd prepare for her death and then she'd wake up. I could see the ways in which she manipulated me but could do nothing to stop it. . . This kind of

one-to-one work for an extended period really wipes you out. When I finished I really needed a long holiday.

When the illness trajectory is "too long" then staff may experience significant stress as they interact with family members. An oncologist commented that:

The most difficult thing about dying is the family not the patient, particularly with the patient who doesn't die who "should"—even worse when it's someone else's patient and you get stuck with the family. You try to do nothing but to do it actively—to seem to be active without really doing anything to keep her alive. Here the family who can manipulate and bring in other doctors presents a real problem.

Artificial Prolongation of Life (12%)

This presented particular problems on intensive care units and for caregivers working with chronically ill children.

One of the most difficult decisions to make in the care of a chronically ill child is how far to treat the child and what types of heroics should continue to be used. A community nurse who works with children with muscular dystrophy said: "We wonder, as we begin to treat these chronically ill kids' infections, still yet another time, 'what are we really doing and why? Should we bother continuing to treat their infections?'"

A physiotherapist working with cystic fibrosis children: "One of the biggest problems is when there really isn't anything left to do, but the doctors decide to keep prolonging life by trying one more thing which they know won't work, but pretend they think will work. It just serves to prolong the kid's dying for 6 weeks longer when it could have happened in a shorter period.

A nurse working with cancer patients:

I worked with a teenager who knew he was dying and accepted it, but they sent him to the ICU. My heart was broken. They knew he didn't want to go, and they sent him anyhow to the ICU where he'd get filled up with tubes in every orifice. He died anyway. I was upset that the doctors wouldn't let kids die. The kids would cry and say, "I want to stay here to die, not on the ICU." I realize that if a patient was dying, sometimes the best thing the doctor could do would be to walk out and then come back a few minutes later, allowing the patient to die with dignity in the meantime.

Keeping people on machines while waiting for their organs to be used for transplants is often difficult. "It's hard to use prolonged life support systems on a 20-year-old 'mess' because he's a potential donor. . . You have to come to realize that you're not nursing a dead person, you're nursing a donor so that someone else might live."

Sometimes this artificial prolongation is stopped without discussion as happened with a gambler who was paralyzed following surgery. Prior to surgery he had said, "If anything goes wrong I'll be the worst quad you've ever seen." An ICU nurse reported that following surgery, ". . . someone shut off his alarms and he was found with a flat monitor."

Stopping treatment that is primarily serving to prolong life also creates problems for all involved. A social worker on a palliative care team commented:

I was called about a woman on renal dialysis. The physicians decided to take her off because they felt they were just prolonging her misery. They took her off and then called us. I knew it was too late to do much but went up to the ward anyway. It was 5:30 p.m. on Friday and my husband was waiting for me. I thought I'd talk with the family because sometimes we've been able to be helpful with bereavement follow-up in this sort of situation. I spoke with the daughter on the weekend who felt they were managing fine and would give me a call if needed.

The head nurse called on Monday. The husband was drunk and abusive with staff. I couldn't talk to the patient—she was really withdrawn so I couldn't find out if anyone had talked to her regarding stopping dialysis. She was becoming more and more toxic at this point. I hoped the husband could fill me in but I would have liked to talk to her.

I thought, "This lady's really been let down and I'm here to bandage." Dialysis doesn't usually refer. They refuse to admit that patients die there. I swear that sometimes they dialyze them after they're dead. They referred in this instance only because the husband was coming onto the ward drunk and scaring the nurses.

The husband said to me, "I needed your help 10 years ago and you have the nerve to come up here now. Get off the ward. . . How could you come here?"

I tried to quietly explain why I was called. He said, "You're trying to calm me down" to which I replied, "I'm sure someone should before you crack up."

His response was, "Well, I don't want to cry now." His son-in-law said, "He's not always like this."

We get the really hard ones that no one can do anything with in a situation like this.

Uncontrolled or Difficult Trajectory (12%)

When caregivers were not able to provide the expected relief of symptoms, especially when they believed this was their mandate, they experienced great stress. Not surprisingly, the specialty in which this was a major stressor was palliative care. Caregivers spoke of patients dying in unrelieved pain despite their best efforts, or dying with unrelieved respiratory problems. Staff working in a unit for cystic fibrosis children were extremely upset one weekend as one of their "favorite" patients was dying a respiratory death and kept gasping, "Please help me, I'm dying." They felt impotent at being unable to relieve the distress she was experiencing. An oncologist commented that she had promised a young woman with whom she worked that she wouldn't die in pain. "She didn't but she died in status epilepticus and there was nothing I could do."

A nurse on a bone marrow transplant unit spoke of a patient

. . . who was always very sweet, always saying, "I'm going to make it." Suddenly he was screaming, it took six of us to turn him. He was bleeding from all orifices and his skin was falling off. He kept begging us to let him die.

The doctors said, "That's what women say in childbirth too." They have horrendous deaths. My family members and friends can't bear my telling them stories of what I see. . . of people passing three litres of diarrhea with large chunks of tissue. . . I no longer plan for a future. I just enjoy today.

REFERENCES

1. Weisman, A., & Hackett, T. (1961). Predeliction to death. *Psychosomatic Medicine, 23*, 232–256.

2. Vachon, M. L. S., & Pakes, E. H. (1984). Staff stress in the care of the critically ill and dying child. In H. Wass & C. A. Corr (Eds.), *Childhood and death* (pp. 151–182). Washington, DC: Hemisphere.

3. Glaser, B. G., & Strauss, A. L. (1968). *Time for dying.* Chicago: Aldine.

4. Adams, D. W. (1979). *Childhood malignancy: The psychosocial care of the child and his family.* Springfield: Charles C Thomas.

8

Caregiver Stress

Physical and Behavioral Manifestations

As the reader has no doubt begun to realize from previous anecdotes, caregiver stress may be manifest in physical, psychological, or behavioral symptoms. Some caregivers reported very few manifestations of stress. Perhaps they were unwilling to talk about their stress, or alternatively, their coping mechanisms were now sufficiently well developed that few of the stressors they mentioned actually resulted in the development of symptoms of stress. Rather, most stressors simply elicited coping strategies that could consciously or unconsciously be evoked at the point at which they experienced strain rather than resulting in a stress response. Support for this hypothesis comes from the fact that the reported symptoms of stress were highest in the youngest group of caregivers and the lowest in the oldest group, while the number of coping strategies mentioned were the highest in the oldest group and the lowest in the youngest group. Caregivers in intensive care units and oncology reported more stress symptoms than the average for the sample.

The manifestations of stress were divided into three major categories: physical, psychological, and behavioral. Of these there were very few reported physical symptoms of stress and more reports of psychological than of behavioral manifestations. The major reported symptoms of stress were: feelings of depression, guilt and grief; staff conflict; job-home interaction, including marital and family problems related to work stress; feelings of helplessness or inadequacy and anger or irritability. Together these accounted for 63% of the manifestations of stress mentioned.

PHYSICAL MANIFESTATIONS

Physical manifestations of stress were divided into major and minor illnesses. These involved symptoms that the caregivers themselves felt were related to work stress. The categories did not include such physical problems as infertility, cancer, kidney disease, pulmonary emboli, hepatitis, and gynecological problems which caregivers reported, but felt were not related to work stress. The fact that few physical illnesses are reported as being related to job stress has been corroborated in other studies (1). A physician was not atypical of the group in his reports of good health. "I can't ever remember missing a day of work. Once I tried to and came home 12 years ago with what I thought was thrombophlebitis. My wife took one look at it and said, 'That's a bee sting you idiot,' so I learned not to be sick."

Minor Illness Problems

Minor illness accounted for two-thirds of the stress-related physical illnesses mentioned and included: constant fatigue, stomach and gastro-intestinal problems, headaches, appetite disturbances involving weight loss and gain, menstrual irregularities, back aches, muscular problems, and urinary tract infections. The reader will recall from Chapter 5 that sleep and digestive problems were found to be associated with shift rotation (2-4). The fact that nurses reported these symptoms somewhat more often than the other professional groups lends credence to the hypothesis that these symptoms may be a manifestation of stress associated with one's work schedule.

A group of emergency room nurses reported that their physical manifestations of stress ranged from being unable to eat or to sleep, vomiting before work every morning, and overeating. A head nurse on an oncology unit commented that the nurses on her ward frequently experienced weight loss or weight gain in response to the fluctuations and the physical status of some of the patients for whom they were caring.

> I have two nurses who don't eat when they're looking after dying patients. One of them found that whenever the floor was heavy she couldn't eat at all. She finally left and became a visiting nurse. Another one finds that she has no appetite if a patient is dying or, if she does eat, it makes her ill so she doesn't feel like eating. Still another is so busy worrying about patients and her role at work that she finds she can fix a meal for her family but can't sit down to eat with them. When two favorite leukemic patients died recently within a month of each other, one of the nurses gained a considerable amount of weight. It was as though for every pound that the patients were losing, she felt that she had to gain a pound.

Changes in eating patterns and sleep disturbances were also found to be a problem in a group of palliative care nurses earlier studied by the author and her colleagues (5). In that group it was found that not only did nurses not "feed" themselves as well as usual, those who cooked for their families found themselves no longer able to "feed" their families and took to ordering deliveries of fast foods from restaurants.

A nurse in obstetrics said:

> When I get off work it takes me 3 days to relax. I find that I'm ruining my health. I'm tired all of the time, I have no appetite for food, and I'm not getting any exercise. Life seems to be nothing but working and sleeping. I'm depressed when I never used to be and I'm having problems with my sex life as a result of my work stress. I've decided that I'm leaving my job and I'm leaving nursing.

As a result of the physical manifestations of stress that caregivers had, their rate of calling in sick is often increased (4). As one nurse commented: "With

12-hour-days we have incredible sick calls and lots of mental health breaks. The nurses aren't physiologically sick but they're just exhausted."

Major Illness Problems

More serious physical illnesses include: hypertension, Crohn's disease, cardiac symptoms including shortness of breath, incapacitating migraine headaches, cluster headaches, ulcers, anorexia, and severe back pain. A nurse on an intensive care unit said: "I probably don't cope very well. I'm a perfectionist. I'm vocal with what bothers me. I've had one ulcer and I don't intend to get another. I have colitis and GI problems at the moment, however."

Ulcers were a symptom that occurred more often than any of the other major physical illnesses mentioned. An oncologist said, "I said to my department head, 'You gave me an ulcer by accusing me of stealing your patients.' " A nurse who previously worked in an abortion clinic reported that after she had worked in this setting for 5 years, she:

> ... developed ulcers and couldn't eat. I was in my early 30s and felt that I was becoming a complete slob. I was going into work early and working late every day and found that the level of stress was very intense. I hadn't had lots of professional training and I was inexperienced and lived with the constant fear of doing or saying something that would ruin the lives of the adolescent girls that I was working with, or their parents and boyfriends with whom I met. The weight of that decision in helping them to come to their own conclusions eventually became something that I didn't want to do.

An oncology nurse reported that in the first 7 months of her new job she constantly had headaches, and was now being worked up for multiple sclerosis. She was aware that some people felt that multiple sclerosis might be stress related and she was wondering if her disease might have been triggered by the emotional stress that she was experiencing because of the unit on which she was working.

> I'm having problems with my left side and I'm now going through a work up for multiple sclerosis. I felt that I couldn't cope with dealing with my work and the symptoms of my own disease at the same time. Recently when I had my first episode one of the young patients with whom I had been working died. His mother called and said, "Where were you when I needed you?" Two more patients died with brain metastasis and it was very difficult on me to know that my symptoms correlated with theirs extremely well. I'm now at the point where I've decided to leave work and find a less stressful job and concentrate on taking care of my own health.

Earlier unpublished work by the author and her colleagues showed that caregivers who had preexisting chronic illness might well find this exacerbated by exposure to chronic work stressors.

BEHAVIORAL MANIFESTATIONS OF CAREGIVER STRESS

A third of the manifestations mentioned were behavioral and involved caregivers' interactions with others in their personal or work environment.

STAFF CONFLICT (33%)

Second only to psychological feelings of depression, grief, and guilt was the behavioral manifestation of stress, staff conflict. This was the major manifestation of stress for caregivers in the specialties of pediatric intensive care units, intensive care units, and palliative care services.

Staff conflict revolved around a number of issues, but particularly focused on the areas of power struggles and rivalry which evolved from role conflict and/or personal questions of adequacy.

These power struggles often reflected a basic lack of trust in colleagues' competence and judgement. Staff conflict would then be manifest as a symptom of stress and insecurity around decision-making or it might be obvious in response to iatrogenic illness or following a patient's death. In the latter situation it was often easier to become angry and have conflict with colleagues than to confront one's own grief, depression, and guilt in response to death.

On many units staff seemed to develop cliques or subgroups that "scapegoated" or blamed one or more people for all of the problems within a team situation. Sometimes groups seem able to function only if there is an identified scapegoat who is seen as being "the current problem" within the work situation. In such a team, one can often get antagonistic pairings; that is, two or more people will team up to complain about others (6). Frequently it will be found that when the group is upset about an issue such as a patient's death, they will choose to focus in on problems with their colleagues rather than focusing in on the death. This displacement helps to avoid the impotence staff may feel with a death. Scapegoating may also reflect a general dissatisfaction with work and life in general and may serve to defuse caregivers' feelings so that they do not have to confront the real issues involved.

Katherine Mitchell, a nurse who works in a teaching hospital emergency room observed that:

> When staff are unhappy with themselves about something what happens is that it gets dumped into the workplace—not focused on the source of unhappiness, but rather displaced onto the system or onto someone else. On our unit I once saw someone scapegoated. Sure she had a few problems but they kept after her until she had a full scale nervous breakdown and had to leave.

Often staff do not understand the dynamics of the situation when people are being scapegoated and rather than looking at the issues involved the problem is allowed to escalate. When the scapegoat finally leaves the situation then usually someone else is quickly recast into the role. It is as though the group cannot survive without being united against someone as opposed to being focused towards a group goal.

A resident who had been going through problems in his personal life reflected on what could happen within a team situation.

> If your colleagues aren't supportive then you aren't likely to tell them about your personal problems. If they then notice that you are looking "down" they'll often begin to "dump" on you. I didn't tell anyone when my brother was critically ill. I was performing okay but probably looked depressed. I found myself getting scapegoated for lots of things. The nurses and staff physicians "dumped" on me. There seems to almost be a need to get you when you are down. Maybe in the future I'll tell people I

am having problems, but if you don't trust your colleagues you're hesitant to open up to them.

Frequently scapegoating occurs when there are cliques or antagonistic pairings amongst staff members. In such a situation it is found that with the pairings that go on within the unit, newcomers may not feel welcome and may quickly leave. This can be particularly common in the group burnout situation. In addition however, when a person who has been part of this group leaves, others may soon follow. As one nurse in a community hospital observed, "With a lot of interpersonal relationship problems with your colleagues, there's a rapid turnover of staff. You can't begin to get close to each other because people leave and you feel unattached. After this has been going on for a period of about 5 or 6 months, you get low morale, which leads to more staff conflict." Yancik constrasted three hospice programs and found that the program that had the greatest amount of staff support stress had the highest staff turnovers (7).

Scapegoating may become particularly severe when it appears that there is an iatrogenic illness.

Rita Pearson, an ICU nurse in a teaching hospital said that:

With an unexpected death there may be some scapegoating towards the doctor, but that's not a general thing. Usually there's scapegoating only if the nurses felt that it's really deserved and that the physician really is incompetent. We have one surgeon around here who has a terrific bedside manner and his patients really love him but he's a lousy surgeon. Recently we had one of his patients die from a mistake that was made in the operating room. The hostility towards this doctor continues to this day, despite the fact that we know it wasn't only his mistake. For a while he was cut off his O.R. privileges but now he continues to perform surgery. I don't know how he feels about the mistakes he makes, but he always looks good, he always has a terrific bedside manner, and his patients continue to love him. . . but the nurses don't trust him at all.

Nurses are certainly not the only ones to have trouble with staff conflict. Physicians often talked in terms of rivalry and the power struggles that went on within their professional group. Dr. Norman Thomas reflected on some of the rivalry that he saw within the oncology profession. He said:

You need to have a lot of arrogance to take on the odds that we've got to take on, and frequently this arrogance doesn't allow physicians to see that they reflect their own arrogance to the patient and their colleagues. As a group I find that doctors are tremendously rivalrous and in turn are very isolated from one another. The sense is that you're only as good as your competition in this hospital and your goals are reflective of how good the others around you are. This competition really isn't very generous.

An oncologist who worked in the same hospital spoke in terms of how his colleagues had frozen out some of the more competent physicians within the organization. It seemed as though if someone was more competent than they were, then they didn't want that individual around. This of course is a manifestation of their own feelings of insecurity but it can become obvious in staff conflicts and communication breakdowns.

The rivalry and tension that exists amongst various professionals can come out in a variety of other ways as well. Dr. Helen Ulysses, an oncologist, found that one of the greatest difficulties that she had was with the fact that her male colleagues frequently had no sympathy for the fact that as a woman with dual roles her stressors were somewhat different from theirs.

I find if I have to leave here because my child is sick, then that means that I have to load someone else with my work. They feel that if I'm a female in the workforce I should have my life organized. Sure I have backup systems, but at times of stress there's often a feeling that the stress that all of this causes for me is not truly appreciated. Many of the men around here don't let their wives work and wouldn't be married to a working woman. Recently when my support people were away I said to my male colleague, "This housework is really getting to me." His response was, "Now you know what life is really like. That's what women are supposed to be doing—staying at home." I feel that there's not a true appreciation for this mixed role and for what I'm trying to accomplish.

At times when numerous work stressors are impinging on department members then it is easy for them to begin to take out their aggression on their colleagues. A nurse in an emergency room commented that a physician had recently asked her in an angry tone, "Why haven't you done this job?" She said her response was, "I haven't done everything because unfortunately I have only two hands, two feet, and one head."

Sometimes staff members come to understand what they're doing when team conflicts arise, but at other times they don't. A social worker working with children with cystic fibrosis said: "We realized that we needed to do team work when the psychiatrists were angry at the physios for beating up on the patients and the physios were angry at the psychiatrists because they were using behavior modification and depriving the kids."

Often staff conflict leads to caregivers leaving the work situation which will be discussed in Chapter 10. When caregivers announce that they are going to leave a unit, however, this can result in considerable stress on the team. One nurse observed that: "When I left the unit it was like a divorce with the physician with whom I work. He had recently gotten divorced from his wife and when I left, he really had a lot of trouble with it."

Frequently it will be found that when staff members are having difficulty with their separation anxiety when a key colleague is leaving, then others will begin to close out that colleague in anger and grief and will begin to give the message that "We really didn't think that much of you anyway; you really weren't that good. We really won't miss you." It is interesting to observe this type of behavior in caregivers who are supposed to be so experienced in dealing with separation anxiety and grief when their own patients die. It is sometimes as though we are accepting of the patients dying because it is not of their own volition, but when colleagues leave us, it is a conscious decision. As a result, much of the anger that we unconsciously would like to express towards patients for dying and "leaving us" may get projected onto our colleagues whom we may feel abandon us by leaving stressful job situations. The reader who wishes more information on staff conflict is referred to Mount and Voyer's excellent article (8) on palliative care stress and to Roberts' article on NICU staff conflict from a house officer's perspective (9).

JOB–HOME INTERACTION (28%)

Job-home interaction increased with age and was reported by men twice as often as by women. This may well be because the males in the study tended to have higher status and independent jobs in which they were frequently on call. They tended to bring work home with them as well. If one looks at the reasons why males might have more difficulty with job-home interaction than females, one might hypothesize that it might be socially more acceptable for men to get away with bringing the job situation home with them until such time as it becomes a big problem and begins to actually seriously interfere with their home and family life. Over time both caregivers and their families may well become less tolerant of the interaction between job and home, and indeed a few caregivers spoke of the fact that they were having severe personal problems because of the way in which they had allowed their job to interfere with their family life. This section will look at why job-home interaction occurs, how it happens, the way in which it is manifest, and the effect it has on caregivers and their families. In addition, we will look at some of the ways in which caregivers have chosen to decrease the job-home interaction that they were beginning to find problematic.

Job-home interaction can occur because of the way in which caregivers have been educated and the role expectations that have derived from their educational systems, their own personality, the personality of their spouses and family members, and the interaction amongst these variables. Dr. Marvin Mendelson, a family practitioner, observed that he felt that:

> Working towards being a doctor is drummed into you at least from university. Once you're into medical school with its systems approach everything is directed towards medical science and not at looking at the total person. This outlook tends to neglect the emotional and psychosocial aspects of one's self and others. Dependency on this system of looking at life is fed within the medical system. Once one gets into the big bad world, then you come to realize that you have to make decisions and you have personal responsibilities that you can no longer refuse to face. When one is in medical school and even in residency, one could make excuses because "I have to study" but when one begins practice then personal and financial problems begin to develop and people have expectations that at last you should be performing.
>
> This is a problem however, because during medical school people have tended to neglect other social supports. They have no hobbies, do no other reading, and have gotten out of the habit of doing anything other than simply focusing in on their work life. When they do become involved, even in a hobby, then they tend to become obsessive with it, in the same way that they have become obsessive about diagnosing, caring, and curing. For example I've seen colleagues of mine become gentlemen-farmers but become absolutely obsessive in all of these activities as well. Everything needs to be completely precise. This just serves to add to the professional stress that they experience, rather than alleviating it. They tend to have a need to see an end product in whatever they do. One of my colleagues has a beautiful farmhouse which he has expended all of his extra effort on furnishing with antiques and making quite lovely, but he can never actually enjoy it. His wife recently told him that she wants a divorce and shocked him when she told him that their most recent child is not even his.
>
> Things are even complicated at the level of choosing a spouse. Here physicians are particularly vulnerable. They often expect to settle down and have a family while at the same time they don't have time to develop a relationship. Often times you see physicians marrying the people that they're most in contact with and these are apt to be secretaries and nurses who may as a group have an artificial image of the physician and his or her role. Doctors as a group tend not to develop their relationships but to focus on developing their careers.

The physician as an individual may also change over the course of his or her training. Dr. Helen Ulysses said that:

> Medical people tend to be bossy and it gets worse as it goes on. I'm simply not the person that my husband married. When I married I was in medical school and was fairly dependent. I changed from believing that the male was dominant and that I

as the female was to maintain a traditional role, to being increasingly more independent, aggressive, and needing to parcel my time all the time. I have a no-nonsense approach at work and I tend to take it home with me. What winds up happening is that work sees my big effort and there, I'm seen as being pleasant and coping well, and then I defuse at home. My family gets short-changed when I've had a hard day at work.

Spouses may allow the caregiver to get away with bringing a lot of job tensions home with him or her. One wife of an oncologist said that she found it particularly difficult to meet with the wives of her husband's colleagues because some of them seemed to feel that it was important that they assume the role of being "a doormat". She observed that she saw some of the oncologists with whom she socialized, treat their wives in a fairly negative fashion. Some of these women appeared quite willing to put up with this because they felt that it was their indirect contribution to treating patients with cancer. They seemed to feel that their husbands were entitled to be demanding at home because they had to give so much of themselves at work.

Dr. Ulysses acknowledged that she sometimes takes job tension home with her, but said that when she's feeling this way she tries to explain to her husband and children that, "Today is really bad, but tomorrow won't be, so let's set time aside tomorrow to do something good." She noted however, that her male colleagues didn't seem to do that, as in their parenting role, she saw them functioning as "non-fathers":

They seem to be the father figure that appears at meal time and sits behind the newspaper, neither observing nor being observed. They seem to primarily focus on making money and participate less and less in raising their own kids. When I see them on weekends in their parenting role, the message is very clear that it's the wife's role to do the parenting because father has worked hard all week and is tired. I have to question how long these wives are going to be willing to put up with this. As a group, physicians have a high divorce rate. Many of these spouses have been dragged through the years of stress in putting their husbands through medical school and they find them getting involved in the job situation and no longer giving at home. The wife has to ask herself, "What am I doing there maintaining the family unit but getting no sense of satisfaction in my relationship."

Dr. Robert Walters, a surgeon, spoke of the father's and husband's perspective:

Medicine involves such a time commitment. You begin to see your family suffer. I used to think that I'd make it up to them and find time tomorrow, but I find that I never do. My children are stressed because they feel they can't keep up to being as perfect as they see me as being, and that's hard on kids. What you do as a physician comes almost unconsciously to you. You have to have such self-control and frequently that means that your kids see you as being almost perfect in your disciplined way of doing things. You tend to then unconsciously demand that your kids perform in the same way. As I get older I find myself making a major effort to avoid pressuring my children, but when I'm busy, it's easy to gloss over and become quite demanding of them.

I find I work so hard and I'm under so much pressure that when I then start to have some free time, I want to do the kind of thing that I want to do and that may not be what the kids want to do. I also find that I need to base everything on priorities and find that it's hard to keep kids as a top priority. I wind up spending a lot of my evening time doing my own work and then the kids ask why I'm not watching TV with them. Usually that means that they're guilty that they are watching TV and it becomes a difficult situation.

Problems with job-home interaction can occur for a number of different reasons.

Dr. Ed Travers, a family practitioner, explained how he felt that it happened in his life.

> Often there are times that one's commitments to work and family life are in conflict. There's no such thing as a perfect family; all of our families are vulnerable. When my kids were younger, they used to count on going to the zoo. Their noses would be pressed to the window on Sunday afternoon and I'd get caught up with something at work. My wife would say, "Oh come on, we've been waiting three quarters of an hour; did you have to let yourself get caught up again?" The little stresses begin to start niggling and I think to myself, "I'll say 'no' more often and I'll delegate more" but often it doesn't work.
>
> On those days we'd drive to the zoo with me white-knuckled to have "family fun." We'd get there and I'd angrily say, "Oh look at the bloody giraffe." It takes its toll. It's easier for me now because the kids are grown but I watch the young residents and I wonder what's going to happen to them.
>
> Even in my present life as I reached middle-age however, I find that I still can get involved in overload which comes with fatigue or vice-versa. There's always too much work to be done in too short a time. Last week for example my office was scheduled to finish at five. At 4:30 I looked around and thought, okay, I'll be finished by 5:30 and I'll get home by 6:30 to take the family to the cottage as I promised. Then the phone rings. It's Mr. Jones saying his wife is on the floor and can't move, can I come right away. I say, "No, I can't." I take enough of a history to know an ambulance should be called and tell him what to do. I call the ambulance myself because if he calls, they'll take her to the closest hospital instead of the one where her records are. Then I call the hospital. By then 15 minutes have elapsed. I know I'll be late getting home and I drive home feeling guilty and angry at my family because I know they'll be angry at me. They don't care if the woman's on the floor. They want to go to the cottage. There have been too many women on the floor over the years. In the car and at home the stress builds up.

In contrast, Dr. Patrick Nelson, an oncologist, reflected that with his increasing age he found that he gradually allowed his work to interfere with his home life much less.

> I almost have two families because I have a 3-year-old who is now a great source of enjoyment to me as I watch him grow up. As I aged, I just stopped bringing work home with me as much and the older kids are pleased that I'm now much more available to them. When they were younger it used to be that I'd get home at 8:00 or 9:00 at night with a tale of woe that I couldn't tell them because if I said anything, they'd say, "Dad, who the hell needs to hear that kind of a story?" I don't think that my not being available to them in their early years did any apparent damage to them, other than the fact that they're fairly indolent which seems to be pretty typical of the age. They don't work very hard in school but at least they appear to enjoy themselves.

A hospital administrator reflected that in his observation, physicians often became locked into their work situation because of the economics involved. He observed that,

> The problem is the fee-for-service system. A doctor gets caught up in needing to do a certain number of procedures or work a certain number of hours to make "x" amount of money. He doesn't get to spend much time with his wife or family; therefore the wife feels she needs to get paid back in material goods for what she's missing in interpersonal satisfaction, so she pushes to get her $300,000 home with an ocean view which makes him need to work all the harder to keep up with payments.

Problems with job-home interaction may be manifest in a number of different ways. A few physicians spoke of trying to sneak time away from their spouses in order to get caught up on paper work, knowing that their spouses would be quite furious if they discovered what they were doing. One oncology nurse in a small community said that her husband complained that patients called her at home too often and so she organized her home visits so as to be able to sneak out to do them when her husband was on his hunting trips.

Dr. Walter French, an oncologist, said that he felt considerable personal stress because he felt inadequate with his family in that he was not seeing his wife or children enough.

> I get home at about 9:30 at night and my kids who are three and six are still up waiting to see me. I got home for dinner twice this week but tomorrow's my son's last T-ball game and my wife is furious because I'm not going to be there to see it. There just isn't a lot of time. When I get home at bedtime for the kids they need stories and won't go to bed without a story, and they really demand that I be the one to read them stories. Recently they don't get a hell of a lot else from me because what time there is, is devoted to other things that need doing. Generally the kids get seen to be primarily an annoyance who are making messes while I'm trying to tidy up. I was trying to fix the driveway recently and my 6-year-old was throwing stones and I just wanted to kill him. I know that's not a very good thing and so I play a little T-ball with him, but it just isn't enough.
>
> Holidays are coming now and the first week the kids will get a lot of attention. By the second week I'm not so interested in them and by the third week I'm thinking in terms of getting back to work. I find it takes me 4 or 5 days of a vacation to come down from working and then the last 5 days, I'm gearing up to go back to work and I get to be a bitch. I worry about what to do and I start working during my holidays trying to gear up. My wife tells me not to bring work home with me so I sneak to do it and I find that I want to work whenever she's not looking at me; but heaven help me if I want to work when others are playing or when she catches me sneaking out to the dock to get in a little bit of extra dictating.

As much as families resent caregivers' absence because of work situations, they seem to be particularly upset (and caregivers felt particularly guilty) around leaving their family members on special occasions such as Christmas. A social worker spoke of feeling uncomfortable when she left her own three young children on Christmas Eve in order to go off and speak with a dying person. A funeral director said that on Christmas Eve one of the women that he knew called him because her son had drowned in the bathtub at home: "What do you do? I left the family to have Christmas Eve dinner by themselves and went to handle her."

Caregivers can disappear just so often before a considerable amount of family strife begins to develop. A woman who had been married to an oncologist said that many factors entered into her divorcing her husband of many years, but one of the biggest difficulties was the tremendous problem the family had at Christmas time. This physician was seen as the model of the caring doctor within the hospital situation. He would show up on Christmas day bringing presents for all the patients and playing Santa Claus, but when he came home he would always be tremendously depressed and feel very guilty at having left all those dying patients behind. His wife said that Christmas for their family was always quite terrible if one of his patients was dying in the hospital. Gradually she decided that she was no longer willing to have her family constantly suffer because of what was going on within her husband's work situation and so she separated from him.

One has to ask what this type of work does to caregivers' interactions with their own family. Some caregivers spoke of colleagues who had managed to create a situation where they spent very little time with their own families and expected their colleagues to do the same. A physician said: "One of the professors is up at 6:00 a.m. to dictate and work. On Saturday he does leisurely rounds and teaching—the residents have to be there and they become furious and their families are angry because they aren't home with them. After a while in this business you come to think that everything you say is teaching." Medical students who were attempting to explore how to have a balanced home life and professional career state that successful physicians said, "Fine, there are lots of people willing to work hard. Don't expect to get onto my service."

Other people spoke of the increased sense of vulnerability they felt because of the work they did. Several caregivers spoke of being concerned that their children had cancer when they had fairly minor symptoms. One nurse from Australia who had begun to develop more of a professional reputation because of some of her research said that she found that when she was traveling for business she had a sense that she would be punished for becoming overinvested in her work and she feared at those times that her children would get cancer since she had become so sensitized to it within the work situation. Still other caregivers said that they changed their feelings about their family members as a direct result of their work. A therapist working with families where someone had suicided said that she felt an inherent sense of vulnerability because of her role:

> I am less trustful of my own relationships and I have less feeling of my ability to judge them accurately. When I see a woman whose husband has suicided after a business failure, then I want my husband to check in with me more often and I put extra pressure on that relationship. I've become very conscious of my child rearing practices. As parents we all have points of regret and I find myself looking at points of regret but trying to minimize the guilt I feel about the mistakes I make. I'm constantly confronted with the fact that I have become a very self-conscious parent and I don't want to have any regrets from my own children.
>
> I have an unnatural focus and preoccupation with my work life. I have to realize that these are people just like me and their kids committed suicide. I don't have the balance of seeing lots of people whose kids don't suicide and after a while I find that it's easy for me and for the volunteers who work with me, to begin to lose perspective from our work.

Family members also experience certain feelings and problems directly as a result of their interaction with the caregivers. Nurses in an emergency room spoke of the fact that husbands of emergency room nurses tended to lose their own sense of personal identity. "We as emergency nurses have a strong identity and we tend to take over with our family. In the early days in my role I found I talked incessantly to my husband about losing a child, the cardiac arrest I had, and I would talk incessantly until I was talked out. Sometimes I'd talk until 5:00 a.m."

Family members sometimes become concerned about what this kind of over-involvement in a professional role is doing to the caregiver and to his or her personality. Several of the younger female caregivers spoke in terms of their mothers being particularly concerned with the kind of job stress they were bringing home. One young nurse in a community hospital said that her mother kept begging her to leave oncology and go into work in the nursery. "I'm so tense when I go home that when she says, 'Hi' I say, 'What do you mean by that?' I find I don't want to talk or to hear a single voice when I go home from work at the end of a shift and sometimes I think I'm going to go crazy. This work takes so much out of me all day long that when I go home, there's just nothing left."

Family members can also find that they become very involved in the job that the caregiver is doing and they may sometimes be fairly ambivalent about this. A physician in a small community said that he found it difficult because he couldn't tell his wife things about the patient-friend that he was seeing and yet, "Total strangers call my wife expecting that she knows everything about them— she feels excluded, but used, because she's a nurse,"

One of the more verbal caregiver family members with whom I spoke felt that her husband's work had really come to bother her.

> We've been married now for 18 years, When we first got together I wasn't afraid of death, but the more I'm with him, the more depressed I get. I read all of his papers and books and talk with him about the patients he sees and about all the meetings that he goes to. I'd say that talk about death absorbs about 80% of our time. About 10 years ago I started getting depressed. The doctors said it was change of life, or hormones but I think it was just too much exposure to death. At this time I feel I just can't hear about it any more.

Some physicians were quite honest about the problems that they were having with their own children as a direct or indirect result of the job-home interaction they had experienced over the years. Others who were not yet having problems with their young families watched their more experienced colleagues' difficulties and wondered what would happen. They talked in terms of suicide in the adolescent children of their colleagues, drug abuse, and an inability to perform reasonably well in school.

> The kids of physicians tend to be the most mixed up crazy kids—they're all over the place. The best family doctor I know is living in a situation where his wife doesn't talk to him, his kids won't talk to him, his daughter is a heroin addict. If you can't relate to your wife and kids, who can you relate to, and does it matter who else you relate to?

Caregivers cope with the job-home interaction they experience in a number of different ways. A few who had younger children talked in terms of bringing their children into the work situation with them and letting them get to know the patients. A social worker said that he included his 3 and 6-year-old sons in his work in the hospital:

> They get to know some of the kids in the hospital and when one girl they knew died, they were noticeably upset for 2 days. They were all choked up and had constant questions about Tammy's dying. My wife also reacts emotionally. She doesn't want to be excluded but if a kid dies, she cries. I haven't cried about a child's death in 3 years.

One has to question what this kind of vicarious involvement in the work situation will do to these children and spouses in the long run. One minister said he had to ask himself this question when he called his 5-year-old daughter to come down for dinner and she said she couldn't come down because one of her dolls was dying that night and she had to stay with the doll so that she wouldn't die alone. Will this preoccupation with death turn out to be a healthy or an unhealthy experience for children? If they come to see their parents placing dying patients as a priority over them, will that come to make death a more enviable status in their eyes and might it in some instances, result in suicidal gestures or attempts in order to get attention in that way?

Some caregivers have learned over the years to avoid bringing their job situation home with them. A head nurse on a busy intensive care unit said, "I used to live with a nurse room-mate and talk shop all the time, but now I don't and I feel that I don't have anybody to discuss my job stress with, so I've learned not to talk about it. Now when there are people around I don't bother to discuss it. Something may flash into my mind, but I don't usually carry my work home with me."

An oncologist observed:

This work takes time away from my family. Whenever possible I try to do as much with my kids as I can but that winds up leaving very little time for me. I don't get to sit and read a nonmedical book except on the occasional holiday. I couldn't do this work if I were married to somebody who wasn't sympathetic to my role. As a result I try to compensate to make sure that my wife is able to do the things that she wants to do like get to her fitness classes.

ERRORS IN JUDGEMENT (12%)

Errors in judgement were a manifestation of stress that were somewhat more commonly reported by the younger group of caregivers and interestingly enough, were mentioned only by physicians and nurses. It is not surprising that younger caregivers would report more errors in judgement because of younger age, correspondingly limited practice experience, and frequently a lack of supervision that may make them vulnerable to stress reactions in which errors in judgement may occur. This problem may be particularly acute in fast-paced environments wherein decisions must be made quickly, such as intensive care units, emergency rooms, and obstetrics. Errors in judgement may be more likely to occur at night when supervisors are not immediately available. A physician commented:

Patients seldom die because of the mistakes I make now, but they used to die and it used to bug me. I can remember one man who was admitted with a ruptured renal artery when I was a casualty officer. I sent him up to the ward with a diagnosis of myocardial infarction with IV morphine—I didn't twig to what was really going on and he couldn't give the history. When patients would die after mistakes like that, I didn't go about resolving my stress by studying; rather I would learn from the incident and would enter that into my next differential diagnosis.

For the older caregiver the problem of being called upon to perform in one's professional role outside the clinical setting can often cause considerable stress.

Making a personal error in judgement really worries me. Having to deal with a coronary in a public place would be a hell of a stress. Recently at a restaurant when they called for a doctor I started to get up and my wife said, "I hope the person has cancer." I vowed to take a CPR course but I know I won't.

Taking responsibility in the area where you don't know what you're doing is a real stress. When you're younger you frequently can't admit when you don't know something and you can't get someone else to do it as easily; now I have people under me to direct so I don't get involved in that kind of situation professionally but any of us can personally.

Older caregivers often questioned if in fact they were getting out of practice with situations such as cardiac arrests that they didn't see too often. A family physician had a visiting resident in his office with him. When he proceeded to treat a patient in a particular way, the resident responded, "Surely you're not doing that."

I was right but I could have been wrong. I began to wonder if I really was wrong and behind. When you make an error in judgement it can just about destroy you. I've seen colleagues of mine make such errors or be suspected of such errors. One of the problems is that you're suspected until you're vindicated even when you're innocent and during that time your work is compromised and spoiled. I saw one colleague go through 6 years of hell until his name was cleared for the particular incident. I watched another colleague who was supervising a physician in the emergency room. He assigned an intern to deal with a woman who came in screaming that her husband had poisoned her. No one said that she was pregnant but within a few minutes she had ruptured an occult tubal pregnancy and died. The disapproval of the doctors and nurses was tremendously stressful for this particular colleague because he always was very conscientious.

At other times caregivers may unconsciously not want to discover problems in particular patients and this may interfere with their judgement. White (10) speaks of denial on the part of health professionals and notes that hundreds of times women have found lumps in their breasts and asked their physicians to do something, only to be told that it was nothing serious. In work by the author and her colleagues (11), it was found that women with breast cancer whose physicians delayed in their diagnosis were much more likely to develop recurrences and/or die, and Holland and Mastrovito (12) commented that patients with physician delay are among the most difficult to treat. White says that in his view, the reasons for physicians not properly diagnosing breast lumps and not performing pap smears or sigmoidoscopies on patients is not laziness, but may well be reflective of an unwillingness to find something unpleasant. He suggests that it may be the old fear of the herald bringing bad news to the emperor. He also notes that it may well be the caregivers' identification with patients and their fear of how they would respond in a similar situation that keeps them from looking to fully discover what is wrong with the particular patient.

One young woman who was dying of cancer spoke of the fact that she had a chronic cough for several months. Despite the fact that she had already had one recurrence of her cancer of the thyroid, her physician said, "I'm so sure that your cough isn't cancer that I won't do blood levels to test if it is." Obviously, when physicians avoid looking to determine the real cause of disease and then the patient goes on to die of the disease, considerable stress results for both parties.

Errors in judgement can also occur because there is not sufficient time to evaluate one's judgement. An obstetrician had a patient come to see him because she was trying to avoid a C-section. He hadn't really had to time to evaluate her when the patient quickly went into labor. . . "with a double footling breech presentation . . . the baby died. . . I knew she probably should have been a C-section but. . . ."

In addition to a lack of time to make judgements, caregivers sometimes do not fully think through the judgements that they have made. A policeman spoke of bringing a patient into the emergency room at a community hospital and being told, " 'He's gone. Get him out of here.' Another doctor came in and started yelling, 'Get me this, get me that' and they brought the guy around. He's out and functioning now." There may also be biases against particular patients that may predispose caregivers to judgement errors. A nurse at another community hospital spoke of problems that her colleagues had with their judgements about suicidal patients. They felt that suicidal patients were inappropriately placed on the ICU and belonged in the psychiatric unit. They tended to ignore the suicidal patients. Nevertheless, the hospital had a policy of placing all overdoses on the ICU.

"A young girl was brought to ICU after an overdose. The next day she had been assessed and found to be still actively suicidal but was left alone. As soon as the assessor's back was turned, she reached over to the bed beside her, grabbed the syringes off the bedside table and injected herself with all the emergency drugs that were there."

Finally, caregivers are frequently more critical of themselves and think that they have made judgement errors when their colleagues in fact feel that their judgements were appropriate. A public health nurse spoke of the fact that she was called by a landlord about an elderly woman who hadn't been able to get out of bed. The nurse had difficulty getting a doctor to do a home visit to assess the patient. By the time the physician arrived, the patient was dead. "The physician told me that this was the woman's choice—to die at home. But I felt guilty and felt I should have called the ambulance myself rather than waiting for the physician's judgement. I felt I erred in my own professional judgement and this is a threat to my self-esteem. I like to be right and this was very hard."

REFERENCES

1. Krakowski, A. J. (1982). Stress and the practice of medicine—The myth and the reality. *Journal of Psychosomatic Research, 26*(1) 91–98.

2. Elliott, G. R., & Eisdorfer, C. (Eds.). (1982). *Stress and human health: Analysis and implications of research.* New York: Springer.

3. Vander-Doelen, J. (1982). Problems and approaches to shift-work. *Occupational Health in Ontario, 3*(1) 37–47.

4. Tasto, D. L. (1977). The health consequences of shift work. *Conference on Occupational Stress,* Los Angeles, CA, pp. 37–41.

5. Lyall, W. A. L., Vachon, M. L. S., & Rogers, J. (1980). A study of the degree of stress experienced by professionals caring for dying patients. In I. Ajemian and B. Mount (Eds.), *The Royal Victoria Hospital manual on palliative/hospice care: A resource book.* (pp. 489–509). New York: ARNO.

6. Edelwich, J. (1980). *Burn-out: Stages of disillusionment in the helping professions.* New York: Human Sciences.

7. Yancik, R. (1984). Sources of work stress for hospice staff. *Journal of Psychosocial Oncology, 2*(1) 21–31.

8. Mount, B., & Voyer, J. (1980). Staff stress in palliative/hospice care. In I. Ajemian and B. Mount (Eds.), *The R.V.H. manual on palliative/hospice care.* (pp. 457–488). New York: ARNO.

9. Roberts, J. L. (1982). Adapting to the NICU: The house officer's perspective. In R. E. Marshall, C. Kasman, & L. S. Cape (Eds.), *Coping with caring for sick newborns.* Philadelphia: Saunders.

10. White, L. P. (1977). Death and the physician: Mortuis vivos docent. In H. Feifel (Ed.), *New meanings of death.* (pp. 92–106). New York: McGraw-Hill.

11. Vachon, M. L. S. (1986). A comparison of the impact of breast cancer and bereavement: Personality, social support and adaptation. In S. Hobfoll (Ed.), *Stress social support, and women* (pp. 187–204). Washington, DC: Hemisphere.

12. Holland, J., & Mastrovito, R. (1980). Psychologic adaptation to breast cancer. *Cancer, 46,* 1045–1052.

9

Psychological Manifestations of Stress

The psychological manifestations of stress in caregivers have been documented in quantitative terms in relatively few studies, although there are numerous anecdotal accounts. Lyall, Vachon, and Rogers (1) found that 3 months after the opening of a palliative care unit, the nurses studied had distress scores on the Goldberg General Health Questionnaire comparable to a group of newly widowed women, and almost twice as high as those found in women newly diagnosed with breast cancer (2, 3). The palliative care nurses had distress scores twice as high as nurses on two other units in the same hospital (4).

More recent work by Gray-Toft and Anderson (5) found that hospice nurses experienced less stress than did those on other units in the same hospital. They hypothesized that this was because of structural characteristics of the different units that affected the amount of role ambiguity and conflict the staff experienced. By the time of that study some of the problems that were noted in our original research were known to those starting similar units. Livingston and Livingston found distress in nursing to be more common in younger, less experienced nurses spending more time with patients (6)—a finding which is of course similar to that of the present study.

This study has attempted to quantify qualitative data and in doing so, found that psychological manifestations of stress accounted for 61% of the manifestations mentioned. Of these psychological symptoms, three symptoms: feelings of depression, grief, and guilt; helplessness and inadequacy; and anger and irritability accounted for 63% of the manifestations.

DEPRESSION, GRIEF, AND GUILT (22%)

Feelings of depression, grief, and guilt constituted the single greatest manifestation of stress across all professional groups and in the specialties of oncology, emergency room, and chronic care. The emotions of depression, grief, and guilt were closely intertwined and were usually experienced in response to a loss situation that involved bereavement.

In order to understand caregiver depression we will discuss some of the psychodynamics of bereavement and grieving. Bereavement presupposes the loss of an important individual or object that had meaning to an individual. One might expect that a caregiver would grieve at the time of the death of a patient with whom he or she had a close relationship, yet bereavement does not always come about through the death of a person, but can evolve through many other losses as well. These losses may involve the loss of a patient through death, the loss of a sense of self-esteem, or the loss of support from one's significant others. The individual meaning that we consciously or unconsciously ascribe to the particular loss that we experience will then in part determine whether we experience grief.

Some caregivers may be particularly vulnerable to situations involving loss. This susceptibility to loss may evolve from an overinvestment in the caregiver role. Such an overinvestment may reflect a lack of other sources of validation of one's worth as a human being which might be derived through other roles and through contact with other people outside of the clinical situation. Those who have allowed their major psychological investment of energy to be in their work are probably more vulnerable to threats to their feelings of professional competence, whether this results from a patient death or from problems with role performance, than are their colleagues who have other interests in their lives that serve to sustain their identity. The response of these overinvested caregivers to a loss may be similar to that of a new widow whose identity was totally tied up with her spouse. With his death she loses not only her spouse, but her sense of self, the sense of meaning in her life and her major role. Caregivers who are overinvested may well have a more difficult grief reaction because of being unable to see themselves as functioning in any role other than that of a competent professional—as the new widow may similarly have difficulty seeing herself functioning outside of the role of "wife."

Although depression, grief, and guilt were often found to occur together it is important to distinguish amongst these emotions. In his excellent book *Grief Counselling and Grief Therapy,* Dr. J. William Worden (7) notes that grief looks very much like depression. Grief may in fact develop into a full blown depression. In both states one finds the classic symptoms of sleep and appetite disturbances and intense sadness, but in a grief reaction one does not find the loss of self-esteem found in most depressions. "That is, the people who have lost someone do not regard themselves less because of such a loss or if they do, it tends to be for only a brief time. And if the survivors of the deceased experience guilt, it is usually guilt associated with some specific aspect of the loss rather than a general, overall sense of culpability" (7, p. 28).

Depression

The depression that caregivers experienced often reflected the loss of self-esteem and guilt not usually found in grief and often involved a sense of guilt. Their depressive symptoms ranged from relatively benign sleep disturbances and feelings of fatigue to more severe symptoms of early morning wakening, appetite disturbances, decreased libido and a preoccupation with illness and death. Some caregivers reported having been actively suicidal and a few reported that colleagues had suicided during a depressive episode which often involved problems in both their personal and professional lives. A large scale survey of over 3,000 nurses revealed that 76% reported feeling depressed either almost always or occasionally when caring for an incurable, terminally ill patient (8). A much smaller study of pediatric residents showed that 7 out of the 13 studied had been obviously distressed or depressed while caring for a terminally ill child, while two consistently had difficulty during and after caring for such a child (9).

The depression that accompanies grief was often obvious in caregivers at the time that a patient died, especially when the caregiver and patient had a long-term relationship or the caregiver felt a major loss with this death. As well, however, the effects of a more chronic depression could become evident at unexpected times. One nurse reported breaking into tears when she went to the vegetable store and the tomatoes were not ripe. Another nurse reported becoming equally teary when she watched an old couple climb up the stairs of a bus. Others reported an inability to plan for the future because of a sense that one couldn't invest in life—illness, death, or disaster could occur at any time. In their depression some caregivers came to envy their dying patients—the fact that they had a "way out" as well as the fact that they were the recipients of such good care. One nurse in oncology said that as she watched the patients with whom she worked dying, she often thought to herself that her life was not particularly valuable and she wondered if she would be able to die as well as her patients were dying. She said that she came to feel that since she had to die anyhow, she might as well die sooner rather than later, as her life had such little meaning for her and society. She commented "After all, I've already lived my life—I'm 30." A physician also spoke of depression that had to do with the loss of self-esteem which accompanied problems in his professional and personal lives.

> I was profoundly depressed in my late 40s. My income was dropping. I was going bankrupt, in part because my wife overspent to compensate for a lack of attention from me. It was most fearsome. My financial status was going down when it should have been going up. I started looking for a new job. I decided that I was finished. Business was dropping off. I started looking for a job teaching ethics in the university and then I found that I could only make $15,000 to $20,000 a year in teaching. I couldn't afford to get out and I wasn't making it in the profession. I didn't realize that I was depressed but one day my wife called me at work to say "do you know what day it is, it's your son's birthday and you're supposed to be at home." I said, "Do you know where your son is—he's had an accident and he's in Emergency." When I got home my family was waiting for me. They said "you're sick. You have to get help."

A young psychiatrist described his bout with a serious depression that occurred when his homosexual lover left him:

> I had been in what I thought was a solid relationship with an older man who left me quite unexpectedly. I had been doing a lot of work with AIDS patients and was caught up in grieving for their deaths when I found myself confronted with this loss. I was angry at being abandoned and wanted to go out and "screw around" to show him that others could still find me attractive, but I couldn't do this because of my fear of AIDS. I became quite depressed and seriously contemplated suicide.

Grief

The symptoms of normal grief are varied and include: sadness, anger, guilt and self-reproach, anxiety, loneliness, fatigue, helplessness, shock, yearning, emancipation, relief, and numbness (11). Most of these manifestations of grief were seen in caregivers in response to loss from death but some of the symptoms emerged in response to other stressors involving feelings of loss as well. The main symptoms associated with grief were as follows:

Shock and disbelief are common responses to grief and were perhaps best exhibited by the physician who had to be pulled off a child on whom he had been performing external cardiac massage for two and a half hours. This cardiac surgeon was heavily invested in the child's living and he kept saying to the dead child, "You can't die on me."

Anger was the common response to grief when iatrogenic illness was involved or when there was a physician delay in making a diagnosis and the patient was dying in response to this apparent delay. At other times caregivers were either consciously or unconsciously angry at patients for dying. If a caregiver had been particularly close to a patient then the death might feel like abandonment. This situation is most likely to occur if a caregiver has had an earlier unresolved loss and has become very invested in patients as a way of avoiding confronting that loss.

In a few instances caregivers had engaged in magical thinking and felt that because of their caring, they were going to be able to save this patient from inevitable death. When this was impossible then caregivers became quite distressed. They sometimes became angry at patients for "breaking their promise" to survive and in some situations, staff members became acutely suicidal in response to patient death. They had fantasies of killing themselves and rejoining the patient "on the other side."

Caregivers could also be angry at patients for putting themselves into a position where they increased their risk of dying. The reader may remember the anger of the nurse mentioned in Chapter 7 when the young woman with cardiac problems deliberately became pregnant. The woman had realized that by becoming pregnant she was risking death but she decided to defy the odds to have a child. When the woman died shortly after delivery, the nurses became aware that they were very angry at her for having put herself into this position and for bringing a child into the world who would be motherless. They realized that their anger was irrational as the woman had made an informed decision to become pregnant—yet they wanted her back to undo her decision. They also projected their anger on to a physician who had misdiagnosed a disease many years ago because it was this undiagnosed disease which led to her death.

Feelings of guilt were common, especially if there was a question of responsibility for a patient's death. In one situation a physician ordered an incorrect drug. When the patient died, the physician went to her funeral and then went home and killed himself. Nurses sometimes experienced a considerable amount of guilt when they gave a final dose of morphine which they were afraid had precipitated the patient's death.

A physician spoke of the guilt that he experienced when he was working in an emergency room as a registrar. "A couple of people died because I didn't twig to the diagnosis. Mostly this happened late at night when I was exhausted and fatigued and when it came out at autopsy I felt really badly." This same physician said that in his current position as a researcher, he felt really guilty if he presented early data at a medical meeting indicating that research was pointing in a particular direction if it then turned out that further analysis of the data proved this was not the case. He felt guilty that other medical colleagues might be making judgements in patient care based on his inaccurate reading of his data. His wife appreciated his feelings of responsibility and questioned if he might commit suicide if he reported inaccurate data which compromised patients' lives.

When patients actually did die as a result of some oversight of caregivers, then the staff involved often had very severe grief reactions. Sometimes this was because of a patient dying for example in response to too large a dose of a chemotherapeutic drug and other times it was the result of people suiciding. In one situation an order for a drug was incorrectly written as staff members joked about "overdosing" the difficult patient on tranquilizers. The drug was given as ordered and the patient died. Needless to say, this type of situation causes extreme grief in staff. A public health nurse said that she was involved with a patient who said that she was going to jump off the balcony.

> I felt that she was going to and I called the psychiatrist who said that this patient might threaten but she wouldn't do it. The woman jumped and I was quite devastated with guilt. I kept asking myself what I could have said to convince the psychiatrist to see this woman again. I kept asking myself how I could have prevented her suicide. The minister called and dumped his anger about her death onto me and a lot of other people who were concerned about the woman were angry at me because she had died. I defended myself by asking people what I could have done. I also empathized with the psychiatrist who cried and said we were faced with these decisions all the time—usually we made the right judgement but this time we didn't.

Caregivers working in the area of abortion also sometimes had difficulty with their grief. In one situation a nurse became aware of her own guilt when she began to analyze a dream that she had.

> I had a dream that I was at home and saw a black figure with a pointed hood. It was winter time and he had a green garbage bag which he put in front of my house in a hole in the snow. I thought to myself, "this is ridiculous to put this garbage bag in the hole in the snow because when the snow melts, the garbage bag will be there." In my gestalt therapy session I looked more closely at this and discovered that this black figure was not actually holding a green garbage bag, but was actually holding something wrapped in a nursery blanket. It took me a couple of years to really work on this dream, but the second time I worked on it, my therapist asked, "What do you want to say to the figure?" I wanted to say, "I'm sorry, I need to grieve, I'm sorry but it needs to be done." I began to come in touch with my incredible sense of loss regarding what we're actually doing by performing abortions.

Other caregivers also reported that their dreams made them aware of some of the guilt they were feeling. A nutritionist working in a cancer hospital said that she found herself dreaming about a train one night. When she looked at the passengers in the train, she realized that each of them was a patient who had died since she had been working in the cancer hospital. As each face floated before her she saw a tray that she had fixed for this patient and became aware that she had left something off each of the trays. She began to see that she felt that she was somehow responsible for these patients dying. A nurse working in an intensive care unit reported dreaming about a young girl her own age who was dying. This nurse felt very guilty that this patient was being kept alive on machines to be an organ donor. In the nurse's dream, the patient came chasing after her down the hall.

Patterns of Grief

Grief in caregivers may follow as many patterns as it follows in other bereaved persons. Caregivers may have anticipatory grief and as well grief may be denied or distorted. It may be exaggerated or it may become chronic.

Anticipatory grief occurs when a caregiver who has had a close relationship with a patient begins to grieve for the patient's death before actual death occurs. Sometimes this means that the caregiver becomes very involved with the patient during the final few days, in such a case the caregiver may become what Dr. Robert Fulton has called a "surrogate griever" (10). In this situation the caregiver comes to grieve almost as much, if not more, than the family member. The caregiver might be completely incapacitated by grief and be unable to actually participate in the care of the person who is dying. In other situations the caregiver who engages in anticipatory grieving may well withdraw from the person who is going to die. A nurse working on a bone marrow transplant unit said: "I feel really badly that I've now gotten to the stage where I sometimes close a patient's chart and say, 'That's it, he's not going home.' I feel guilty that I've given up on a person like this before he's actually dead." In an important paper on caregivers' plight Weisman (11) notes that occasionally caregivers may become impatient, irritable, and even antagonistic should patients exceed predictions as to their life span and live longer than the anticipatory grief of caregivers requires.

Denial of grief is difficult to assess because the cultures in which we work often attempt to define how much grief caregivers should experience. In some instances caregivers became quite concerned about their response to death because they felt they were unable to grieve. A physiotherapist who worked in a chronic care hospital said: "I've worked here for a year and I've never grieved for a patient. I feel that maybe there's something wrong with me as everyone else seems to get upset. I've never had a personal death and so I wonder if this means that when someone really close to me dies I won't grieve either—that really upsets me."

Other caregivers reported that they did not grieve in their professional roles but their grief was displaced onto other losses. An emergency room nurse said: "It's a weird thing with death—it just doesn't bother me. I didn't cry with deaths in my own family—they just didn't bother me. Recently when the hospital chaplain died and I had to care for him in emergency, I didn't cry either. I cried however when my dog died."

Caregivers need to be able to decide how much grief is appropriate at a particular point in time. In addition they need to come to realize that not all deaths will cause them to experience grief. Caregivers will not grieve equally for all patients because not all grief situations involve equal losses. However caregivers who never grieve and are never able to acknowledge the constant losses to which they are exposed may have difficulty. Sometimes a caregiver will find that he or she almost never grieves but will be surprised when grief unexpectedly occurs with the death of a particular patient; perhaps one with whom the caregiver particularly identifies. This grief may be quite extreme. In examining this grief a caregiver will sometimes become aware of using the grief experience as a way of grieving for many other deaths. This may be particularly obvious in specialties such as palliative care wherein within a short period of time caregivers may experience the death of many patients with whom they have close relationships.

Sometimes instead of being expressed, grief may also be *distorted or masked.* In this response there is no obvious manifestation of grief but there may be manic or "life-affirming" behavior that masks grief. A few caregivers spoke of becoming sexually involved with colleagues in a way that seemed to show, "We are alive and let's celebrate life. We don't know when we might be in the same position as our patients." Caregivers may also become physically ill in response to grief. In an earlier study my colleagues and I found that nurses in a palliative care unit who had preexisting physical problems had exacerbations of their illness while working in palliative care (4). Another way that grief may be distorted is with substance abuse. A priest from the West Indies spoke of the fact that on two occasions when he had dealt with particularly difficult deaths he dealt with the pressure that he felt by drinking.

> I was quite guilty with one death. I had been asked to go to the country to substitute for a sick priest. He didn't need me to come and so I took the time off. I had been dealing with an Indian woman and her son of mixed blood. The day I was away she looked everywhere for me and when she couldn't find me she killed her son and then killed herself. I went off with a bottle of rum and got completely drunk when I found out what had happened. The people in the community said to me, "If you were here this wouldn't have happened." The chaplain that I had gone to relieve came up to see me the next day and he helped me to look at this. He said to me that I couldn't take that kind of responsibility for people as it wasn't mine to take.

Grief may also be *exaggerated* as is the situation with the caregiver who grieves openly and for an extended period of time with each and every patient who dies. Such a caregiver needs to question whether this is the appropriate job situation and/or whether there is unresolved grief for a previous loss that is best resolved before continuing in the present job.

For other caregivers, grief may become *chronic* because they experience so many losses either close together or over a long period of time. They may become preoccupied with death and patients' failure to thrive (11). This may result in the sense of generalized depression which has already been mentioned and misgivings about their own competence (11). Occasionally caregivers working with the dying experience a chronic grief reaction that precludes their being invested in any relationship outside of work and may particularly preclude a "life affirming" sexual relationship. An oncologist described the chronic grief that he experienced in his early days of practice.

> With the leukemia patients we used to just be able to get a remission for about 6 months. You used to know that you'd lose every patient that you worked with but each time it was wrenching. I was a 35-year-old demigod who was supposed to have all the answers and I felt I couldn't tell anyone that I didn't really know the answers. I was really blue and withdrawn and couldn't explain anything to people at home about what was causing this.

For other caregivers their experience with chronic grief becomes an issue that is shared openly with patients to the detriment of their performance in their professional roles. In one instance a young woman was referred because she was going to die and felt the need to make plans to prepare her husband and child for her impending death. The referral was rather surprising as she came from out of the province and was being treated in a hospital that prided itself on excellent psychosocial support services. When asked why the particular nurse who was assigned to this role had not helped her to prepare for her death she responded, "But I didn't know that nurse was supposed to help me organize my death....We're friends and we cry together about me, about the fact that I'm going to die, and about all the others who've died recently."

A priest in Newfoundland attended a workshop and at the end came up with tears in his eyes and said:

> Doesn't all this work with dying people get you down? I didn't want to come tonight but I made myself. As I listened to you and the panelists, each story you told reminded me of someone I knew or someone I'd buried. I carry them all with me all the time. I don't have anywhere to put them. I don't have anyone to talk with. I can't even go to a movie because it might be about death.
>
> I sat there listening tonight to the woman whose baby died and it took all I could do to sit and listen. I didn't want to be there. It just reminded me of too many stories.

Some caregivers choose to deal with their chronic grief by leaving the work situation. An oncology nurse said:

> I want to get out of oncology because now it's too depressing for me. I feel like it's a continual state of mourning. It has given me a terrible fear of death for myself, for my family, for everyone. The thought of death troubles me a great deal where it didn't before. I tend to get phobic and I often think that I'm going to get cancer myself.

Grief as a Group Phenomenon

Individuals may have certain expectations as to the appropriate manner in which grief should be expressed. So too might the cultures in which they work have predefined ideas as to the appropriate expression of grief. Within a given ward or unit or particular culture, grief may be exhibited in a number of different ways. Some unit cultures have a stoic approach to dealing with dying. The message is, "Here, there are no tears. We say that this death was for the best or we say that we feel relief that his suffering is over." Often these are units with minimal involvement with patients and/or a short patient stay and quick turnover. There are few references to people who have died. The deaths may begin to pile up however, and individual caregivers sometimes get a delayed reaction when they have engaged in this stoic acceptance of death. For example, a dialysis nurse said that she worked quite well on the dialysis unit until three deaths of long-term patients occurred within one week. At that point in time she decided that she was going to get out of the work situation and promptly began to look for another job.

Even on the most stoic units, however, grief can sometimes be accepted if it is kept within certain limits. A clergywoman who worked in a hospital in Sweden said, "One day a young patient died and I cried. I felt so bad because you're not supposed to do this, but when I could finally lift up my eyes I looked into all those other eyes around me and they all looked sympathetic." At other times even this much grief cannot be accepted. The same clergywoman said that when a resident had tears in his eyes when a patient died a senior staff physician handed him a valium and said, "Here, take this. It's what the rest of us around here use to deal with these situations."

As a professional group, physicians often have difficulty expressing their grief.

They sometimes have the feeling that they should not experience grief or else they feel that their patients and families would not really understand the grief that they're experiencing. Many years ago my colleagues and I were called in to work with a group of oncology nurses. They complained that they were dealing with difficult, dying patients and the staff physicians were not being supportive. Further investigation revealed that the reason that the doctors weren't being supportive was that they were down in their own offices crying alone.

Not only may colleagues, patients, and families expect caregivers to be very stoical, this expectation may come from members of their outside social support system as well. A hospital chaplain said that she had a great deal of difficulty when a 22-year-old woman died when she was first starting her work. She said:

We had been very close and involved. A priest friend of mine called and I started to cry. He said, "*You*, the pillar of strength are crumbling? I don't believe it." I got furious and said, "Who the hell are you to say this to me? I'm human like the rest of the world." I thought he'd understand. He works in a hospital and I would have thought that he'd understand. I feel that God talks to me in problems and maybe he was saying to me, "You have to be more careful who you talk to."

Some of the faster paced units such as the intensive care unit or emergency room which have a stoical acceptance of death as a part of the ward milieu may still acknowledge that it is appropriate for staff members to grieve but expect that it will be done outside of the immediate work environment. In addition, caregivers who are uncomfortable with grief themselves might realize that others have a right to grieve and may facilitate this process. One chaplain said:

In the ICU when a patient dies, I have to deal with the patient, the family, and the nurses who are crying. With long-term involvement the nurses have a right to their grief but they often can't share this with their co-workers or with their own family so they come to share their grief with us. The doctors too like to see us at the time of death. Some are very good. They come in and sit down and explain to the bereaved what has happened. Sometimes they're very technical which isn't good, but others are able to give condolences. Some, especially some surgeons, send residents to make announcements when patients have died. When a death happens in the operating room, the surgeon will often tell the staff to call the chaplain. One of the surgeons here will come and tell the family that the person has died but he'll want me to be here as well. Another surgeon will send the resident. Some surgeons are so horrified that they come in and make the announcement to the family that the person has died, and run. They can't face their own grief and are really glad to see a chaplain at that point in time.

In other settings *open expressions of grief are expected.* The message that colleagues give is that "Here, we all grieve openly. In this department four buckets of tears are expected for every patient who dies and anyone who doesn't grieve openly is not considered part of the group."

The young physiotherapist already mentioned, who wondered if in fact she would be able to grieve when people in her own family died, said: "Sure I miss some of the patients, but I just can't get terribly upset when they die. I return from a day off and see all the glum faces. I ask what happened and they say, 'Haven't you heard that Mrs. X died?' I say, 'Oh, I'm sorry.' But I can't really feel upset at the news. She was old and we knew she was going to die eventually."

Another physiotherapist questioned why staff members cry so openly when someone dies: "We don't really know them—but we have related to that person and we have the sense 'it could be me.' Sometimes I think we have to ask ourselves,

'Am I crying because I miss this person, because the family will be alone, or am I crying for myself?' Sometimes asking these questions helps caregivers to clarify their feelings."

Other unit cultures give the expectation that *"we all grieve privately in this setting."* Here grief is acknowledged but caregivers are expected to bring it home rather than express it at work. This expectation creates job-home interaction difficulties.

Finally, there is the *normal acceptance of grief* within a unit. In this type of situation, it is accepted that it is alright to grieve for patients, but it is expected that grief will pass over time. This type of unit recognizes that not all caregivers grieve in the same way, that grief is acceptable, and that not all caregivers will grieve equally for all patients.

ANGER, IRRITABILITY, AND FRUSTRATION (17%)

Anger was the most common manifestation in obstetrics and it was the second most common manifestation of stress in intensive care units, where it was second only to staff conflict (with which it obviously had an interactive effect). It was reported equally by males and females and across all age and professional groups.

Some rather extreme manifestations of anger were observed with caregivers. In one intensive care unit the nurses became upset because a resident would yell and scream and had gone so far as to pull the phone out of the wall on two different occasions. What was interesting to observe however, was that despite the nurses being extremely upset with this resident's behavior, they all agreed that in fact he was an excellent physician and in many ways his behavior was sanctioned because of this. It would appear that at least within some hospital systems the phenomenon of physicians or other high status people having temper tantrums is tolerated and even subtly encouraged as long as the people are seen as being highly skilled practitioners. A nurse on a busy intensive care unit said: "The clinical fellow gets angry and yells and screams, his face turns red and his neck veins stand out. I've complained to our chief who says, 'We need manipulators in the profession.'"

In a conversation, a noted psychoanalyst who has examined issues related to death for many years reflected on the medical "temper tantrum." He noted that the operating room is called the "theatre" within the British medical system and reflected that this open tolerance of medical "temper tantrums" is comparable to the stage, opera, or film which also allows for and in fact encourages prima donnas within the system. Acting out behavior then becomes an accepted norm. An intern became aware that once he was identified as being particularly competent within the hospital in which he worked, "I can get away with being an 'enfant terrible.' It's only when you've attained the reputation as being a good doctor that you're allowed to have these temper tantrums and that people no longer cross you when your behavior seems to be something other than they expected."

While the competent intern and resident sometimes attempt to role model on the behavior of more experienced physicians who have such temper tantrums, this system does not always work. A fourth year medical student was concerned about the behavior that he was observing in his classmates:

There's a lack in medical school in helping us to handle the stresses of maturation during the process of becoming a physician. We're given lectures and books but it's a massive maturing process during which you're abandoned. We have advisors and a progressive faculty who've offered to be educational and personal counsellors to students, but the people who need it the least will be the ones most likely to take advantage. I have some very seriously disturbed classmates who probably won't be able to maintain their integrity over the next 2 years. With the slightest stress they have to run out and scream. The faculty often don't pick up what's going on and the student is allowed to finish and break apart with no support.

A medical administrator in a hospital dismissed the observation about the acceptability of medical temper tantrums within the system with the following comment: "When I see temper tantrums, I'm aware that the physician is playing a role instead of really reacting to being stressed and relieving it in an appropriate way. This is very childish behavior and I have little sympathy with it. It's not to be encouraged and I will make sure that such a person is not considered when promotion time comes around."

Needless to say, much of the anger that some caregivers experience in response to observing others openly displaying their anger at work may be repressed for the caregiver who is unable to express his or her rage publicly. This anger may then be displaced elsewhere. An ICU nurse said: "After a hard day at work, I go home and get angry and dump on my husband. I can't get angry with the people at work because I have to work with them. . . I guess that sounds kind of strange because I have to live with my husband for a long time to come." Anger has been reported in several other studies including those by Baider and Porath (12) and Vachon, Lyall, and Freeman (13).

An Australian physician observed that surgeons often take their aggression out on nurses and a surgical oncologist said, "We, the surgical oncologists don't have stress. We take it out in the O.R."

Caregivers who had some insight into the anger and feelings of aggression that they experienced were often able to say that it was reflective of other aspects of job tension. An intern observed that when working within a particular system that had totally unrealistic expectations of what interns and residents should do, that,

I found I was always angry and I'm usually very overcontrolled. When I worked within this hospital, no one ever crossed me and got away with it. I started to observe that my colleagues who were generally quite easy to get along with also were doing the same thing. One of the women with whom I had been in medical school was always very competent but within one week in this hospital she began to look really haggard and got really chippy with the nurses. She really blew up at them one day when I was called to do an admission that she should have done. It was clear that the nurses had decided to call me because she was so busy but she just blew up at them because she felt it was her responsibility to do these extra admissions and didn't want to lay it on me. She tore the hell out of the nurses despite the fact that they were trying to spare her. She's usually not like that and I have to ask what it is about the system that gets everybody feeling that way.

Many caregivers reported that they were able to realize that much of their anger towards their colleagues or towards patients came because they were feeling frustrated and didn't know what to do with their feelings. Nurses and social workers reported having difficulty dealing with physicians if they were angry because they felt that the physicians had delayed a patient's diagnosis and now the patient was going to die.

Holland and Mastrovito (14) have noted that such patients may be very bitter about their earlier problems and this may then of course interfere with the care the nurses and social workers would like to provide. Caregiver anger was sometimes taken out on patients because their value system was different from that of the caregivers. A nurse reported hearing a physician walking by the room where four young women were having abortions and saying, "This is the slut room." She suggested that in work with abortion patients, the system made the whole experience very difficult for caregivers and then their anger was displaced onto the patient who was "flip" or didn't seem to appreciate how hard the caregiver was working in order to get the abortion done.

When a patient dies then anger can frequently be expressed in personal tension with our colleagues or else it can be reflected onto interactions with others. A man who had a cardiac arrest in the emergency room and then recovered had an interesting observation to make of the tension, anger, and frustration that his physician had obviously experienced. "I heard the doctor say, 'He's gone. Where's the wife?' Someone answered, 'She's right outside.' He said, 'Get her the hell away from here. I don't want her seeing what's going on. I'll go talk to her and let her know he's gone later, but get her as far away from here as you can now.' " Obviously it is the rare patient who comes back from such a situation to speak with caregivers about their obvious manifestations of stress. Indeed, this man had never mentioned his experience to his personal physician.

Patients who attempted suicide often generated a great deal of anger in caregivers in emergency rooms who were simultaneously dealing with people with other "real" medical problems. This may then be reflected in interaction with patients. A nurse in a community emergency room said:

> There's a patient who came in for the third time in 6 months with a suicide attempt. He was lying there pulling out his IV and catheter and I was trying to deal with him and with a new M.I. at the same time. I found myself getting really impatient and wanting to say to him, "Look if you're going to do it, then do it right. Let me know the next time and I'll write up the directions for you." I try not to let my feelings show but sometimes it's really hard.

When caregivers are in a setting in which many people are dying and many systems problems exist then their stress and feelings of anger can really escalate. One oncologist observed:

> One of my colleagues and I used to really spend a lot of time laughing. We'd discuss all of the problems of the hospital and we'd gossip and tear everyone apart. As I traveled to meetings with some of my other colleagues, I found that they too had similar problems and we could give one another support without feeling too isolated. Only recently however, I'm beginning to feel a real weariness and a sense of "will the situation ever improve"—there's a more subtle and complex feeling of physical weariness that I'm experiencing now which is reflected in irritation with patients and families. I begin to lose perspective and think to myself, "Why don't they realize how busy I am, why do they keep hassling me?"

Finally, the noted hospice physician Dr. Robert Twycross has written of the anger he experiences in his role (15). He speaks of the fact that in this type of role one must absorb a considerable amount of other people's negative emotion. He suggests that some of this negativity can be absorbed and evaporated in the business of life. Larger quantities can be released through physical exercise, activity, or hobbies. However, there is a limit that can be dealt with neither by evaporation nor by exertion. He suggests that this excess negativity can result in tiredness and stress and in many caregivers will lead inevitably to lost temper and angry words that may well be displaced onto family members. Dr. Twycross says that for his anger he turns to the Bible to David's Psalms and vents his anger on God.

For David, described as a man after God's own heart, and for me, there was and is no other way. I did not ask to be born. I did not ask to be a hospice doctor. I cannot cope with so much negativity. *Damn it, God, I cannot cope.* [Italics in original.] There is so much suffering, so much apparent unfairness. . . Being angry at God is a necessity for me. Without this avenue of release, I could not continue as a hospice physician. (15, p. 14)

FEELINGS OF HELPLESSNESS AND INSECURITY (17%)

Feelings of helplessness and insecurity were the most common manifestations in pediatric chronic care. These feelings were fairly equally distributed across all age groups, were the same between sexes, and were fairly evenly distributed across professional groups, with a slight tendency for feelings of helplessness and insecurity to be greater amongst the counsellor group.

Feelings of helplessness, insecurity, and hopelessness can come about in part because of caregivers' unrealistic expectations of themselves (16). One intern has suggested, "Rather than problem patients we have problem staff because our expectations of what we should be able to do are unrealistic." A nurse administrator said, "We have the feeling of wanting to be all things to all people. To be available to patients, nursing staff and medical staff. Our self-expectations of what we can do are not in line with the reality of what it is in fact possible for us to accomplish."

These feelings of failure can begin to eat away at people and seriously interfere with their ability to maintain an outside life. A nurse in a community intensive care unit said, "Everyday when I go home I think about all the things I didn't do or all the things I did wrong. I never feel that I've done a good job."

It is perhaps not surprising that caregivers suffer feelings of failure and insecurity in situations where patients die (12, 13). A palliative care physician commented, "Sometimes it hurts because what we have to offer just doesn't work. People really suffer at their point of strength—we're really vulnerable there." When deaths happen and caregivers are unable to understand what is occurring, then the feelings of helplessness and failure really begin to mount. A nurse in a community hospital intensive care unit said:

A patient with peritioneal dialysis arrested during a simple procedure. His potassium level was 9. We started resuscitation. For 3 hours we kept it up with the doctor saying, "But he shouldn't die of this." We went through the supplies on two crash carts and all the soda-bicarb we had on the floor. Eventually I said, "Why are we doing all of this?" Gradually they stopped but the feeling was one of failure and it never should have happened.

Nurses in an intensive care unit in another setting became quite upset when many of the patients that they transferred to the medical units started dying. They began to lose confidence in their judgement and began to question what was wrong with them that they were judging patients to be alright for transfer to the ward and then they were dying. The nurses began to feel incompetent and ward nurses around the hospital were asking, "What's wrong with you that you don't know how to evaluate people? Why are all these patients dying?" When it was then discovered that in fact some of the patients might have been murdered by someone within the hospital, then feelings of panic began to ensue as staff members attempted to make sense of the situation.

All professional groups can experience feelings of failure. A nurse who worked in a cardiovascular surgical team said:

> We had three pump deaths in 2 weeks. Certain surgical teams would no longer work together. Certain anesthetists and residents wouldn't work together anymore. They rotated everyone so they wouldn't have the same teams performing together. They got really superstitious. The head nurse and I were the only ones who remained constant. It was the first time I ever saw grown men swapping O.R. partners because it might bring them better luck the next time.

Physicians who made possible medical errors spoke of the tremendous difficulty they had with feelings that they were complete failures as physicians. One oncologist spoke at a medical meeting about feeling really stupid and inadequate because she was unable to discover the primary cancer of one of her patients who was dying. She broke into tears with one of her colleagues who said to her, "You didn't make a mistake. None of us could have picked it up. I'll take you for a drink." When in fact a physician was responsible for an error in medical judgement that then resulted in death, then the physician often experienced an incredible amount of stress. Perhaps the ultimate example was that already mentioned of a resident who made an error in prescribing a particular drug. The patient died and the resident attended the patient's funeral and then went home and committed suicide.

There may also be feelings of failure and inadequacy when one is working with a disease with which it is impossible to do very much. A resident said, "It's hard to work in the solid tumor clinics because the response rate is so low." An oncologist said,

> I hate the feeling that I'm not able to do anything. When I go to the G.I. clinic I feel that there's so little I can do. After one of these clinics I come up and tear my heart out because I want to be able to give patients more sense of hope. I want to be able to tell them that I can do something other than simply saying that it's inevitable that they'll die. It takes away all of your feeling of worth as a physician to feel that you can't do anything specific to cure the patient. Sure I know I can involve community facilities and bring in a visiting nurse, a homemaker, provide a walker and help the family; but as a physician I think to myself, "Anybody could do that, what can I do as an individual?"

In research units where patients' prognosis is fairly negative and experimental procedures are being carried out, caregivers may also have considerable feelings of helplessness and insecurity. A head nurse working on a bone marrow transplant team said:

> Working here may not be that much more stressful than in other settings where we work with acutely ill patients with leukemia, but somehow I think it is. When we're working simply with acutely ill leukemic patients, we know they stand a chance of getting better, but when we're working with transplants and they start to get acutely ill, we can't think back to the thousands of other successes that we've had. We don't have the same experience with them. At this point in our experience, if you're a nonresponder to a bone marrow transplant, then you're a nonresponder. We have the feeling "if this doesn't work, then what?"

In situations where caregivers have come to expect a response and then don't get one, they may also experience considerable feelings of helplessness and impotence. Another oncologist said: "Over time the prognosis of the people I've worked with has changed. We can now do more for patients and it's hard not to do better. It's hard when you don't get a good remission because you've come to expect that you should be able to get one."

Finally, in the intensive care unit the sense of standing by helplessly and watching people die can cause caregivers to have an incredible sense of helplessness and futility which may be manifest in a variety of ways. A head nurse spoke of the fact that her staff had two young renal patients, both of whom were having horrible deaths.

One of them had had two failed transplants since age 12 and she was a very difficult person anyway. She developed a seizure disorder and we could do nothing. Her kidney became even more shut down and she was hard to dialize. She blew up like a balloon and started having constant seizures. The nurse watched this for 5 days and finally reached the stage where she couldn't stand it. In the early hours of the morning of one night shift she put up a sign on the patient's door saying "Seizure City." The nurses started dancing to music and acting as though they too were seizuring. A supervisor going by reported this to me the next day and when I spoke with the nurse, her response was, "How would you like to be in this room with no one able to make a decision about the patient? How would you like to be there for 12 hours watching the family come in, cry and go out?" I was able to see that in this situation nurses would need to have some kind of relief and it wasn't that surprising that they would have this fairly unusual response.

OVERINVESTMENT AND OVERINVOLVEMENT (8%)

Overinvestment and overinvolvement either with particular patients or with one's role in general, can occur at any point in a professional career; but the former is generally more commonly found in fairly inexperienced caregivers while the latter may be equally found in inexperienced or in very experienced caregivers. In the early stages of one's professional career, overinvolvement and overinvestment (in particular patients or in one's role) is frequently associated with inexperience in being able to set limits on one's own personal abilities and boundaries, whereas later in a career, it is often reflective of long-term difficulty in setting limits. Such overinvolvement is frequently associated with a lack of sufficient stimulation in one's outside life and a sense that it is only through identification with patients or with the professional role that one attains a true sense of self-esteem and well-being.

While overinvolvement may well prove to be a major manifestation of stress for some caregivers, it can also be an important learning experience, particularly for those who are reasonably new in their career. Several people have spoken of the fact that being "burned" in the early stages of their career taught them how to set limits on future occasions. Dr. Kevin Templeton, an oncologist, looked back at an earlier point in his career and spoke of the way in which his early involvement with a patient had been constructive to his long-term career development, although at the same time it created problems.

I became quite involved with an appealing young patient and I found that once engaged in the relationship I couldn't abandon him. This did things to my career in the hospital and even at a later point in time people remember it and feel that I have a tendency to get too involved. As he began to deteriorate, I found that it was hard to work at nonpatient related things. This relationship taught me a great deal although it was quite wearing physically but not emotionally. I was really glad when he died that I was then able to be uninvolved. I knew that it was the wrong thing to do professionally to get so involved but I couldn't get out with any sense of decency and I wasn't so involved that I couldn't make decisions.

Numerous caregivers who did not feel that they themselves were overinvolved or overinvested with patients gave examples of colleagues who did have difficulty and they questioned the effect it had on decision making. A nurse who worked on a gynecological oncology unit said that she found that the female physicians were more likely to get overinvolved and identify with patients than were male physicians.

They (female doctors) have the power to do things to get them overinvolved with patients that nurses don't. Frequently I find that the women doctors who get over-involved do not have any outside relationships. One physician often calls the unit at 4:00 a.m. to check on how her patients are doing. I feel that she's getting overinvolved but whenever there are any problems with her patients, she does comes in and always tries to think of the best thing for them. She's a single woman and her work is her whole life but I question sometimes if it interferes with her judgement. Usually she seems to know when to quit with patients but sometimes when she's really emotionally involved she needs to be pulled back. At the moment for example, we have a 39-year-old woman dying of metastatic cervical cancer. The patient is practically moribund with a nephrostomy and on active chemotherapy. The physician keeps pushing her to have more treatment. Earlier when the patient first got sick she said she didn't want any treatment and would rather go to Hawaii and make trips and enjoy her life. Now she's not enjoying anything at all. She tells us that she doesn't really want to continue with her therapy but the physician is pushing it.

I try to support both the patient and the doctor in this situation and I try to say to her, "Hey look, what are we really doing here? Who are you really trying to make feel better?" She'll listen sometimes but other times she just can't.

At times caregivers who become involved in such relationships begin to develop magical thinking. It is as though by investing so much of themselves they come to believe that they will be able to save the patient from an inevitable death. In these instances caregivers sometimes become closer to patients who are dying than they are ever able to be with people who are living. It is as though they are able to risk themselves with dying people in a way that they would be unable to do if the person were to live and in a way that they are unable to do in their normal relation-ships with other people. Sometimes this can happen even with very experienced caregivers as they come to see this particular patient as being different. In these instances as people begin to die, the caregiver can become very angry at the person for abandoning them and may withdraw and become depressed or even suicidal in response to the impending death. As was mentioned in the section on anticipa-tory grief, sometimes the staff members are unable to help the patient at this point in time because of their overinvolvement. At other times they want to spend all of their time with a dying patient and resent anyone else's involvement. In this situation the message is sometimes given "You can't die on me. You promised me that you wouldn't die." In one such situation when the patient died the nurse involved with her took her body to another state to be buried and then became acutely suicidal herself in an attempt to rejoin her much-loved patient.

At times these relationships with patients become sexual and intense personal relationships develop to the extent of caregivers either bringing patients home or moving in to live with them. Some caregivers have even gone so far as to leave their own families to move in with dying patients. One physician commented on a nurse colleague who had become very involved with a patient.

> When Susan became so involved everyone watched what was going on and made fun of the situation that she got herself into with getting so overinvolved with this patient and taking him home, organizing his funeral, etc. People didn't support her, they just watched what was going on. No one said to her, "Hey, this happens to all of us to one degree to another at one time or another." We don't share that sort of thing. It made her a better nurse and more understanding of patients by going through this . . . but it creates real problems with her credibility with staff members now.

When caregivers are overinvested in particular patients they frequently feel that their loved patient is not getting the proper attention from their colleagues. One radiology technician who fell in love with a young man with a brain tumor had a great deal of difficulty following his death because she felt that she should have pushed her physician colleagues to treat him more. These unresolved feelings then create ongoing stress in the relationship between colleagues and frequently the caregivers involved feel that they must leave the work situation to escape from the source of grief.

One of the real problems that happens in this type of situation is that caregivers who are having such relationships frequently attempt to hide them from their colleagues who do not believe in getting "overinvolved with patients." This then leads to "secret" relationships. These relationships can become much more dangerous because caregivers are unable to set limits on their personal involvement. When they find themselves getting deeply involved, they do not know where to turn for help. They fear being severely criticized by their colleagues and even losing their jobs as a response to this overinvolvement. This type of involvement frequently extends to developing or maintaining relationships with family members after the patients have died. This may lead to the expectation that family members will in some way reward one for the care that was given to the person who died. A physician who worked with a child who died of leukemia found that she became quite close to the girl's parents following the girl's death. The doctor developed symptoms of a debilitating physical illness and began to fantasize that she would become the parents' surrogate child and would be cared for in the loving way in which she and they had cared for their daughter. This physician's own lack of early mothering had caused her to have a vacuum in her own personality structure for which she then overcompensated by mothering children in a way in which she was never mothered but in a way that she subconsciously wished that she had been mothered. When her own dependency needs surfaced in this grief situation and with her own physical illness, she became very vulnerable and felt a great need to be cared for. Because these parents had been able to be so loving to their own daughter and because there was a vacuum in their life, she turned to them expecting them to love her as they had loved their daughter.

When the role of a caregiver changes to that of someone who wishes to be cared for, severe problems occur and often both caregiver and family members come to feel angry and betrayed. It is the rare relationship between caregiver and bereaved family members that can evolve into the reciprocal relationship that characterizes a true friendship.

ANXIETY AND DIFFICULTY
WITH DECISION-MAKING (6%)

According to Elliott and Eisdorfer (17) anxiety typically develops when individuals believe that circumstances are making or will make demands that exceed their abilities. White (18) has suggested that anxiety is probably the least tolerable of the unpleasant feelings that caregivers experience. He suggests that many of us will substitute anger for anxiety.

Other authors such as Campbell (19) and Price and Bergen (20) suggest that the anxiety that caregivers experience is frequently a reflection of constant exposure to death, uncertainty about decision-making, and questions regarding who is ultimately in control. Price and Bergen found that in working with nurses on an intensive care unit there was often anxiety present as a result of the unconscious confusion between the feelings of being responsible for the care of a dying patient and the feeling of being responsible for the occurrence of the patient's illness or death. Many of the caregivers interviewed spoke of escalating feelings of anxiety within the health care team that led to increasing difficulty with decision-making.

Feelings of anxiety can be contagious within a health care team. As one nurse in an intensive care unit noted: "I take on the feeling of the environment. If it's hyper, then I am too. You get the feeling when you walk in the door and hear the respirators. If it's already a busy day then for sure there will be more crises. If it's quiet. . . well. . . "

Physician anxiety was most often reflected in difficulty with decision-making. Helen Cochrane, an ICU head nurse said that one of her medical colleagues seemed to be having a lot of difficulty making decisions. As they began to talk about this, they both realized that this had begun to occur following the death of a patient who had been taken off the respirator. The patient was a young woman with very poor lung functioning who had been weaned from the respirator and made the decision that she did not want to be put back on the respirator when her condition deteriorated. The woman later died in respiratory failure and the caregivers still questioned if in fact they were justified in not putting her on the ventilator at the end. Ms. Cochrane said:

> I have difficulty criticizing my physician colleagues for their ability to make or not make decisions. The longer you work in a situation like this and the more you realize their difficulty the less apt you are to criticize them. I come to think that if I can make a decision quickly, then it's probably not a problem. I think that nurses often arrive at the point of decision-making earlier than physicians do because of the fact that they're under a different kind of pressure of being in the room with the patient and family for up to 12 hours a day.

The most severe case of anxiety that was presented by the caregivers surveyed involved a head nurse on a community hospital intensive care unit. She said:

> I quit after 5 years of being the head nurse on the ICU when the stress really began to get to me. At that time I was having palpitations and difficulty breathing fairly regularly. I began having panic episodes when I was going home if I became stuck in traffic or had to stop at a stop sign. I was fine if I could just drive right home, but if I had to stop for traffic, then I'd be unable to breathe and would have to be opening the window and leaning out. Not only was I dreaming about my patients, I was shaking my husband in my sleep and telling him to go check on certain patients. He'd have to wake me up and it really began to get to him as he was losing sleep.

The more pressure I felt inside, the more patient I was with everyone else because I didn't want them to see. I finally broke down completely in a supermarket. I wondered why everyone was shouting. I had to leave because I knew if I didn't get out, I was going to die right there. I got to my car and a man came and asked me if I was okay. Usually I'd smile and say I was fine but for once I didn't. I let him drive me home. To this day I don't even know what he looked like. I went home and wrote my resignation that night.

BURNOUT (4%)

The term "burnout" is one that is frequently used in the literature on stress these days. Burnout has been defined as, "The progressive loss of idealism, energy, and purpose experienced by people in the helping professions as the result of the conditions of their work" (21, p. 14).

Burnout is generally seen to be the interaction between the needs of a person to sacrifice him/herself for a job and a job situation that places inordinate demands on an individual. Burnout in a large study of hospice staff was found to be associated with high educational levels, long tenure, and full-time status (22). In a study of NICU nurses it was found to be associated with a head nurse leadership style of low consideration—high structure (23). Edelwich (21) has noted that burnout can come about not only in an individual but as well within a system. Despite the fact that burnout is such a popular concept, it constituted only 4% of the psychological manifestations of stress that were mentioned. Usually the manifestations mentioned were more specific than the broad term burnout implies. Caregivers made comments such as: "We go through burnout on this ICU about every 3 months and I feel 'burned out' and would like to change jobs but feel trapped within my job because I can't get another with the same pay."

One nurse suggested that her colleagues had come to label many of their feelings as being burnout when in fact they were simply looking for a reason to leave the work situation. She noted that, "Nurses will change work areas regardless of whether or not we call it burnout." There were some fairly clear examples of burnout that emerged from interviews and then other situations in which the term burnout was being used to describe anxiety reactions or reactive depressions (see 24 for the distinctions). A fairly clear-cut case of burnout was the case of Dr. Walter French, a 37-year-old medical oncologist in a large teaching hospital. He found himself feeling increasingly frustrated with the political problems that were emerging within the institution and in addition found it increasingly difficult to continue with the amount of research, clinical work, and administrative responsibilities that he was having to carry. As usually happens this burnout did not occur suddenly but developed over an extended period of time (25).

I found myself feeling really burned out. I was working 10 to 12 hours a day and no matter how hard I worked, I had the feeling that I was never on top of it. At the end of a 12-hour day I'd carry home a briefcase which weighed 30 pounds and would then arrive home at night at about 10:00 o'clock and find myself just too exhausted to begin the work that I'd brought home. I came to think that I'd be much happier if I could get clear of my workload but I never felt that I was out from under—I was always backlogged, I was always behind. I'd have problems returning phone calls because I'd have a zillion messages. I'd take these home with me and then think to myself, "Shit, I'll do it tomorrow." When I'd finally get to call a patient, he might say, "Gee, you're hard to get" or "It's nice to finally talk to you." It got so that I just wanted to go somewhere and die. Lots of the calls were from family members simply wanting more information.

I'd already talked with the patient and felt that I just didn't have time to talk with six family members as well.

One day it just got to be too much for me. I went into the office of the chief of medicine and said, "I've had it, I quit, I'm leaving and I'm never coming back again." I went home and arrived at my front door at 11:00 a.m. and said to my wife, "I've had it, I'm leaving work and I'm never going back again." It took me about a week of just doing absolutely nothing at home and then I bounced back to the point where my boss said to my wife, "Gee, he bounced back quickly." I've come to realize that I'm probably going to burn out a few times in my life because I work very hard. I think it's worth it though because I have the feeling that I am better than many of my colleagues. As a result of my yelling and screaming, I got a bit more help than I had before and so it may be a while before this happens again.

Not only do individuals burn out but entire groups of caregivers can experience burnout. Edelwich (21) described a group state of "apathy," that may lead to an antagonism towards anyone new who comes in and attempts to change the general apathetic atmosphere of the organization. Carol Graham is a 45-year-old experienced emergency room head nurse. She said,

I've worked in lots of emergency rooms but recently I was a head nurse in one and burned out after only 7 months. There were about 15 staff members who had started together and they provided a really negative influence on the group. They were friends inside and outside of work. They were really good clinically but had lost their enthusiasm and just came to work for the paycheck. One of them had wanted the job as head nurse and it was decided not to give it to her. As a result, they blocked everything I tried to do—every change I tried to make.

This, added to the fact that I never knew in this emergency room when someone might walk in off the street and put a knife to my back and decide to smash up the windows, made the job impossible. I got to the stage where I didn't know what was happening to me. I felt like I was outside of myself and looking down on myself and everyone else. I was unable to make the simplest decision about myself or the unit. I didn't know what was happening to me—no one else did either. My friends were good but they didn't know what was going on. It was quit or be fired so I quit. For weeks I couldn't do anything. Then I heard a television show about burnout and thought "That's what happened to me." I was angry for a long time. Now I'm not but I can't go back to that hospital ever again.

I'm leaving nursing now. Many of my friends are feeling the same way. I'm getting a job in the human relations field. I've often been a trendsetter in my group of friends. My bet is that if I can manage to make it outside nursing, they'll soon quit their jobs too.

OTHER PSYCHOLOGICAL SYMPTOMS (13%)

This category contains a variety of symptoms that while too small in number to be categorized specifically, are certainly worthy of mention. Some of these symptoms while occurring in a fairly small number of caregivers indicated severe problems while others were less incapacitating but still worthy of note. The symptoms can be seen to be reflective of depression, grief, and guilt or anxiety, they will be mentioned separately because they are often not recognized as such.

Sleep disturbances took a variety of forms. One director of nursing said, "You need to know your own symptoms of stress. Mine is that I start being unable to sleep. When this happens, I know I need to break the stress cycle." A nurse who was working directly with a cardiovascular surgeon doing heart transplants, said that she was finding it difficult to sleep at night because she couldn't calm down. "When I told the surgeon with whom I worked, he said 'I'm not sleeping nights either—go home and take a sleeping pill. That's what I do.' " He justified the personal stress that they were experiencing by saying, "Remember, surgery is an act of man, not an act of God as in medicine." Often times sleep disturbances were reflective of anxiety concerning patient management. An ICU nurse spoke of waking up at 2:00 a.m. remembering that she forgot to chart her medications and TPRs. Frequently she would call the floor in the middle of the night to tell them about her oversights. Other ICU nurses spoke of talking in their sleep telling their "bed partners" to go and check on "Mrs. Smith." A few even awakened to find themselves doing external cardiac massage on their husbands.

An oncologist said that: "On bad weeks I think about patient management all night. I can't sleep and then I wind up getting up and working. My wife can tell what kind of night it was by the volume of work that I've accomplished in the morning."

The same physician's wife said that she frequently wakes up in the morning and finds that her husband is not in bed. On those nights she knows that after going to bed with her, he has gotten up and started to work, then showered, fallen asleep again, and gotten up early to continue working.

One oncologist said that while he used to have sleepless nights, he found that by changing his practice to include patients who would live as well as those who would die, that his sleep disturbances had been significantly altered.

Frequently sleep disturbances were the result of either having to rotate shifts or else being on call. Nurses who had to rotate from one shift to another often found that they were unable to sleep when they were on the night shift.

Sleep can also be used as a way of escaping from some of the stress that care-givers experience. A hospital chaplain said that when he is on call all night in the hospital,

> It's a real drainer emotionally. Deaths seem to go in rashes. At 11:00 p.m. there may be a D.O.A. in the emergency room and that's good for at least an hour. You stay with the person who's died until someone comes, or else I try to sleep until the relatives come. Then at 2:00 a.m. I may have the experience of being with the patient who's dying after a long lingering death. Then at 5:30 a.m. I'm on the ICU for a sudden death. By 8:00 a.m. I'm almost falling asleep. It's not physical—it's being exposed to the bad side of life for so many hours at a time.
>
> I have to get out of the hospital as frequently as I can. Here we have four chaplains and when I'm on call, I go to bed early and leave the number where I'm sleeping. As long as you know you're on call however, you're vulnerable and you don't sleep very well. If you did only this kind of work it could really be emotionally draining after a while and you really would burn out.

Dreams also reflected caregiver stress. The most commonly reported dreams were those in which caregivers dreamt of being placed in the role of "patient or victim" in which they developed the same symptoms as the patients with whom they were working. A few physicians who worked in oncology reported having dreams of developing cancer, while caregivers in other units had dreams of developing the particular illness with which they were involved. A social worker in a chronic care hospital said that he and a colleague both had very similar dreams in which they were patients on the tuberculosis unit where the head nurse is a very domineering woman. He said: "I felt that I had lost my adulthood when I saw myself as a patient on her unit. I felt put back to childhood and kept repeating, 'Yes Miss Smith, I'll do it.' "

Other social workers working in the same chronic care hospital reported having dreams about having amputations. They reported hearing the sound of the saw and dreaming of themselves without a limb and going through the experience of rehabilitation. A nurse on an intensive care unit said that she and some of her colleagues had dreams of being pavulonized and being unable to move with their eyes being closed. An ICU nurse who developed a serious illness lived in dread that she would wind up on the ICU and would be seen as being such a difficult patient that she would be pavulonized as a way of her colleagues coping with her behavior problems.

Terri Roberts, a 25-year-old nurse working in gynecology said that this work had changed her self-image and had begun to impact on her dream life as well.

> I came to feel very unclean. I talked about it with my friends who said it was ridiculous but I found that I felt much differently about my own sexuality than I used to before starting to work in gynecology. I'm now much more reserved and careful regarding my sexuality. I used to think that women's vulvas were beautiful; now I feel that we're okay but no longer beautiful. I found that putting tents in for D&Cs and working with medical students affected my sex life. I've now become quite a militant feminist and have developed a real distrust for physicians. I had a dream that women had teeth in their vaginas and could do whatever they wanted with them. This came about because I began to develop a sense of how defenseless women were with surgery and how often after gynecological surgery they felt raped.

Other dreams that caregivers reported involved continuing to relive the day. "I work 16 hours here and then I go home and dream about my job all night." Or: "I know I've done something that needed to be done, but in my dreams I haven't done it and I live through all the repercussions of what would happen if I hadn't managed to do that." Sometimes the work that caregivers do not only affects their dreams but can be responsible for sleep walking: "As a new nurse when I was working nights on the ICU I used to sleep until 2:00 p.m. and then start sleep walking down the hall of my apartment giving out medications."

Caregivers also dream about particularly disfigured patients whom they have. A nursing supervisor who worked on a neurosurgical unit said that many of the nurses working with a young 17-year-old quadraplegic had nightmares because they had never seen anyone looking quite so ugly. They didn't want the head nurse to know how they felt about this patient because they were afraid that they would be judged incapable of coping. When caregivers get beyond the physical appearance of patients, they can also have difficulties with this involvement as well. A nurse on an intensive care unit said:

> Sometimes I get very angry. We had a girl of 20 who had become a "gork" after an accident. They were ready to declare her dead but wanted her kidneys. I had to watch the blood and plasma running into a body that was essentially dead for 3 days. Her family kept thinking that maybe she'd live, but I knew that they were just keeping her alive for her kidneys. I felt that I couldn't treat her as a human being until I talked to her family about who she was as a person. When I then came to know who she was as a person, I had a nightmare in which I saw her following me down the hall of the hospital with the pins sticking out from her head and all the facial disfiguration that was so evident with her. I woke in a cold sweat wondering who was going to fill her IVs if I wasn't taking care of her.

Dreams can also be reflective of guilt that caregivers feel after someone has died as we already saw with the nutritionist previously mentioned who dreamed of dead patients and food she had forgotten to put in their trays. They can also serve as a barometer of one's stress level. A medical oncologist said that whenever he had a recurring dream of having acute myelogenous leukemia he knew it was time to slow down. "I think to myself if I had AML I wouldn't be able to do all these things so maybe I should give them up now before my overwork makes me sick."

Finally, dreams can serve as a way of caregivers coming to terms with the death of patients.

> I worked with a grandmotherly patient who had had a radical vulvectomy and her wound broke down so that her groins were involved. When she had to come into the hospital her husband was admitted to a nursing home. The day before this woman died, her gynecologist had told her that she was too sick to go home and she would have to go to a nursing home as well. She was afraid that she wouldn't be with her husband and became quite depressed. I got her up to go to the bathroom and she sat on the bed and died in my arms. I realized that she just didn't want to go to the nursing home. I had a dream about her dying and then she sat up again and was alive. Everyone was shocked when this woman died but I realized that she was depressed, ill, and uncomfortable. After my dream I was able to rationalize it out and I became glad that she'd died in such a quiet and peaceful way.

Suicidal fantasies were related by a few of the caregivers who were interviewed. One bereavement counsellor who worked with the survivors of suicide felt that both she and her staff were at increased risk of suicide, not because of depression but because of constantly seeing this option in their daily professional lives. "When I have a fight with my husband, I think, 'Now I'll kill myself and leave a note that the people in the suicide program shouldn't help him to cope with his guilt.' "

When colleagues actually did commit suicide, there was often a considerable amount of guilt and a feeling that this could have been prevented. One nurse in a small community spoke of the feelings that she and her colleagues had when one of the nurses in the chronic care hospital committed suicide by hanging herself when she was 7 months pregnant.

> Evidently she tried to cut her wrists a few months before and was treated at the psychiatric hospital for a short time and then came back to work. Many of us feel guilty even though we knew that it wasn't really our fault that she had suicided. Some felt that the staff should have had sessions to get their feelings of guilt out of their system, but it never happened and many of us still feel that we let this woman down.

A physician spoke of a colleague who had suicided:

> We all knew that he was prone to manic-depressive illness and had been in one of his depressive periods. He was under stress with his chief and was advised to take a vacation. He seemed okay and told his wife that he was going to go out to play golf and then suicided. The staff were all quite shocked and subdued and we were unable to talk about it very much. Some of us became angry at the chief feeling that if he hadn't upset him, this wouldn't have happened, but even there we weren't comfortable expressing our anger outright. We knew it wasn't completely his job stress but it was job stress added to an underlying psychiatric problem. We all felt guilty because we didn't notice anything coming on this time and we were so relieved when we saw that he seemed to be feeling somewhat better.

Caregivers with experience working with suicidal people realize of course that it is often when people appear to be better that they have the energy to commit suicide.

Drug and alcohol abuse have been noted to be a major problem in caregivers. Despite these statistics, only 2% of the manifestations of stress involved any kind of alcohol or drug abuse. For the most part, caregivers commented that they had some concerns when they found themselves beginning to rely too much on either alcohol or drugs and they were often apt to cut back. One woman whose father was director of an intensive care unit said, "My father always copes with his work stress by coming home and pouring a stiff drink as soon as he comes in the door. I'm beginning to think that it's a real problem." A surgeon said,

> When I'm really under stress I swear and drink. With two drinks before dinner my brain turns off. When I relax then it's easy to drink too much. It's easy to have two drinks before dinner plus two with dinner, plus a few after dinner as a method of turning off. I used to smoke too much but I stopped cold turkey when I started to have a chronic cough. To die of cancer wouldn't be a problem to me but to die of bronchiectasis would be the pits. Therefore I just stopped cold.

An anesthetist commented that in his career he had only seen one colleague who was involved in drug abuse. He said that this stemmed from stress and the physician decided to get out of the intensive care unit environment and now has a very successful practice in anesthesia: "Generally you don't see it. If you're doing a job as much as we are then we can't be out drinking."

REFERENCES

1. Lyall, W. A. L., Vachon, M. L. S., & Rogers, J. (1980). A study of the degree of stress experienced by professionals caring for dying patients. In I. Ajemian & B. Mount (Eds.), *The Royal Victoria Hospital manual on palliative/hospice care: A resource book,* (pp. 489–509). New York: ARNO.

2. Vachon, M. L. S., Lyall, W. A. L., Rogers, J., Cochrane, J., & Freeman, S. J. J. (1981–1982). The effectiveness of psychosocial support during post-surgical treatment of breast cancer. *International Journal of Psychiatry in Medicine, 11*(4), 365–372.

3. Vachon, M. L. S. (1986). A comparison of the impact of breast cancer and bereavement: Personality, social support, and adaptation. In S. Hobfoll (Ed.), *Stress, social support, and women* (pp. 187–204). New York: Hemisphere.

4. Lyall, W. A. L., Rogers, J., & Vachon, M. L. S. (1976, October). Professional stress in the care of the dying. In *Palliative Care Service Report.* (pp. 457–468). Royal Victoria Hospital.

5. Gray-Toft, P., & Anderson, J. G. (1981). Stress among hospital nursing staff: Its causes and effects, *Social Science and Medicine, 15A,* 639–647.

6. Livingston, M., and Livingston, H. (1984). Emotional distress in nurses at work. *British Journal of Medical Psychology, 57,* 291–294.

7. Worden, J. W. (1982) *Grief counselling and grief therapy.* New York: Springer.

8. The right to die. (1984). *Nursing Life, 4*(1) 17–25.

9. Sahler, O. J., McAnarney, E. R., & Freidman, S. B. (1981). Factors influencing pediatric interns' relationships with dying children and their parents. *Pediatrics, 67*(2) 207–216.

10. Fulton, R. (1979). Anticipatory grief, stress and the surrogate griever. In J. Tache, H. Selye, & S. B. Day (Eds.), *Cancer, stress and death.* (pp. 87–93). New York: Plenum.

11. Weisman, A. D. (1981). Understanding the cancer patient: The syndrome of caregiver's plight. *Psychiatry, 44,* 161–168.

12. Baider, L. & Porath, S. (1981). Uncovering fear: Group experience of nurses on a cancer ward. *International Journal of Nursing Studies, 18,* 47–52.

13. Vachon, M. L. S., Lyall, W. A. L., & Freeman, S. J. J. (1978). Measurement and management of stress in health professionals working with advanced cancer patients. *Death Education, 1,* 365–375.

14. Holland, J., & Mastrovito, R. (1980). Psychologic adaptation to breast cancer. *Cancer, 46,* 1045–1052.

15. Twycross, R. G. (1984). *A time to die.* London: Christian Medical Fellowship Publications.

16. Vachon, M. L. S. (1979). Staff stress in the care of the terminally ill. *Quality Review Bulletin, 5*(5) 13–17.

17. Elliott, G. R., & Eisdorfer, C. (Ed.). (1982). *Stress and human health: Analysis and implications of research.* New York: Springer.

18. White, L. P. (1977). Death and the physician: Mortuis vivos docent. In H. Feifel (Ed.), *New meanings of death.* (pp. 92–106). New York: McGraw-Hill.

19. Campbell, T. W. (1980). Death anxiety on a coronary care unit. *Psychosomatics, 21*(2) 127–136.

20. Price, T. R., & Bergen, B. J. (1977). The relationship to death as a source of stress for nurses on a coronary care unit. *Omega, 8*(3) 229–238.

21. Edelwich, J. (1980). *Burnout: Stages of disillusionment in the helping professions.* New York: Human Sciences Press.

22. Mor, V., & Laliberte, L. (1984). Burnout among hospice staff. *Health and social work, 9*(4) 274–283.

23. Duxbury, M. L., Armstrong, G. D., Drew, D. J., & S. J. Henly. (1984). Head nurse leadership style with staff nurse burnout and job satisfaction in neonatal care units. *Nursing Research, 33*(2) 97–101.

24. Vachon, M. L. S. (1982). Are your patients burning out? *Canadian Family Physician, 28*:1570–1574.

25. MacBride, A. (1983). Burnout: Possible? probable? preventable? *Canada's Mental Health, 31*(1) 2–3.

10

Coping with Occupational Stress

An Overview and Personal Coping Mechanisms

There is an extensive literature on coping and adaptation that this chapter cannot begin to review (1-14). Here we shall draw most heavily on the work of Lazarus and his colleagues, particularly as reviewed in Folkman and Lazarus (6) and the work of Pearlin and Schooler (13).

In the cognitive-phenomenological (6) approach of Lazarus and his colleagues previously discussed in Chapter 1, the person and environment are seen in an ongoing relationship of reciprocal action, each affected and in turn being affected by the other. This relationship is then mediated through two cognitive processes: appraisal and coping. The degree to which a person then feels stress—that is feels harmed, threatened, or challenged—is determined by the relationship between the person and the environment in that encounter. Thus perceived stress is defined both by the evaluation of what is perceived to be at stake and the evaluation of coping resources and options available.

Coping is defined as "the cognitive and behavioral efforts made to master, tolerate or reduce external and internal demands and conflicts among them" (6, p. 223). Coping efforts serve to either manage or alter the person-environment relationship that is serving as the source of stress (problem-focused coping) or to regulate stressful emotions (emotion-focused coping). Coping efforts are made in response to stress appraisals that are continuously interactive throughout an encounter.

Coping processes occurring within a particular encounter may alter this encounter, or coping may occur across episodes that are part of common stressful encounters. Little research has been done on how individuals cope or change their coping mechanisms over time. One of the advantages of the present study is that it not only asks caregivers what they do to cope with specific stressful events, but in general asks them to reflect on the coping mechanisms that they have found to be effective over time.

OVERVIEW OF FINDINGS

The caregivers surveyed reported 3,297 coping responses or an average of 10.08 per subject. This constituted 39% of the total anecdotes in the study. A content analysis was performed, looking for coping themes that represented coping techniques caregivers used in specific situations, those they had developed over the years to deal with stress, their most common coping mechanisms, and their response to the question, "All things considered, what is it that keeps you functioning in your job?" Sixty-four percent of the coping mechanisms identified were personal and 36% were environmental. This proportion was roughly equivalent across all specialties, professions, age groups, and both sexes. The number of coping techniques reported increased with age in both personal and environmental categories. Table 6 in the Appendix shows the 17 major coping processes identified; each of these will of course have subcategories.

Previously it has been found that when a situation is appraised as having potential for amelioration by action then the person will use problem-focused coping to alter the troubled relationship that produced emotional distress. If there is a threatening or harmful situation that is appraised as holding few possibilities for beneficial change, then the person will employ emotion-focused ways of coping (6). In the present study there was a trend towards individuals reporting themselves as primarily employing emotion-regulating ways of coping and their organizations as using problem-solving ways of coping. The individual responses indicated that caregivers learn their jobs and develop some sense of control over what they were doing. Their personal coping mechanisms seem to reflect the fact that they both knew what they were doing and why they were doing it. They developed some special areas of expertise in their practice and sought ways to decrease some of the stress they experience by having relationships, activities, and effective lifestyle management outside of the work situation. When they were not satisfied with a particular job, then they left that job situation.

The environmental ways of coping that caregivers reported their organizations as using seemed to reflect, first of all, an attempt to act on specific identified problems and then to provide an outlet for sharing feelings regarding problems that either could not be solved or else were perceived as being unchangeable. It is of course clear that although individuals primarily used emotion-regulating ways of coping, they also used problem-solving coping processes and emotion-regulating processes were also used in organizations where the primary focus was on problem-solving approaches.

Some of the coping processes identified can be seen as serving both problem-solving and emotion-regulating functions. The coping techniques that were primarily problem-solving were: team philosophy—support-building, staffing policies, administrative policies, formalized ways of handling decisions, good orientation and ongoing educational programs, job flexibility and mobility, developing control over certain aspects of practice, leaving the work situation, and getting increased education.

Coping techniques that were primarily emotion-regulating were: having a sense of competence, control or pleasure in work; developing a personal philosophy of illness, death, or one's role; avoiding or distancing from patients either physically or psychologically; developing support outside the work situation; lifestyle management; having a sense of humor; talking to colleagues at work; and participating in support groups.

Although it has been found in previous research that men are somewhat more apt to use problem-focused coping processes within the work situation, this did not hold true in the present study, as the two sexes were equal in most of their responses.

Lest there be any judgement on the part of the reader that one type of coping process is better than another, it is important to note that it is crucial to maintain an equilibrium between problem-solving and emotion-regulating types of coping. Any individual who relies on either one type of coping technique or worse yet, one technique, is very much at risk (1).

Pearlin and Schooler (13) have noted three types of coping responses: those that change the situation out of which strainful experiences arises, those that control the meaning of the experience before stress occurs, and those that function to control stress. It was found that the caregivers coped by changing the situation out of which the strainful experience might arise by: developing control over certain areas of practice; having a personal philosophy of illness, death, and one's role; increasing education; team philosophy—support-building; staffing policies; administrative policies; formalized ways of handling decision-making; good orientation; and job flexibility. A coping response that *controlled the meaning of the experience after it occurred* but before the emergence of stress was the development of a sense of competence, control, and pleasure in one's work. Responses that functioned more for the *control of stress* itself after it emerged included: leaving the work situation, developing support outside of the work situation, lifestyle management, having a sense of humor, avoiding patients or families, using colleagues at work, and support groups. Table 7 in the Appendix shows the top ten coping mechanisms that were identified by caregivers. From this list it can be seen that six out of ten of the top coping mechanisms were problem-focused coping techniques and six out of ten involved attempts to change the situations out of which strainful experiences might arise.

One of the two most common coping techniques however, that of having a sense of competence, control, and pleasure in one's work, served primarily to control the meaning of the experience after it occurred but before the emergence of stress. In other words, it served to appraise a situation as being potentially strainful but not stressful. For example, the caregiver dealing with a dying patient might think to herself, "I know what I'm doing, I will be able to handle any situation that might arise with this patient, and having encounters like this are a very important and rewarding part of my work." Thus an individual takes a potentially stressful situation and by consciously or unconsciously appraising it in a particular way uses an effective coping technique, thereby decreasing the strain associated with the situation. It may well be that caregivers were not inclined to rate dealing with dying patients as much of a stressor in this study because they have developed just this type of personal coping technique. On the other hand, dealing with impersonal organizational stressors may be appraised or perceived as being much more difficult because the caregiver feels impotent to change the situation or may not feel personally competent in response to this type of stressor. One might then use emotion-regulating ways of coping, but if these do not serve to enhance the sense of competence, self-esteem, or membership within a caring community, then one may well experience symptoms of stress such as depression or feelings of helplessness or impotence. This would be comparable to Pearlin and Schooler's finding that coping efforts in the occupational area were least effective because it is an area of life in which the person may well be confronted by issues that are beyond his or her control. Personal coping techniques are discussed below.

A SENSE OF COMPETENCE, CONTROL, OR PLEASURE FROM WORK (19%)

When caregivers were asked what made it possible for them to continue in their work situation despite all the stressors that they experienced, they often responded in the following manner: "The bottom line is that I know what I'm doing and I love my work." Over and over again this sense of competence and having a sense of control over what one was doing was seen as being directly responsible for one's enjoying the work situation. This sense of competence is quite comparable to Antonovsky's sense of coherence (1). He describes a sense of coherence as: ". . . a global orientation that expresses the extent to which one has a pervasive, enduring though dynamic feeling of confidence that one's internal and external environments are predictable and that there is a high probability that things will work out as well as can reasonably be expected" (1, p. 23).

It is a crucial element in this concept of coherence that it is an aspect of one's basic personality and not something that occurs simply in response to a particular stressor. Nevertheless when caregivers were asked how they coped with stressful situations, this sense of competence and pleasure in work which is similar to the sense of control, coherence, or of Kobasa's Hardy Personality (15) emerged. Whether in fact this was an initial personality trait of the caregivers or whether it is something that has evolved as a coping strategy over time would bear further investigation. Yancik (16) has hypothesized that the similar psychologic resources of self-esteem and mastery seemed to be effective in sustaining hospice workers against the emotional distress that might result from their work.

Individuals may have a stronger or a weaker sense of coherence. Someone with a weaker sense of coherence will tend to anticipate that things are likely to go wrong, while with a stronger sense of coherence, one is able to see reality and is able to judge the likelihood of desirable outcomes in view of the countervailing forces operative in life. Antonovsky stresses that this does not mean that one is blinded by confidence but rather that one expects that things will work out as well as can be reasonably expected.

Within this framework caregivers for example, come to understand that they will not always succeed in saving patients' lives but as long as they have the sense that they have performed well professionally and that they have done "As well as can be expected, given the circumstances"—that the patient has had "a good-enough death," there is a sense of competence even if a patient dies. Antonovsky stresses that with the sense of coherence there is not the sense that life is easy—rather, life may be seen as being full of complexities, conflicts, and complications but the individual understands what these are.

Antonovsky distinguishes between a sense of coherence and a sense of control which implies that "I am in control." He states that a sense of coherence doesn't imply that one is in control, rather that one is a participant in the process of shaping one's destiny as well as one's daily experience. In the present framework this implies a sense that one has the capacity to make decisions and to have a sense of competence within the clinical situation. Antonovsky also says that with a sense of coherence the location of power is seen as being where it legitimately should be. That may involve the individual being in a position of power or it may involve power being vested in someone else, but in any event the sense is that power is where it belongs.

Caregivers who described this sense of competence, control and pleasure in their work often talked in terms of functioning within a team of one sort or another in which they received validation for their sense of self-worth.

Marta Cavanagh was a 33-year-old nurse who was beginning a new role as director of nursing at the time that she was interviewed. She spoke of leaving a previous job as a nurse because of various feelings of impotence and lack of role satisfactions within the environment in which she was functioning. Her comments integrate much of what has just been said about developing a sense of competence, control, and pleasure, but within a social system. In addition, they reflect the growth that happens with increasing maturity and a variety of life experiences.

> What I see and think are different now from the way they were when I left nursing 2½ years ago. As I've grown older and been away from the profession for 2½ years going to graduate school and thinking what I want, I have now become more philosophical about what I can and can't do. I now know what type of stressors interfere with my judgement. I've just come out of 2½ years of unstressed time but I'm conscious of where I might find stressors within my new role. I still find things threatening when patients want to know everything that's going on in a given situation. I know however that I feel a sense of confidence in my theoretical background. I feel competence in my new professional role and I'm starting to get my self-image together. Although I may hesitate in a specific instance, I feel that I'm as competent as anyone else to deal with these problems. I get a lot of support from my administrator. She realizes that this new position is going to be a learning experience for all of us, but I've been carefully chosen and I'll get good support.

It has been said by John Ruskin that, "In order that people may be happy in their work, these three things are needed. They must be for it, they must not do too much of it, and they must have a sense of success in it" (17, p. 375). This section will explore the ways in which caregivers developed a sense of competence in their work, the ways in which they began to get some sense of control in it, and the manner in which they derived a sense of success from what they were doing. Three major categories will be discussed: gaining and maintaining a sense of competence, developing a sense of control, and deriving a sense of pleasure from one's work.

Gaining and Maintaining a Sense of Competence

Caregivers developed a sense of competence through the following stages: they developed their professional skills, set goals for themselves, had frequent tests of their competence, developed ways of ensuring that they were competent, proved their competence in a number of situations, learned that because they were secure in their own competence that they could share that competence with other people, and eventually were able to report being comfortable living with a sense that they were competent within their work situation.

The development of skills was a process that took place both in undergraduate educational programs as well as throughout one's professional career. Frequently caregivers reported developing skills within the team in which they functioned.

The skill development that took place in caregivers involved developing a professional knowledge base planning and judging which aspects were important, comparing and contrasting courses of action, and eventually deciding on what was appropriate. Periodically they needed to redefine personal and professional goals. Pines (18) states that an effective way of avoiding burnout is for caregivers to set their own short-term goals and to be willing to acknowledge achieving them. An ICU nurse said, "My goal is for my patient to look comfortable and be comfortable. It takes a lot of planning. You need to be a good organizer."

A physician shared an early experience that revealed some of his inadequacies as a professional but also caused him to set new goals.

> On Christmas day when I was a third-year medical student I rode with an ambulance and by noon time had pronounced five people dead. The only problem was with a man with sudden death. He was okay at the top of the stairs and walking down had a heart attack and was dead at the bottom of the stairs. When I arrived it was clear to me that the man was dead and I expected that the wife realized this. It was only when I'd worked on him and said, "Well yes, he's dead" that I realized that she'd really expected me to make him okay.
>
> It was the first time I'd had to tell a family that someone had died and I realized afterwards I'd been too brusque and hadn't realized this was a shock to her.
>
> I decided I'd have to do better the next time and I did, and I've continued to get better and more comfortable over time.

Dr. Ed Hines, a gynecologist, spoke of how a sense of competence develops over a professional career through a series of confrontations with stressors in which one tests one's competence and how one can eventually become comfortable with proven competence.

> Your ability to handle problems is in a linear line from one's first exposure to patients in third year meds. Training isn't a big deal, it's just hard work and learning to make decisions. Residents are in the early stage of their career and they tend to focus on the technical aspects of what's going on and making their decisions. If they've done everything correctly, they have no real qualms about what happens to the patient. One of my colleagues and I recently reminisced about when we were residents. The more blood and calamity, the better we liked it. Any complication that we didn't create ourselves, we loved to deal with it. If there was a placenta previa, then we felt "let's go to it." As you become more mature you begin to realize the impact of these situations on patients.
>
> At this point I cope by being as good as I possibly can in a technical way so that when I meet an unforeseeable problem I realize that I'm not perfect but probably no one else could have been more perfect than I was in this particular situation. Now when I have a stillborn or a problem with a baby dying, I attempt to look at whether or not I've done everything I could have done. The sadness of dealing with death is manageable by the physician or nurse provided they know they're doing everything possible. If a baby dies and I know I have already ruled out mycoplasmosis, septo-defect, an incompetent cervix, and anything else I might have been expected to know about, then I'm okay. I find that it also helps that I'm a surgeon. If for example, I have a woman with an incompetent cervix, then I have a surgical tool that can deal with the problem and that makes me feel that I can do something. When I feel better and the patient sees that I feel better, then she feels, "He's confident therefore I feel better." Being a surgeon and being able to do something like a bit of plumbing, makes both me and the patient feel better.

In work with dying patients it sometimes happens that as caregivers it is no longer possible to plan for patients to have an extended life span. At that point in time, it becomes important for caregivers to redefine goals that extend beyond simply the prolongation of life. Dr. John Nielson, an oncologist who performs bone marrow transplants says:

I have my own rule. I never say I can't do anything for you. The patient understands that I can't cure him, but I can go in and listen and do simple sorts of things for him. If I have stopped active curative treatment of a patient's disease, I have as my goal decreasing the problems that patients have with sleep, nutritional difficulties, pain, pain medication, or whatever. I make it a point never to remove all hope from patients, even when I can't cure them. When it's clear that patients are not going to survive, I look to determine what I can have for goals in this particular situation. For example, maybe I can decrease the pain that the person experiences. This may sometimes get me into difficulty with my colleagues if I don't carefully explain what is going on. For example, if someone has extreme bone pain then I may give him chemotherapy, not for cure, but because it's the best analgesic for his pain–the approach is being used not to cure but for pain–I'm using one modality for two purposes. If the nurses don't understand however, they get angry and feel I'm still trying to give patients curative treatment. If a patient is bleeding then the nurse may ask me why I'm still giving him platelets and antibiotics. I explain to her that my goal is that I don't want the patient to bleed all the time. My goal is to provide as much comfort and relief as possible. I also have as a goal, to find out more about what is helpful for this particular patient. I find I know lots more about patients when I've spent time with them and I can make better decisions when I know them better. That means that for some, my goal is not to do anything and for others I may go full out, but that's determined on the basis of what I feel that they want and need.

Developing a Sense of Control

In situations where caregivers sometimes question their own competence they may attempt to cope by gaining control over the situation in one way or another. Karen Irish, a gynecological nurse in her early twenties talked in terms of redefining a potentially stressful situation as a controllable situation in order to give herself a sense of competence:

I had a woman with a radical vulvectomy. It was very foul and really stank so much that I wound up gagging much of the time. To cope with it, I threw myself into the situation and became meticulous with her hygiene. I tried to make it a challenge and made nursing care plans so everyone would regard this as a challenge, as opposed to a terrible situation. We changed her dressing every hour instead of just once a shift and used baby powder, vaseline intensive care lotion, and made sure we had lots of pleasant smells in her room. We said to her, "Let's make it a habit of freshening you up." Sometimes it seemed almost as though we made a comedy out of our routines with her as a partner in this comedy, but we had to face it. This is a reality that we have to deal with, and we had to do something to make it possible for all of us to be comfortable and feel some sense of control in this situation.

An example of gaining and maintaining a sense of competence and control in a very difficult professional role came from a priest who was in the unusual situation of working with executioners and people about to be executed in the West Indies. When I asked Reverend Edward Connors how he handled being the priest assigned to be present when someone was executed, he spoke of how he initially had great difficulty in this role but was helped when he gained some control by redefining his role and involvement with people.

I come in in second gear in these sorts of situations and I realize that the executioner needs my ministry as much as does the man on death row. The hangman is someone who no one knows and he wears a hood and is dropped off in a different place each time he executes someone. I don't approve of capital punishment but I had no choice in this role. I had to perform a ministry to people being executed. After an execution I'd have diarrhea and I'd have to have a few drinks and would find myself unable to sleep for a few days. If I had two in a row, then I'd try to get someone to help me. Long ago I had to participate when they cut down the man's body and annoint him right after the death. Now I annoint him before death and I find that this can be a very rewarding part of my ministry.

A physician spoke of the way in which he had gradually evolved more control over professional situations over the course of his 20-year career.

Professionally my antennae are sharper and I'm good at sensing where patients are at. I don't act the same way with a guy off the drilling rigs with testicular cancer as I do with a newspaper editor. In my professional role I act. I consciously play a role. I use my person. I have a physical advantage—I can stand up tall with the person who wants God almighty—or not emphasize my height with someone who wants to be more of an equal.

I'm more conscious of playing a role and do it better than I did ten years ago. I feel myself snapping into a role. I used to find it difficult to deal with sexuality but now I don't because I snap on my role. The armor becomes more comfortable and finally becomes tailor made. I'm probably less personally involved with my patients than I was ten years ago when each one of them felt like a brother or a sister—but I think I'm now more effective.

As alluded in this incident the competent professional is often able to relinquish control to patients when that seems to be appropriate. This may be particularly relevant in dealing with people who are dying, in that people have a right to make choices involving many aspects of their dying process. One of the myths that has developed around death and dying is that everyone must be open about the process and what is going on, and that it is the role of the "competent" professional to ensure that this happens. It is sometimes thought that patients have almost an obligation to openly talk about their dying throughout the whole course of the illness. This may not be what they want or need. Reverend Patrick Illingsworth, a 62-year-old Catholic priest, worked in a small community where he became very active with his dying parishioners:

The last person I was really involved with who died was my friend Jack. The doctor spoke to me ahead of time. He said, "This is what the story is, these are what the problems will be. I'm going in to tell him now so he'll probably want to talk with you later." I went in to see him that afternoon. He said, "Well, in view of what Dr. S told me this morning, there are some things I want to talk with you about, and I have some things I want to get in order." We talked about his faith and how he thought that his illness was God's will. I called his family and as many as were up to it came to the hospital and participated while I gave him the Sacrament of the Sick to which they and he all responded. After that was over, he looked at me and said, "You know and I know that I know what's going on. We've talked about what needs to be talked about, you know I've made my preparations, and now let's talk about the Red Sox." And that's what we talked about until he died.

Shared decision-making and sharing control with patients can also take place earlier in the illness process. An oncologist commented:

With the cancer patients I work with I have my own set of ethics and I always inform them that there are other options beside the treatment that I'm suggesting. I say that other treatments might be better than mine and I'll try to recommend the best treatment possible. In this game one's ego must always be kept out of decision-making but you can only do this with insight. I find it difficult when I'm following a university study protocol because I like to be able to involve the patients in decision making. This sounds a lot more noble than it is—there's really no way of not projecting your biases onto patients as you're helping them with their decision making. My bottom line though is that I use an emphasis on ethics as one of my ways of coping with my job stress.

And he thereby gains control over at least some of the stressors to which he is exposed. While it is always important to negotiate with patients or clients in decision-making situations, sometimes caregivers have a sense that they know more about this particular situation and the long-term implications than do the clients with whom they are involved. In this situation they may decide to try to exert some control by pushing to some extent in order to ensure that the client is making the best possible decision in this situation. Kevin Nash, a young funeral director, said that he finds it frustrating if clients refuse to have an open casket, unless this is something that they've been used to all their lives.

> Whatever customs are their own social practice are fine with me. But when someone who traditionally would have had an open casket decides to have a closed casket, then I get concerned. In that situation, we'll often tell them that we want someone to identify the body. We don't really need for them to identify the body, but we want the closest person to the deceased to see and acknowledge the death. Recently we had a very prominent man send in his housekeeper to make arrangements following his wife's sudden death. I refused to deal with the housekeeper and told the man that he would have to come in himself. He went from one extreme to the other. Initially he wanted a closed casket with no visiting, and said he didn't want to see her because he didn't want to remember her pain. I asked him to come in before her service which was scheduled to be at 3:00 p.m. I suggested that he come in to become familiar with the surroundings. Once he came in he asked if I minded if he had a quick look at his dead wife. The staff in our home always fix up the bodies just in case the family members should ask to see the deceased, even after they've insisted that they won't. He was taken aback at how peaceful, calm, and out of pain his wife looked. He cancelled the funeral arrangements and postponed them until the next day. He invited his friends to come in and see his wife with an open casket. He was a very prominent man who spoke about this situation for several months after the event. I know that pushing him a bit helped him so much that I believe in it well enough to push other people in a similar sort of situation.

Caregivers who pride themselves on their competence and enjoy a sense of control sometimes find it difficult because in order to really effectively perform in their role they must share some of the glory with other care providers. A nurse and physician on a palliative care team were asked if other physicians became resentful when they were able to control pain that the physician had not been.

> Sure we have that, but we try to help the other doctors feel that they not us, have controlled the pain. Recently we had a really bad situation—the kind we haven't had in a long time. The patient was screaming in pain and the resident had ordered only 5 milligrams of morphine. The chief knew it was a problem but said that the resident had to learn his own way about pain control and he'd give him a couple more days before he stepped in. The resident felt strongly that he should be able to do it himself and shouldn't need any help. As we were talking outside the patient's room, she screamed in pain and the staff man decided that on teaching grounds, he could transfer her case to the clinical clerk who followed our directions and upped her morphine to 84 milligrams within 2 days. He then said to us, "Now that I've controlled the pain. . . oh, I mean, now that we've controlled the pain. . . " but it's important that he feel that he has controlled the pain so that he develops a sense of competence and a sense that it's important to give good pain control to patients.

Deriving a Sense of Pleasure from One's Work

Over time, professionals who have effective coping mechanisms gain a sense of competence in their professional roles and often manage to develop some sense of control either over their work situation, or over their role within the work environment. At that point one is able to develop a real sense of pleasure in the work situation or in a job well done. This analysis implies that a sense of pleasure in one's work takes time to develop, although caregivers may have early experiences from which they derive similar satisfaction. Therefore, most but not all, of the anecdotes in this section will be from experienced caregivers.

The sense of pleasure in work may evolve either from one's work with individual patients, from pleasure in the utilization of professional skills, or satisfaction with the indirect impact that one's work can have on groups of patients and families that one might influence indirectly through teaching or administrative roles. Often caregivers allow themselves to derive pleasure from a "job well done." A surgeon reflected on these feelings when he said, "I enjoy what I do and find it stimulating and exhilarating. Stress is the fee that you pay for the rest of it. I'm constantly putting myself in the position of more stress because I want the challenge of meeting it."

Staff in a palliative care unit reflected on the ways in which they derived pleasure from their work:

> The staff don't object to stress as long as there is satisfaction to go along with it. We feel it is a privilege to work with the dying. Sure we get stressed, but we feel that we are giving something and that we are making a difference to patients. We cope by knowing what the alternatives are for patients before we start. . . . We don't have the ideal now but it is better.
>
> We have tremendous satisfaction and get a lot of good feedback. Sometimes it's almost embarrassing to get told that you're wonderful so often. To have someone come and say, "You people are so good" doesn't hurt a bit.

Caregivers in acute care settings derive pleasure from seeing patients get well. Nurses in a pediatric intensive care unit reflected on the pleasure they received:

> Having a child come down to see us right before a discharge is incredible. Last week a little girl we never thought would make it came running through the unit just before going home. There wasn't a dry eye in the place and that included the doctors. It makes everything you are doing so worthwhile and gave us what we needed to carry on because three other children died that weekend.

An older nurse in an adult intensive care unit had a similar story.

> People in the ICU often need a push to get out of bed. I try to push nicely but to be firm. A few years ago I had the brother of one of the doctors as a patient. He kept saying, "No, I won't get up." I said to him, "You wouldn't let your employees tell you how to run your business. I won't let you tell me how to run mine." He was a real miracle and I can see myself as having played a part. He still comes back to visit and to bring gifts.

Several caregivers reflected on the pleasure they derived from the letters and gifts they received from patients. These served as symbols that their personal satisfaction was also reflected in satisfied patients and families. In talking about their personal satisfaction with their work, many caregivers took out letters that were kept close at hand or pointed to objects in their offices that reflected the appreciation of patients—most of whom were now dead—or their family members, who took the time to acknowledge the effort the caregiver invested.

Even without the tangible rewards of gifts and letters, caregivers received pleasure from their patients acknowledging the impact they had on their lives. An oncologist reflected: "I'm in oncology because it is an area in which I can do something. The idea of treating patients with incurable disease didn't bother me because I could see past the issue that if you couldn't cure then you couldn't do anything. Patients were appreciative and would acknowledge that what I thought was worthwhile, was."

When patients don't acknowledge the role of caregivers, sometimes it hurts and decreases some of their pleasure in their work, perhaps because it threatens their self-esteem and makes them wonder if they really are doing anything worthwhile. "I've saved this woman's leg for 5 years and she doesn't even say thanks. Should I expect more? Probably not, but those to whom you've given so little give the most back, while sometimes those to whom you've given the most think that it is your duty."

CONTROL OVER ASPECTS OF ONE'S PRACTICE (19%)

Closely aligned to a sense of competence, control, and pleasure in one's work is developing control over certain aspects of one's practice. This coping strategy differs from the sense of control described above. The latter form often comes from a knowledge of one's role and expected role performance, which evolves over time. Developing control over one's practice is a more active coping mechanism that implies actively seeking to change a part of one's work environment. Unlike a sense of competence, control, and pleasure in one's work, this coping mechanism was one that did not increase with age; younger caregivers were in fact slightly more apt to report using this coping mechanism than were other groups.

Operationally, this coping mechanism involved setting limits on one or another aspect of one's clinical practice and organizing one's work to decrease stress and to give one a sense of personal satisfaction. Sometimes this involved developing multiple roles that could bring satisfaction and having special "treats" in one's practice. It involved having at least some idea of what one wanted to achieve from one's work and of having a sense of what one was capable of doing.

Friedman (19) has reviewed the stress literature as it relates to intensive care unit nurses and concludes that "top-of-the-ladder" individuals have a greater degree of control over their schedules. This in turn favors career advancement and is beneficial in that it allows time to be managed more flexibly. With this ability often comes an increase in status and the ability to delegate to subordinates. This section can perhaps best be summarized in the words of Theresa Little, a 33-year-old social worker who commented, "You have to know who you are... what you can and cannot do, get your resources together... admit what you can't do, and take a stab at what you might be able to do."

One of the most important ways of gaining control is of course to know what you are doing and to set up certain routines for your clinical practice. Dr. Ed Travers, a senior family practitioner commented that one of his ways of developing a sense of control was to always carefully review the charts of any of his patients that a consultant diagnosed as having cancer. "Insist that you confirm and stage the disease and go through the charts yourself. I've picked up mistakes in diagnoses. . . . Then know the patient and family and the awareness that they have of the illness. . . . Keep good records of all important interviews. . . . Find something special that you like about each person you see and get all the help you can."

Tessie Gans, a 30-year-old former intensive care nurse who was now attending university and doing some part-time work said that with increased experience she was much more willing to admit when she did not know something and to ask for help.

> I was working with a neurosurgery patient who had to be given all kinds of treatments I didn't know. I said to the head nurse, "You come here and help me to sort out this patient. I haven't done many of these things in 2 years. . . so you sit with me for 40 minutes until I get it all straight, dosages, etc." . . . I know that I'm a perfectionist. Other nurses will give drugs when they don't know what they're doing, but I've seen too many things happen.

Many caregivers spoke of the way in which they organized their clinical practices in order to give themselves personal satisfaction or to minimize their stress. Several spoke of working part time in order to decrease stress and to maximize their sense of satisfaction with life, both personally and professionally; others chose a specific specialty area because that gave them high personal satisfaction or maximum control over their work schedule. For example, a young newly married nurse who very much enjoyed working in the intensive care unit found that the constant shift rotation, even with 12-hour shifts, really affected her personal life. She therefore took a course and transferred to the operating room where, while the work was not as personally satisfying, she felt more in control of her life. Eventually she began working with the cardiovascular surgery team where she was able to utilize her previous experience and her personal satisfaction increased.

Other caregivers evolved a specialized role for themselves wherein they were acknowledged as having expertise and from which they derived great personal satisfaction. An ICU nurse in her sixties said: "I used to do active cases but as the younger kids come on they enjoy the challenge and the machines. I enjoy just getting the chronic ones that they think won't make it. . ., I've had my day of that other kind challenge. The doctors tease me and say, 'If I ever wake up here and see you standing over me, I'll know I'm in trouble.' "

Some staff members set limits on the type of patient with whom they will work or with the length of time they will spend with a certain patient who is difficult either physically or emotionally. Caregivers who, for example, had difficulty working with women having abortions handled the situation in a number of different ways. Physicians sometimes gained control by doing only certain types of abortions, such as first trimester D&Cs, wherein they did not have to be aware of the fact that there was a fetus. Others would do second trimester abortions but would then do only saline abortions where they simply had to inject the saline and did not have to be present to see the fetus expelled. That then left the nurses to deal with the aborted fetus. Thus, one profession's seeking to gain control left another profession feeling out of control and under stress. Nurses then sometimes decided to gain control by leaving the work situation.

At other times caregivers may feel the need to set limits on what they feel they can competently handle at a certain point in time. For example, psychotherapists who work with people with life-threatening illness may seek to limit the number of people in their practice who are in the terminal phase of their illness at any one point in time. One approach is to strive to have a balance of people recently diagnosed; others living with recurrences or in the chronic phase of their illness; some who may be approaching or be in the terminal phase, others who are recently bereaved; and a few who have resolved much of their grief and are becoming invested in new lives.

Other practitioners develop control in different ways. Dr. Sarah Barlowe, an oncologist, said,

> I limit the number of patients I'll see in a clinic. I have another physician to pick up the overflow but I refuse to simply see people as bodies coming in and out. I feel that I should be able to walk into a room and make people feel that this time is theirs and it's unlimited. I can't always do this but in the clinic I have a card which I give to people who seem to need more time. I tell them to call my office and make an appointment for a time to talk which is often first thing in the morning or last thing at night when the phone stops ringing.

Caregivers, such as chaplains in hospitals, who are exposed to multiple deaths will sometimes say that they can only deal with a certain number of deaths a day. After three deaths, for example, they may leave for the day. A funeral director commented:

> Some don't feel pressure from the kind of work that we do. They've formed a steel shell around themselves and nothing gets in or out. . . . For the rest of us we have to learn that there will be times when you'll be so down that you'll be no use to yourself or anyone else. At those times when I've had lots of rough calls with family problems I no longer feel guilty saying, "Okay you take it Charley." I don't care if I am the senior person, I'll go and embalm the body. . . . I don't have to talk to it. . . . I'll do the mechanical things where I don't have to give—I've given all I have to give until I get recharged. . . . That is of course presuming that you have a choice.

A pediatric oncology nurse found that she had to set similar limits:

> You have to learn that you can't be equally involved with everyone. I tried to be at first. It was incredibly draining—I'd be on the brink of tears when I'd be in the grocery store and the tomatoes weren't ripe enough. You have to come to the realization that, "I can't go in to see this dying child at this point in time. I can help the staff but can't be with this child."

Other caregivers set limits by working fewer hours and redefining areas of stress. A medical administrator commented,

> I don't work the long hours that I used to and I find that I waste less time spinning my wheels. I organize my time better and find that I have more people to help me. . . . I just feel less anxious about things, more relaxed, and take things as they go now. I refuse to let administrative problems worry me and I just won't personalize administrative hassles. If I start worrying about personal aggrandizement and start confronting colleagues with these issues, I just get into trouble. So I usually let it just blow over. As an administrator, I do react sharply and harshly though if people are being really nasty. I'll let them go because their behavior will otherwise create just too much of a morale problem.

Another way of gaining control is to have the power to function in multiple roles or to develop special "treats" in one's practice. Dr. Walter French spoke of the ways in which his multiple roles gave him great satisfaction.

I see myself as curing, palliating, and doing research. The biggest satisfaction is in curing. Now after 5 years in the business I can look at the cures who come back to the clinic. We pat each other on the head. They tell us how great we are and we tell them how great they're looking. With palliation, it's good to see a good response and keep working ... even if they do succumb they've often had a pretty good extension of life and we're satisfied that we've done a good job. Then research functions as a distraction. You can depersonalize and handle the data which you know represent people simply as numbers, trends, response rates and curves—just a bunch of numbers showing something that is at least as good as any treatment being offered anywhere else. My results are now as good as anyone's internationally and the international group comes to think of you as knowing something. You get a little personal satisfaction in the research vein that gives you reason to exist.

LIFESTYLE MANAGEMENT (13%)

One hears a great deal about effective life-style management these days and yet it is often difficult to find people who actually practice it effectively. Caregivers mentioned a variety of approaches that they had found to be effective in helping them to manage both occupational and personal stress. Lifestyle management consisted of a variety of approaches that were both problem-solving and emotion-regulating and included attention to proper diet, sleep, exercise, avoiding the use of cigarettes, and judicious use of alcohol, caffeine, and other drugs.

Those in emergency rooms, intensive care units, and oncology rated lifestyle management as their second most commonly used coping strategy. Males reported using lifestyle management more than did females and of particular interest was the fact that males were more apt to report separating their work from home as an effective coping strategy. Those in the 30–45 age category reported using lifestyle management more often than did either their younger or older colleagues and social workers were more apt to report using lifestyle management than was any other professional group.

A director of nursing typified a small group of caregivers who were consciously trying to practice lifestyle management using a multipronged approach. She had problems with job stress in the past and in a new career she was trying to avoid a repetition of previous patterns. She had recently become involved in transcendental meditation and had decreased her alcohol intake, now avoided "junk food" and red meat, had stopped drinking coffee, although she still drank tea, and was beginning an exercise program.

Exercise was a very effective coping strategy employed by several caregivers. Probably the most commonly reported exercise was squash but other activities such as mountain climbing, tennis, walking, running, curling, skiing, dancing, and skating were also mentioned. Several caregivers reported finding it helpful to have a "decompression routine" to use on the way home from work. Nurses in British Columbia said they drove home along the ocean to allow themselves to unwind, while a medical engineer said he followed his wife's advice and stopped at the "Y" ... "As a 'buffer zone' between work and home. It's relaxing, invigorating, and a painless way of keeping in shape to music and I don't carry all the tension home with me. It was that or start going out for a drink every day after work and that didn't seem like a very good idea."

A clinical nurse specialist had a more involved approach that worked for her:

When I come home from work feeling either angry or pressured it helps to play the piano. I can play angry music and get lots of tension out. If it works and I feel better then I'll go for a run to celebrate feeling better. If the music doesn't get the tension out then I'll go for a long, hard run and try to run the tension out of me. Usually that works. If it doesn't then I know I'm going to either have to take the time to think things through, or else find someone to talk to. A real problem is what happens when I need to talk and there's no one around or else the people in my life are too invested in their own lives to be able to listen to me.

Other methods of lifestyle management include: consciously pacing one's life to avoid multiple stressors or lifestyle changes simultaneously; becoming aware of one's psychophysiological threshold or the particular symptom or set of symptoms one gets in response to stress, e.g. palpitations, headaches, rapid pulse, insomnia; avoid overloading one's time budget (20); massage therapies of various types; meditation techniques; visualization and hypnosis (21) and leaving at least an hour a day for oneself. Get to know what causes you stress and learn to change the stressors you can alter, and to cope more effectively with the ones over which you have no control. A head nurse said that when she knew that things were going to be bad at work, she coped by cutting back on her social life, ate well and slept well so that she would be up to dealing with her work stressors.

Hobbies such as gardening, music, pottery, woodworking, house renovation, or anything else that interests one and provides an extra incentive to get away from the work situation is helpful. Caregivers spoke of the most important aspect of lifestyle management as being to clear one's mind of work-related issues and to provide a recognition that "I count too and I deserve to take care of myself, not just the patients with whom I work." This was well articulated by a priest chaplain who said:

> In dealing with the sick and dying I recognized that I had to have some contact with the healthy and the living. I went into refereeing soccer football. I figured better football than women. That and a weekly game of golf with the guys became sacrosanct. I had no compunction about leaving the hospital at 4:00 p.m. and saying I won't be back until 6:30 p.m. This is my relaxation. There's no one to substitute for me until 11:00 p.m. but I need my relaxation. They understand and expected it.... The transition from grief to football was difficult at times but I did it.

The final and very important aspect of lifestyle management involved being able to separate work from home. While one might expect that the ability to separate work from home life might be a skill which would develop with time, it in fact was equally common across all age groups although some of the older caregivers had only learned the skill with time. For some the coping strategy was reasonably easy: "Now I shut my mind off when I go through the door. I used to carry it home with me but now I shut off. Most of the time I can talk things over with a colleague when I'm there then I leave it behind." Others learned from previous experience as was the case of a surgeon who was asked to be on the trauma roster for the emergency room in his community hospital. He said "I'd love to do it, but I lost one marriage and family because of overcommitment to patients and the hospital and I'm not going to lose this marriage." One large study of physicians found in fact that the most contented group of physicians were those who spent as much time as possible with their families (22).

Sometimes family members were helpful in pointing out that caregivers needed to separate more effectively. A funeral director said that when he worked in a busy home with more than 750 funerals a year he was under:

> . . . an incredible amount of pressure of numbers which left me emotionally and physically exhausted. I was dealing with people and handling all kinds of detail all day and would go home completely zapped. My initial response was just to turn off when I got home until my wife pointed out to me what I was doing. I realized that I was holding myself in check all day not reacting to impulses or stimuli, not permitting myself to have any feelings. I had to keep the ship running at work and when I got home I didn't want any more problems but when I realized I was making things hard for the family we talked about it and we're better off for it. Now when I get home the kids say, "Hi Dad, what kind of a day have you had?" If it's been bad I won't get their problems then. But can now respond, "I've had a rotten day but what about you?" having set the stage for openness.

Other caregivers have also devised methods of spending time with their families without work pressure. An oncologist attends a weekly bible study with his wife and they also set Friday nights aside, put the kids to bed together and have a romantic, candlelight dinner by themselves at which he is not "allowed" to bring up work or conflict-laden subjects.

Finally, some caregivers learned to reassess their job-home interaction as a result of serious illness experiences. A general practitioner reported that he changed after a coronary during which he faced his own mortality.

> We changed our family life and family goals and the family became much more important. It brought it into focus. I looked at the rest of my life and gave it definition which focused around my wife and me. My wife became much more liberated and self-sufficient in her career which has taken the heavy financial burden off of me. She's much more supportive to me now and I no longer feel that the weight of the entire family is on my shoulders.

A PERSONAL PHILOSOPHY OF ILLNESS, DEATH, AND PROFESSIONAL ROLE (12%)

Caregivers who work with seriously ill and/or dying persons may well need to have some type of philosophy to underpin the work that they do and to explain the suffering to which they are exposed.

Statements of personal philosophy were not a variable for which I searched; rather, they often surfaced at the end of an interview when I would ask caregivers, "Given all the stressors which you have mentioned and the symptoms of stress which you have acknowledged, what is it that gets you to work in the morning? What is it that keeps you going?" Often the response had to do with the sense of professional competence and pleasure in work already discussed; but alternatively, or in addition, the response involved a personal philosophy of life and death that gave meaning to the suffering to which one was exposed, put life and death into perspective, gave value to what one was doing as an individual, or undergirded one's professional role.

Not surprisingly, the likelihood that one would mention being sustained by a personal philosophy increased with age. Males were marginally more apt to mention having a personal philosophy and physicians were somewhat more likely than were other professional groups to mention this coping mechanism. One might speculate that the fact that physicians have a more independent role wherein they are often responsible for making major decisions might have caused them to reflect on the meaning of life, suffering, and death and their involvement in these issues. Alternatively, it may be that the physicians who were willing to be interviewed for the book were as a group more introspective than their colleagues who were not approached.

Of interest was the fact that although a personal philosophy was mentioned by caregivers in all specialties, those in emergency rooms were much less likely to mention having any type of philosophy to undergird their work. Perhaps this is reflective of a personality type that might be found in that setting; alternatively, it might be possible that the stressors to which caregivers were exposed were such that they were difficult to put into a philosophical framework.

Personal Philosophy of Illness and Death

Many of those interviewed said it would be impossible to do this type of work without having some type of philosophy about death. A middle-aged physician who had directed an intensive care unit for several years spoke of the way in which such a philosophy could evolve:

> In an ICU the younger staff suffer more than the older because they haven't come to terms with their own dying. If they have come to terms with it then there is less stress. . . . Staff need to come to accept the fact that they are going to die. They need to talk about the reality of their own death. This is best done at the time of another's death. To get them to talk, however, the experienced clinician needs to have talked about death and his feelings about it before that so that he can talk to them when it happens.

Many years ago I heard Dr. Avery Weisman speak of the philosophy that he tried to impart to young medical students who were going to interview dying patients. As I recall, he told them, "When you go to see these people don't feel guilty that they are dying and you are living. Remember, your time will also come and it may be sooner than you think. As you speak to these people ask yourself, 'What can I do now when it's not my turn that I hope someone else would do tomorrow when it may be.' "

Weisman suggests that for professionals the realization of personal death is very difficult to accept. We reach for ways to avoid confronting our distress regarding our personal death and often cover our fear with bold and pretentious talk. "Nevertheless, the presence of death is unmistakably a part of being alive, and even being fully alive. But unless we achieve mutual respect for our individuality, death will remain an abstract symbol, dehumanizing mankind" (23, p. 110). "The ultimate test of coping effectively with our deaths, yours and mine, is a type of transcendental despair, a process of creative acceptance of limitations and possibilities, without relying on linguistic or theoretical legerdemain" (23, p. 114). Dr. Phyllis Palgi writes from the Israeli experience that each individual needs to struggle to find ways of accepting the inevitability of death that can then help them to find meaning in their lives which extends beyond their own biological existence (24). She quotes the work of Lifton (25) who writes of five general modes of giving alternative means of experiencing a sense of immortality: through one's children and one's children's children; transcending of death through spiritual attainment; the theme of eternal nature; creativity; and finally with a psychic state of experiential transcendence. With regard to creativity Lifton points out that "physicians and psychotherapists associate their therapeutic efforts with beneficient influences that carry forth indefinitely in the lives of patients and their children. Thus, lack of success is often traumatic" (24, p. 36).

A German nurse who had practiced nursing during World War II speculated about the type of personal philosophy that might be helpful in dealing with the dying:

> The ideal person is someone who has come to conscious recognition and acceptance of one's finite existence and has not yet developed the fear of "How is my own death going to be" which is so common to older people. Otherwise constant exposure to death is too frightening to be accepted without growing callous and indifferent. . . . There is nothing quite like death in an old-fashioned Catholic hospital. During a bombing a nun said to her patients, "If you have to die, I'll be with you." After helping to evacuate those she could, she walked back to her patients in body casts and died with them. If one stopped cursing God at that point, her death was meaningful.

Caregivers who had arrived at a personal philosophy of life and death had a variety of approaches. One of the more common was a religious philosophy. A nurse in palliative care said: "Death is not a problem for me because of my faith, a belief in a Supreme Being, a belief that there is something better in the after-life— a just reward. As a Salvationist my conversion experience brought me to believe that there is something else. I try not to use my religious beliefs with patients, however, unless they have similar beliefs."

A very different philosophy was espoused by an oncologist:

> I've given lots of thought to what I'm doing and I've had to come to terms with my personal thoughts of death and dying. I see death as being inevitable but you don't really know how you'll deal with it until you have to face it yourself. My philosophy regarding the meaning of life is that all forms of life are interrelated—humans are only one fragment of life. The purpose of life is evolution—the physical plane you can't do very much about, but the social and emotional you can change with certain limitations. Life is a situation in which there is an opportunity for evolution. Life doesn't end with death because it is a return to the universe. There may be incarnation, . . . there may be a fragment of life manifesting itself as a structural form—returning to the whole.

The caregiver who wishes more specific information about dealing with personal confrontations with death is referred to the very helpful book *Personal Death Awareness,* by Dr. J. William Worden (26). Such confrontations with personal philosophies of death are sometimes best done through dialogue with other team members, social workers, clergy, or in support groups (27) rather than in isolation.

Philosophy Regarding One's Professional Role

Some caregivers had very clearly articulated philosophies regarding their professional roles while others were struggling to determine what type of philosophy might sustain them. Helen Young, a 28-year-old palliative care nurse was very much involved in the struggle: "With all this talk about staff stress, I wonder if we're too self-indulgent. . . the product of the 'me generation,' rather wrapped up in our need to be fulfilled. We become too focused on our work. Our satisfaction then ultimately has to be focused on the team or on the patient. In some ways this isn't a reality. You can't expect that kind of satisfaction from work."

For many caregivers their philosophy involved what religious persons might call "a ministry of presence." They primarily attempted to help to lift the burden with which patients and families labored. They wanted to feel that because they were there the suffering was less than it might have been had they not been present. They made comments such as the following:

A palliative care physician: 'I'm not out to save anyone but to meet people's needs at a time when they're needy and in a way that's dependable. This involves the family almost more than the patient because if the family is well cared for then it's good preventative medicine.

A palliative care social worker: I say to myself when a patient comes in we promise freedom from pain, optimal quality of life, someone to be there with the crises or with death. These are our mandates. If I can look back and say that to the best of my ability these things were done then it was a victory, not a loss. That's what I'm here to do. If I've done it well and contributed to the team effort, then I have to say that we've done a good job.

An oncology nurse: The bottom line is that I know that these crises and disasters are happening. I'm not here to keep them from happening but I can do lots to make it easier—dealing with bureaucratic red tape, system failure, symptoms. I can do something or give it a try. That's what keeps me going.

A nurse working with patients with bone marrow transplants: I can be like people who buy lottery tickets and take a chance. I feel that we're doing well. The patients who are doing well come in and we get letters back from some of the others. I can tell myself, "It worked for someone," "I did this for someone." You don't stop buying lottery tickets because it didn't work. You may have to treat 100 patients to get one success story, but that may make it worthwhile.

An intensive care nurse: Every day when I go home I say to myself, "I really helped someone." You have to, otherwise I couldn't get up and face myself in the mirror every morning. This way I get up every morning and say, "Good morning Theresa, it's a new day. Let's get going."

LEAVE THE WORK SITUATION (11%)

A number of caregivers coped with their work stress by leaving the work situation either temporarily or permanently. This coping mechanism was most common in emergency rooms and both adult and pediatric intensive care units, was more common in females than in males, and was more likely to be used by nurses than by any other professional group. In addition, those under thirty were more likely than were other groups to report leaving the work situation. Previous studies of nurses were similar to this one in that they showed that nurses were apt to leave the work situation because of difficulties with the system rather than because of specific personal complaints and that nurses who were between 25–35 stayed in their jobs only one third as long as nurses in the study who were over 45 (28). The present study differs from previous work by other authors who found that intensive care unit nurses were no more likely than were other nurses to either leave or think of leaving their jobs (29–31); however, the present study surveyed nurses from a wider variety of ICUs than did other studies, as well as surveying people who had in fact already chosen to leave their jobs.

Some caregivers mentioned leaving their jobs only briefly for a mental health day, a long weekend, a conference or course or a vacation as a way of coping with, decreasing or avoiding job stress. Many of these mentioned that regular holidays such as taking one week off every 4 months was an effective stress reduction mechanism. Some volunteers working in palliative care units or bereavement services found that a periodic 2-month break or "mini sabbatical" was effective as a coping strategy.

For others, there were fantasies of leaving their jobs, while many spoke of planning to leave or referred to jobs they had left specifically because of job stress. People transferred jobs within the same organization, changed jobs, left a career within a particular specialty, and in some instances left their profession. These

changes evolved because of pressures within a job situation, because of systems
difficulty, as a result of the interaction between personal and job stress, because
of concerns about career choice implications or career path progression, and rarely
because of a specific incident.

The most dramatic example of leaving a job came from an emergency room
physician who decided to leave the teaching hospital and practice in a smaller
community.

> I began looking at the lifestyle of the people around me when I was training to be a
> teaching surgeon. I looked around at my senior colleagues and saw that at 40 and 50
> they were still underlings. It was a feudal system and they were the [serfs]. They were
> coming in at 3:00 and 4:00 a.m. and working 80-hour weeks. Often they weren't
> allowed to operate but just stood around supporting the chief. There was incredible
> stress and pressure to perform.
>
> I enjoy my family, a more relaxed lifestyle, sports, writing. It wasn't possible within
> that framework. It came together for me one day when we were in doing a gall bladder
> at 3:00 a.m. on a Sunday morning. The scrub nurse who had been there for a while
> suddenly threw down the instruments. She said, "Do you know what's going on here?
> It's 3:00 a.m. Respectable people are home in bed or out doing something they enjoy.
> You're here with your hands inside someone's abdomen and I'm helping you. I've had
> it." She walked out and never came back.
>
> We talked about it for weeks. That she just walked out. That incident in itself didn't
> cause me to leave but it made me think.
>
> Here I was in this intense teaching environment. A colleague had just been diagnosed
> as having a terrible stress ulcer. I sat down and said, "No way. This isn't the life I want."

Oftentimes staff members blamed "systems problems" for their need to leave
a particular setting. Not infrequently this type of complaint came from those
in intensive care units who felt that their units were inadequately staffed—either
in terms of quantity of staff or quality of staff.

In such situations the decision of one or more staff members to leave will often
then precipitate several other staff members making the same decision. Often senior
caregivers would speak of staffing units where no one had been on the unit for
more than a few months. At other times the unit had seemed to be running well
with experienced caregivers, but when one key person decided to leave for personal
reasons or as a way of managing stress, then others would soon follow, feeling, "If
she can do it, so can I." This loss of several people simultaneously, while perhaps
a good coping mechanism for those who leave, can precipitate grief reactions,
resentment, anger, and sometimes feelings of inadequacy in those who remain.

Sometimes the leaving was precipitated by personal problems of which the
caregiver might or might not be aware. Someone who was not fully aware of the
impact of personal problems might focus on job stress as the source of discomfort
and leave a job only to find the same problems surfacing in the next position. A
director of nursing said, "I've known good nurses who ran into serious personal
problems and become totally nonfunctional and actively dangerous. When they
recognized it, they got out. When they didn't, they had to be taken out."

Sometimes working with incompetent colleagues who did not recognize their
inadequacies caused others to leave the job situation. A former nursing instructor
said that she left nursing after she saw one anesthetist make his third mistake which
led to a patient death.

This nurse was not alone in leaving the profession. Some of the others who had
left had also felt impotent in various situations and decided they were not going to

allow this to continue. A few planned to enter medical school because as one nurse said, "I've seen so many problems in medicine I feel that I can do a better job. I want to do something without the powerlessness of nursing. . . . A physician can do more within the system."

Being a physician was no guarantee of professional happiness however, and a few of the physicians spoke of reconsidering their choice of career or specialty. A medical intern commented, "Two-thirds of the medical interns are not reapplying for internal medicine residencies. They're looking to get into radiation, pathology, dermatology—areas that don't demand a lot of extra time or emotional involvement with patients."

A senior ICU physician said that his unit was doing a survey to find out what percentage of the residents they had trained were still working in ICU. "I bet fewer than 5 out of the 20 we've trained in the last 10 years are still doing ICU full time today. With the time and the stress involved—many more hours than anesthesia, with many more hours on call—they're leaving ICU."

Nurses also questioned whether or not to stay in jobs that required long and/or irregular hours. "The younger ones are leaving after less than 5 years in the field. They have the attitude, 'Who needs it. My friends are out having a good time and I'm stuck with 12-hour shifts and working weekends.' People come to feel, 'To heck with it. I'll go on the Registry and have a normal home life working when I want to.' "

Others who left their jobs left the profession as well. I heard of nurses who were selling real estate, cosmetics, drugs, and medical equipment. Others had opened their own business, were driving ambulances, had become funeral directors, ministers, and engineers. A nurse who was now selling cardiac catheterization laboratory computers observed: "As women most of us never expected that we'd be working for the rest of our lives. The Women's Movement gave us so many new options that I for one decided to take advantage of them. . . I'm 36 now and I felt that if I was going to make a career move I should probably do it before 40 because by 46 it becomes a bit late."

A social worker from South Africa was in the same age group and made a career change for somewhat different reasons.

> After 5 years in oncology I began to find the work was really heavy. I'd be drained after a difficult interview. This was particularly marked because of working in South Africa where we have lots of problems around cultural and racial issues. I had to deal with the realities of what people had to return home to. . . . I didn't burn out but I've left the field completely and have gone into the insurance industry.

AVOID OR DISTANCE FROM PATIENT OR FAMILY (11%)

Caregivers coped with their stress by physically avoiding or psychologically distancing from patients for a number of reasons, but generally either consciously or unconsciously they were trying to protect themselves from identifying with patients and experiencing the feelings that such identification might precipitate.

The fact that caregivers tend to avoid dying patients and their families has been documented from the early work of Glaser and Strauss (32, 33), Quint (34), Sudnow (35), and Feifel (36).

Weisman points out that even experienced therapists may feel threatened by annihilation when near a dying person. Some may be put off by the sights and smells of disease; others may become infected by an atmosphere of hopelessness and helplessness (37).

In the present study nurses reported avoiding and distancing from patients more than did the other professional groups. Those caregivers working in specialty areas wherein they had short-term contact such as emergency rooms, ICU, pediatric ICU, and obstetrics were most apt to report using this coping mechanism. At times caregivers were aware of the fact that early in their career they had become very involved with patients who had died. The caregivers then made a conscious or subconscious decision not to again allow themselves to experience that same degree of pain. A young nurse working on a bone marrow transplant unit said: "I got really close to the first person I worked with here who died. Since then, I feel myself withdrawing from people I know are going to die. I feel badly about that because it's not what I saw myself doing as a nurse, but it's happening and I don't know what to do about it."

A gastroenterologist said:

> I never let myself get close to anyone who is going to die. I just block off my feelings. I'm nice to them and ask about their family but then I concentrate on today and don't talk about the future. You can't have two or three people a week that you're close to die and still survive. I'd be glad to have someone paramedically trained to handle these patients and I'm sure most of my colleagues would too.

A paramedic spoke of avoiding family members so as to minimize the risk of confronting their grief. He said, "The first time I saw a dead patient I said to the wife, 'Now dear, step out of the way. Everything will be all right.' She screamed at me that nothing would ever be all right again. Her husband was dead. For weeks I replayed that scene. Now I don't say anything to families because I don't want it to be repeated."

In other instances it may be the culture or milieu of the unit or of society as a whole that keeps caregivers from being involved. A clergywoman from Sweden said: "In our culture one must try not to show tears but to always appear as though nothing really bothers you, so our nurses carry around the problems they feel by themselves."

Such isolation then of course tends to cause caregivers to distance from patients to avoid experiencing this pain.

Staff may also cope with the stress they experience in dealing with patients by developing certain client typologies. This then allows patients to be lumped into categories and to be seen as "types" rather than as unique persons (38).

Intellectualization is a fairly common mechanism that professionals use to distance from patients and thereby to cope with their stress. Several nurses spoke of the difficulty that they had when physicians made rounds and discussed vagaries of the patients' illness within the hearing of the patient. One ICU nurse observed that she found it particularly difficult when physicians "forgot" that a particular patient with Guillian-Barre Syndrome was a nurse and spent a lot of time discussing what her illness meant while in the woman's room. She observed: "One doctor will do rounds outside the door of patients who are conscious, but most don't and forget that there's a human being there. Even with conscious patients they hear discussions of other patients' illnesses and get upset—so much for confidentiality."

A few caregivers spoke of the fact that the patient was not seen as a person but much more as an intellectual challenge. An ICU nurse said, "It's really interesting when you know how the body works and see it totally wracked. I become really impressed by how the body has worn down and how it eventually stops functioning. It's fascinating to watch a heart in congestive failure with no myofibrils contracting anymore."

It is also possible to depersonalize patients through the use of technology. An IV nurse spoke of the days when she used to use her technological role as a way of coping and protecting herself from involvement with patients. "I came in and gave chemotherapy and got out. Some of my colleagues were aware of how we distanced from patients and lots of us deliberately put up fronts to protect ourselves."

Asken (41) observed that nurses working in intensive care units often maintained emotional distance from patients by relating more to their medical equipment and procedures than to the patients. It was suggested however that this detachment might be threatened when caregivers were forced to deal with the patient's family or when the patient's human characteristics were highlighted. A similar observation was made by Dr. Chuck Cartwright, a physician in an intensive care unit who said:

> It's often hard to respond to patients as people in the ICU. It's particularly difficult when we're having problems weaning a patient from a ventilator. Physicians, especially the young ones, tend to avoid having to deal with these decisions. We have an older nurse on our unit who says to these residents, "Look him in the eye and make your decision." "Don't you think we've done enough here? This patient has end-stage lung disease and his lungs are completely obstructed."

Caregivers in oncology also talked in terms of avoiding patients. Within the oncology group, patients also spoke of their concerns that caregivers might abandon them at a time when they were dying. One young woman asked the question, "Will my doctor have trouble and withdraw when I start to die? Will you stick by me as I get worse?" A young man whose wife was diagnosed as having advanced uterine cancer said,

> I see in the eyes of all the doctors who come in to see us that they're scared and they want to get out as soon as they can. They say, "Don't take chemotherapy—just realize that you're going to die—nothing can change it and don't wreck the time you have with chemo." They give the message that she should enjoy the 6 months to 2 years that she has. They're hiding things. They aren't telling me what I want to know. And I'm angry.

Avoidance can be more than a physical phenomenon and can often be disguised as "truth-telling"—but without emotional involvement. An oncologist said that he observed residents going in and telling patients that they were going to die soon after they were diagnosed as having advanced disease: "The junior medical staff seems to be resisting psychological involvement with patients. They seem to be carrying it too far that they are normal, healthy people and that the patients are the sick ones. They talk with patients regarding their prognosis quite casually. I think sometimes it's easier to tell people at day one that they're going to die, but. . ."

A 24-year-old woman who was dying of breast cancer at the same hospital spoke of what it was like to be on the receiving end of such views. The young female resident her first day on the service came in and told this young woman that she was going to die. The resident then left without telling anyone that she had told the young woman of her impending death and without providing any support. The resident never came back to continue this discussion. This avoidance may in part have been because the resident was a young woman close to the patient's age and yet the anxiety that the patient experienced was such that the role of the resident in bringing her this news and then avoiding her must really be questioned from an ethical perspective.

INCREASED EDUCATION (7%)

A coping strategy mentioned by several caregivers was to increase their information base with regard to both professional and personal matters. This did not always involve taking formal courses, but involved learning from others as well as taking responsibility for personal learning needs. This coping strategy was most common in emergency rooms and palliative care units and was more apt to be found in those over 30. Increased education involved a variety of approaches to learning that did not necessarily follow traditional learning models. It involved first of all being willing to learn from others—both in one's own discipline as well as from other disciplines.

A consultation-liaison psychiatrist commented on the oncologists with whom he worked. "These guys are all fierce competitors—that's great. They really know their stuff—they learn so much from their colleagues."

Learning from other disciplines can even come about through negative experience. A nurse in a chronic care hospital observed that at a lecture on palliative care and symptom relief, ". . . some of the physicians started reading to show that you weren't right about pain relief in palliative care and to justify what they were doing. They found new information through their reading which they now see as being their own discovery and pain relief is changing around here."

People often learn through nonverbal communication. A nurse in an emergency room said, "After the first crib death in which I was involved the doctor had tears in his eyes. I learned that it's okay to shed a tear—but you can't get out of control. That doesn't help the family, but a few tears are okay."

Other caregivers set about learning more technical information in an independent fashion, setting their own learning goals. A chaplain said that her usual pattern in all of the areas in which she worked was ". . . to do reading about technology and treatment plans so I know what is going on and what the patient can expect will happen. But the actual technical procedures are not my concern, other than knowing the emotional impact they may have on patients and what they may expect."

Attaining the type of information one needed could not always be done through independent study. Many caregivers took courses to increase their professional learning and several also took courses of broad general interest such as computer science, managerial study, theology, or courses for purely personal interest such as pottery. For several their real learning experiences did not come from formal courses, but, rather, from attending conferences. A nurse who worked with people with cardiac pacemakers observed that, "It's good to get away to meetings where I can sit around and discuss things with others in similar jobs. I want to talk with people who really do pacemakers. That kind of real sharing doesn't happen at the hospital level."

Several people spoke of going on for additional education, either in their present field or in another. An ICU nurse who felt that she was constantly dealing with ethical dilemmas for which she had no answers went to graduate school, "... to gain control, keep myself from being compromised, and to learn about ethical decision-making. I had been there for 8 years and could no longer work there without questioning and disquiet."

A 28-year-old staff nurse said that she was, "Tired of shopping and the disco scene and so I decided to use my time constructively. I'm now in my third year of studying entomology. It's stressful but good. I really enjoy the positive parts of the program and the interactions with my fellow students."

Caregivers have not always decided where such an additional education should lead them. One nurse who decided to do an MBA said, "It was a way of exploring options but I could still come back to health care work if I wanted to."

Oftentimes the education of which caregivers spoke had to do with coming to terms with their personal feelings about death and grief. A palliative care physician commented that with her mother's death,

> I got an increased understanding about what loss is all about. It stretched my coping mechanisms so that the weak ones fell away. It was rather like a postgraduate course in what not to say. Comments like, "You must be so relieved," or from my religious friends who were told of her death: "It's joyful news," felt like real betrayal. ... I learned as well that to be a good physician I'll need to learn more about psychiatry. I've learned to let my emotional response be one of my professional tools, along with my stethescope."

Harper (42) speaks of the stages, through which caregivers pass in learning about death. These include: knowledge and anxiety; trauma; pain, mourning and grief; moderation, mitigation, and accommodation; and self-realization, self-awareness, and self-actualization.

Finally, caregivers spoke of coming to terms with other issues that were of relevance in their lives. Some spoke of needing to learn to be more assertive; others learned to set limits to decrease the job-home interaction problems with which they were confronted; still others learned successful stress management techniques or dealt with issues of self-awareness of one type or another. This was put well by a palliative care nurse who said, "I've studied self-awareness and I have learned what interferes with what I am doing and with what I am capable of doing. I've also learned to look at when I am interfering with patients. ... The person has a right to have control over his or her life and sometimes it's my role to sit back and not to interfere with the decisions of another."

OUTSIDE SUPPORT SYSTEMS (5%)

Newlin and Wellisch (43) comment that the time to begin to ensure the emotional stability of the oncology nurse is when he/she is hired. The same can be said of any caregiver entering a potentially stressful position. These authors suggest that there are two prime attributes or supports that will be required: a supportive family or peer network and the ability to "unplug" from work. Given that so many authors speak of the importance of a personal support system in dealing with work stress, it was interesting that social support outside of the work situation was not mentioned more often than it was.

As we saw in Chapter 3, social support systems can serve as both a hindrance as well as a help. Many caregivers reported feeling that they had to spare their family and friends exposure to the stressors with which they were confronted. An emergency room nurse who had a particularly abusive patient on the night shift said, "I often call my mother to talk after a shift but when I started repeating all the names this man called me I could sense her getting more and more upset. I thought to myself, 'she's 64 years old, why am I doing this to her?' But I have to dump somewhere."

The use of outside social support did not vary much across the specialty areas but was slightly more apt to be reported by those who worked with chronically ill patients such as those in palliative care, oncology, and pediatric chronic care. Counselors and nurses were somewhat more apt to report using this coping mechanism than were physicians, women used it more than men, and younger caregivers used outside social support slightly more than their more experienced colleagues.

An ICU nurse spoke of the need for social support. "You need someone to talk to when you get out—maybe just the cat, but someone. We see a lot and a lot of what we see isn't nice. I can talk about it for hours. You need someone—a boyfriend, a husband, someone."

Some caregivers worked at developing support networks of colleagues with whom they could discuss issues so they didn't have to bring them home. An enterostomal therapist spoke of calling a colleague in another setting which she found to be far more helpful than speaking with others within her own work setting. Others worked at developing a variety of networks to fulfill various needs. A chaplain had one parish group that he used to help with practical problems and another to give him emotional support. Some caregivers spoke of prayer groups. Others developed support networks of colleagues in similar work situations—such as oncology social workers, critical care nurses, emergency medicine groups. One palliative care group that met to discuss professional issues found it very helpful to have a weekend retreat wherein they shared their concerns regarding working in a fishbowl environment with their work being subject to the scrutiny not only of colleagues, but of the community and the media as well. They shared the isolation that they often felt professionally as well as personally as a result of their work and were able to derive support from one another. One physician who was experiencing stress both in her personal and professional roles said that she found that "I received wisdom from the group and the courage to take a major jump which would leave me more alone. I wondered why I had never noticed many of the things people mentioned. I learned much more about working alone, group dynamics, multiple grief, and personal suffering."

A middle-aged internist consciously worked to develop a support system because of certain deficits in his life.

My wife and I felt a big hole in our lives which sent us into a growth group. We developed a support group basically at church which was composed of people we had previously not known, none of them in medicine. This group has now been going on for 12 years and is composed of 6 or 7 couples. I tell them that my growth began the night that one of them pulled me out from underneath the piano. We can be deep with each other. We can be shallow but we care. . . . As a result of this group I'll now lean on someone else to recount an episode—my wife, a fellow staff member, someone to whom I can expose my weaker side—just to be able to say, "I hurt, I'm sad, I'm joyful." That's a freedom that was not mine originally.

Family and friends who were helpful were often seen to be able to set limits on the caregiver by restricting unnecessary dwelling on work situations and by demanding a certain reciprocity in the relationship as was the case with the support group of the physician above. It may not in the long-run be terribly helpful if caregivers just "dump" on their support people without some limits being set and without the expectation that the caregivers will have enough energy to be able to turn around and be able to give to those in their personal support system as well as to their patients.

Pines, Aronson, and Kafry (44) refer to this type of support as providing emotional support and emotional challenge. Emotional support implies being willing to be on an individual's side and to provide unconditional support at least occasionally, even when the other may not completely agree with you. It implies caring more about the individual than about the particular issue being espoused at the moment.

Emotional challenge is also necessary, however, and this implies a trusting relationship in which another can question your approach and behavior in particular situations with a view to helping you to determine whether you really are doing all that you can to fulfill your broader goals and overcome obstacles in a particular situation. Alternatively, it may involve another helping you to use logic to cut through an emotional situation in a rational way.

A palliative care nurse described the emotional help and emotional challenge that she received from her group of friends.

> I talk to my friends surprisingly little about my job. They will tell me to "shut up" in a loving way. They are quick to keep me from becoming pietistic and placing my whole being into my job. They listen to real problems, however. When I applied for my recent job for which I didn't have the paper qualifications, they said, "You know you'd be the best person, so apply."

A palliative care physician also reported that her support system restricted the amount she could talk about work by saying, " 'We're interested in you as a person and not what you do professionally. Your patients are dead and we're alive.' But I can get the time I really need from them. I have the sense that I can take my work stress to prayer. By choice I can go to church daily and have an hour a day of personal prayer."

Organizing a personal support system may not be easy and may require careful planning. A bereavement counsellor who directs a program for survivors of suicide said:

> In an isolated job you may have to plan your support meetings 3 weeks in advance. When I've just seen a 23 year old who is 6 months pregnant and whose husband just suicided I have to talk then, but working in isolation there isn't always someone available. You need to be able to self-initiate support and to identify your ways of coping with this kind of stress.

For several caregivers who worked in fairly isolated positions it was helpful to have a therapist with whom they met regularly on an individual basis. As one British social worker said, "There's often little support when you are in a high level independent position, so I cope by having my own psychiatrist."

SENSE OF HUMOR (3%)

Authors such as Hay and Oken (45) and Asken (41) have noted the use of humor in intensive care units. They observed that humor can be used as a defence against the overwhelming stressors to which caregivers are exposed as well as serving as a natural by-product of the friendly behavior of young people working together. It has even been hypothesized by some that the intensive care unit or emergency room that does not have a friendly banter or black humor going back and forth may in fact be one that is experiencing considerable stress.

Caregivers spoke of using humor when they felt inadequate to the tasks at hand or when they had been severely challenged in dealing with a particular incident. Nurses in one community intensive care unit said that their nursing administration was extemely upset at the level of humor that was exhibited by the ICU staff.

> In the ICU humor is looked upon with disdain. That nurses would fool around is really upsetting to nursing administration but they need to realize that it's a coping mechanism that we use. You can't come back to deal with a dead kid on a ventilator day in and day out until someone has made some kind of decision without some kind of acting out. What does a nurse do when she doesn't use humor? She winds up turning inside out or taking it out on herself or other staff members.

Other staff spoke of playing "water games" over the bodies of patients on ventilators while several spoke of laughter that occurred following a cardiac arrest. "Often at one end of the unit we're really busy and at another end there'll be laughing. We can't leave the ventilated patients alone and we feel helpless and wind up laughing. There's always laughter towards the end of an arrest, no matter what the results. We use joking and humor on our unit to decrease stress as the acuteness is over and you're waiting to see what happens."

Sometimes this use of humor extends to other areas of one's life. Nurses in one intensive care unit said that when they saw young adolescents walking carelessly across the street, they would often call to them, "Watch what you're doing. You wouldn't want to wind up on our unit." They also begin to identify with patients and to realize that they too might wind up in a similar situation, and speak of how they would want the situation handled. "We joke about arresting and how we wouldn't want what we do to others done to us. We laugh about getting ourselves tattooed, 'Do not resuscitate, do not intubate, do not ventilate.' " There are often jokes about the possibility of cardiac arrest as well. In one community emergency room when I was interviewing a number of nurses, a physician walked into the conference room as we were about to begin our discussion. All talk stopped and he said, "I feel embarrassed, . . . like I've stopped something or I'm in a place where I don't belong. . . . I take it as a personal affront like the last time someone coded as I was drawing blood gases."

Humor may also involve the use of labels for patients. McCue (46) observed that the use of such terms as "tubing out" or "gork" by residents is seen as an attempt to develop group support with code words. He suggests that such terms reflect the hopelessness that residents feel as they work with such patients and furthermore states that although dry humor persists in private practice, the ironic name-calling that occurs so often within a teaching hospital is virtually nonexistent outside of educational programs. The reader who is interested in the use of humor in educational programs might refer to Shem (47) and Bosk (48).

A chaplain had the opportunity to observe the way in which staff used humor to allow them to function in particularly difficult situations.

> I remember during our revolution a man was blown up from his knees to his stomach. The fourth year medical students who had admitted him were horrified and started laughing and talking about what he'd had for dinner saying things like, "Here's some rice. I see some green peas." Another time a patient jumped from the fifth floor of the hosptial. The nurses were photographed peeking under his sheets and laughing. They didn't know what to do with how they were feeling.

Humor can form a bond between two people or a group that has just gone through a stressful experience such as a cardiac arrest or the above anecdote or it can in fact be used to prepare people for an upcoming stressful situation. Two oncologists reflected on how they used to engage in very bizarre humor regarding death and disease before beginning to run the head and neck cancer clinic where they would see people whose diseases and treatment had left them quite disfigured. One of these physicians observed that his humor frequently involved a lot of sexual overtones. "This sex thing is a life affirmation. I get sometimes so I want to screw all healthy females and I make these comments. Sometimes when I hear the sick comments and lewd remarks I'm making, I wonder how they mesh with the person that I really am and I'm amazed by my own complexity. I feel badly about this sexual preoccupation and looking at things in the lewd fashion that I do but sometimes it seems I have no choice."

Humor can also serve to keep caregivers from acknowledging the truly painful situations in which patients find themselves. A prominent businessman was told that he probably had only one year to live. He was quite adamant about wanting to do as many things as he possibly could and was very upset when he was told that he wouldn't be able to play baseball that season. "I played my first game and won and broke into tears for the first time in my life. When I told the physician how important this was to me, his immediate response was, 'Who were you playing with—the geriatric unit?' "

Humor can also serve to unite a group of caregivers against everyone else in their environment. On one ICU numerous humorous cartoons and phrases were posted on the bulletin board. Two seemed particularly reflective of the stress under which these caregivers operated: "We, the willing, led by the unknowing, are doing the impossible for the ungrateful" and "We have done so much for so long, with so little, we are now qualified to do anything with nothing." It is interesting to reflect that this was a unit that was in the process of being revamped and they frequently felt that they were inadequately supplied with equipment and that they were ill prepared to deal with the new equipment they had.

Finally, it must be noted that while humor can be an effective way of coping with caregiver stress, it must be carefully used in front of family members. Several caregivers spoke of the fact that they tried to be careful with how humor was exhibited but that sometimes they got caught making inappropriate remarks. Some units handle this by explaining to families ahead of time that when they were laughing, it was not that they were laughing at the patients or at the family members, but, "We're laughing because it's easier to laugh than to cry and you have to laugh to maintain some sanity around this place."

REFERENCES

1. Antonovsky, A. (1979). *Health, stress and coping.* San Francisco: Jossey-Bass.

2. Burke, R. J., & Weir, T. (1980). Coping with the stress of managerial occupations. In C. L. Cooper & R. Payne (Eds.), *Current concerns in occupational stress.* (pp. 299–333). Chichester: Wiley.

3. Coelho, G. V., Hamburg, D. A., & J. E. Adams. (1974). *Coping and adaptation.* New York: Basic.

4. Coyne, J. C., & Lazarus, R. (1980). Cognitive style, stress perception and coping. In I. R. Kutash & L. B. Schlessinger and Associates (Eds.), *Handbook on stress and anxiety.* (pp. 144–158). San Francisco: Jossey-Bass.

5. Ellis, A. (1978). What people can do for themselves to cope with stress. In C. L. Cooper & R. Payne (Eds.), *Stress at Work* (pp. 209–222). Chichester: Wiley.

6. Folkman, S., & Lazarus, R. (1980). An analysis of coping in a middle-aged community sample. *Journal of Health and Social Behavior, 21*(3) 219–239.

7. Ilfeld, F. W. (1980). Coping styles of Chicago adults: Description: *Journal of Human Stress, 6* 2–10.

8. Kobasa, S. C. (1982). Commitment and coping in stress resistance among lawyers. *Journal of Personality and Social Psychology, 42*(4) 707–717.

9. Lazarus, R. S., Averill, J. R., & Opton, E. M. (1974). The psychology of coping. In G. V. Coelho, D. A. Hamburg, & J. E. Adams (Eds.), *Coping and Adaptation* (pp. 249–315). New York: Basic.

10. Lazarus, R. S. (1983). The costs and benefits of denial. In *The denial of stress.* (pp. 1–30). New York: International Universities.

11. Monat, A., & Lazarus, R. (Eds.). (1977). *Stress and coping.* New York: Columbia University Press.

12. Moos, R. H. (1974). Psychological techniques in the assessment of adaptive behavior. In G. V. Coelho, D. A. Hamburg, & J. E. Adams (Eds.), *Coping and Adaptation* (pp. 334–402). New York: Basic.

13. Pearlin, L. I., & Schooler, C. (1978). The structure of coping. *Journal of Health and Social Behavior, 19,* 2–21.

14. Valliant, G. E. (1977). *Adaptation to life.* Boston: Little, Brown.

15. Kobasa, S. C. (1982). The hardy personality: Toward a social psychology of stress and health. In J. Suls & G. Sanders (Eds.), *Social psychology of health and illness.* (pp. 3–32). Hillsdale, NJ: Erlbaum.

16. Yancik, R. (1984). Coping with hospice work stress. *Journal of Psychosocial Oncology, 2*(2) 19–35.

17. Todres, I. D., Howell, M. C., & Shannon, D. C. (1974). Physicians' reactions to training in pediatric intensive care unit. *Pediatrics, 53*(3), 375–383.

18. Pines, A. (1981). Burnout: A current problem in pediatrics. *Current Problems in Pediatrics, 11*(7) 1–32.

19. Friedman, E. H. (1982). Stress and intensive care nursing: A ten year reappraisal. *Heart and Lung, 11*(1) 26–28.

20. Howard, J. H. (1979, November 18–22). Stress and the manager. Paper presented at the 2nd International Symposium on the Management of Stress, Monte Carlo, Monaco.

21. Mount, B. M., & Voyer, J. (1980). Staff stress in palliative/hospice care. In I. Ajemian & B. Mount (Eds.), *The R.V.H. manual on palliative/hospice care.* (pp. 457–488). New York: ARNO.

22. Time-Out. (1981, May 15). *Physician's management manual.*

23. Weisman, A. D. (1977). The psychiatrist and the inexorable. In H. Feifel (Ed.), *New meanings of death.* (pp. 108–121). New York: McGraw-Hill.

24. Palgi, P. (1983). Reflections on some creative modes of confrontation with the phenomenon of death. *The International Journal of Social Psychiatry, 29*(1), 29–37.

25. Lifton, R. J. (1977). The sense of immortality. In H. Feifel (Ed.), *New meanings of death.* (pp. 273–290). New York: McGraw-Hill.

26. Worden, J. W. (1976). *Personal death awareness.* Englewood Cliffs, NJ: Prentice-Hall.

27. Hale, R., & Levy, L. (1982). Staff nurses coping in an NICU. In *Coping with caring for sick newborns* (pp. 103–130). R. E. Marshall, C. Kasman, & L. S. Cape (Eds.), Philadelphia: Saunders.

28. Nursing plagued by high dropout, turnover rate. (1980). *American Association of Critical Care Nurses, 7*(4) 32.

29. Duxbury, M. L., & Thiessen, V. (1979). Staff nurse turnover in neonatal intensive care units. *Journal of Advanced Nursing, 4,* 591–602.

30. Nichols, K. A., Springford, V., & Searle, J. (1981). An investigation of distress and discontent in various types of nursing. *Journal of Advanced Nursing, 6,* 311–318.

31. Dear, M. R., Weisman, C. S., Alexander, C. S., & Chase, G. A. (1982). The effect of the intensive care nursing role on job satisfaction and turnover. *Heart and Lung, 11*(6), 560–565.

32. Glaser, B. G., & Strauss, A. L. (1968). *Time for dying.* Chicago: Aldine.

33. Glaser, B. G., & Strauss, A. L. (1965). *Awareness of dying.* Chicago: Aldine.

34. Quint, J. C. (1967). *The nurse and the dying patient.* New York: Macmillan.

35. Sudnow, D. (1967). *Passing on: The social organization of dying.* Englewood Cliffs, NJ: Prentice-Hall.

36. Feifel, H. (1959). *The meaning of death.* New York: McGraw-Hill.

37. Weisman, A. D. (1972). Psychosocial considerations in terminal care. In B. Schoenberg, A. Carr, D. Peretz, & A. Kutscher (Eds.), *Psychosocial aspects of terminal care* (pp. 162–172). New York: Columbia University Press.

38. Rosenthal, C. J., Marshall, V. W., MacPherson, A. S., & French, S. E. (1980). *Nurses, patients and families.* New York: Springer.

39. Margolies, R., Wachtel, A. B., Sutherland, K. R., & Blum, R. H. (1983). Medical students' attitudes toward cancer: Concepts of professional distance. *Journal of Psychosocial Oncology, 1*(3) 35–49.

40. Neimeyer, G. J., Behnke, M., & Reiss, J. (1983). Constructs and coping: Physicians' responses to patient death. *Death Education, 7*(2–3) 245–264.

41. Asken, M. J. (1979, November). Psychological stress in ICU affects both patients and staff. *Pennsylvania Medicine,* pp. 40–42.

42. Harper, B. C. (1977). *Death: The coping mechanism of the health professional.* Greenville, SC: Southeastern University Press.

43. Newlin, N. J., & Wellisch, D. K. (1978). The oncology nurse: Life on an emotional roller coaster. *Cancer Nursing, 1,* 447–449.

44. Pines, A., Aronson, E., and Kafry, D. (1981). *Burnout: From tedium to personal growth.* New York: The Free Press.

45. Hay, D., & Oken, D. (1972). The psychological stresses of intensive care unit nursing. *Psychosomatic medicine, 34*(2) 109–118.

46. McCue, J. D. (1982). The effects of stress on physicians and their medical practice. *The New England Journal of Medicine, 306*(8) 458–463.

47. Shem, S. (1978). *The house of God.* New York: Dell.

48. Bosk, C. L. (1979). *Forgive and remember: Managing medical failure.* Chicago: The University of Chicago Press.

11

Coping with Stress in the Workplace

Given the fact that stress evolves through the interaction between an individual and the work environment, it is not surprising that the avoidance or resolution of work-related stress will involve institutions making provisions to decrease some of the stressors to which workers are exposed and/or providing resources for workers to use to facilitate their present ability to cope with work stressors. The individual worker also has a role to play in decreasing organizational stressors, in that he or she can choose whether or not to use the resources made available. In addition a worker has a responsibility to identify deficiencies in the system that might be alleviated or eliminated through concerted effort on the part of individuals, teams, interest groups, or administration.

Not all human problems that occur within the occupational field are amenable to individual coping responses. Such stressors may stem from arrangements that are deeply rooted in social and economic organizations and may be impervious to individual personal efforts to change them (1). "This perhaps is the reason that much of our coping functions only to help us endure that which we cannot avoid. Such coping at best provides but a thin cushion to absorb the impact of imperfect social organization. Coping failures, therefore, do not necessarily reflect the short-comings of individuals; in a real sense they may represent the failure of social systems in which the individuals are enmeshed" (1, p. 18).

Factors associated with a healthy work environment include: talking with each other informally, being supportive to one another, consulting among each other, working through interpersonal dissatisfactions, recognition of a job well done, inservice staff development, working together, socializing with one another, and pursuing personal interests within the work setting (2). Such an environment acknowledges three major areas of staff needs: recognition, support, and enjoyment (2). In this chapter the reader will find that it is many of these areas to which care-givers referred when they spoke of the organizational coping mechanisms that they found to be effective in helping them to deal with work stress.

TEAM PHILOSOPHY, BUILDING, AND SUPPORT (31%)

The most important environmental coping mechanism was the sense of belonging to a team that knew what it was doing (team philosophy); knew how to get team members to work towards defined professional and personal goals (team building), and knew how to support one another through professional and personal stressors (team support).

Table 7 in the Appendix shows that this coping mechanism was endorsed twice as often as the next most commonly reported environmental coping mechanism and accounted for one third of the environmental coping mechanisms mentioned. It was the most commonly reported coping mechanism in obstetrics, oncology, palliative care, and chronic care. It was more common in those in the two older age categories, than in their colleagues under thirty, was somewhat more common in community hospitals and chronic care hospitals than in university hospitals or community agencies, and was endorsed equally by physicians, nurses, and social workers.

Beckhard (3) states that an effective team must have the following components: (a) clarity of objectives, mission, and priorities that should be shared by all team members; (b) clear role expectations that need to be realistic and clearly defined when they overlap; (c) good decision-making and problem-solving processes that allow them to look at problems systematically and analytically, collect appropriate facts, adequately define the problem, and generate alternative solutions so as to arrive at the "best" solution; (d) norms that support the task; (e) concerns for each others' needs; and (f) the ability to optimize resources for growth and the enlarging of individual jobs.

Team Philosophy

A team philosophy is sometimes clearly articulated, known, and followed by all team members. At other times, however, it is not clearly formulated but may exist primarily in the minds of leaders. Often there is no obvious team philosophy at all. Speaking of a unit that did not have a clearly articulated philosophy, a nursing director commented, "On hemodialysis they don't talk about the 'team' but they do it. The medical director understands and respects the roles of different professions. The head nurse has profound respect for both nursing and medicine. They all concentrate their thinking on the goal of the patient rather than on the goal of the team."

Other units had more clearly articulated philosophies involving patient care some of which involved a considerable effort to put into practice. A physician who directed an intensive care unit commented on the way in which he attempted to get residents to understand the unit philosophy.

The residents and I stand at the x-ray view box and the resident gives a summary of a patient's history, physical examination, progress, and treatment protocol. He says for example that the patient has pneumonia and is getting worse. He's 70 years old, has been on antibiotics for 3 days and he's going to die. We then do walk-rounds and come to that patient. The residents all begin to walk past the patient and go to the next bed. I continue on rounds with them; then at the end I'll say, "What about that patient who's going to die? What are his needs?"

"Oh yes," they'll say. "He'll need an IV, pain medications, we'll continue antibiotics, and daily cultures."

Then I'll say, "If I'm right and the patient is dying, what else does he need?" The nurses know what else he needs. The residents change feet and aren't quite sure what to say, so what comes out, usually comes from the nurse. A nurse will say, "The patient needs company."

I'll tell them that dying is a lonely business. A person needs someone to talk to if he wants to talk. He often can't talk to his relatives because it's too painful. He needs to be able to talk to a doctor or a nurse—usually a nurse because they are quite prepared to stay with the person, listen, and be part of dying. I tell the residents that to divide themselves from the dying person is to abandon the person when he needs you the most. I tell them to go back, talk to the person, touch the person, and leave the person with some hope. Never leave the bedside of a dying person without letting them know that there's a chance that things might get better. Give the person the opportunity to think things through alone or with others. Ask if the relative needs to talk, particularly if the person is denying. The relatives may need help with facing reality.

A team where there are rotating people with positions of responsibility such as often happens on an intensive care unit, has to evolve a team philosophy that allows for the fact that their approaches may vary. Hayden (4) states that because people have been trained in a variety of clinical approaches, it is often possible that when one person is in charge, that person will prescribe a treatment program that might be different from that which the patient's own treating physician might have prescribed. He states that only with a strong relationship with one's colleagues and the knowledge that there are several successful ways to approach any particular clinical problem will it be possible to continue working together without finding the group splintered by people of various disciplines trying to get the treatment program changed more frequently than is appropriate.

Several caregivers commented that the role of the head nurse was critical in the articulation and carrying out of a team philosophy. A head nurse on a bone marrow transplant unit spoke of the type of philosophy that undergirded her treatment team.

We try to keep people actively involved in life. If they want to do something and we have some questions about it, we'll tell them that they may have problems doing it, rather than telling them not to do it. We feel that even if people are dying, they can be actively involved in life. For example, why not have the television on for someone to get baseball scores. Even when someone's dying, that may be what they want. Talking regarding their feelings about dying doesn't need to be the only thing they get here. Recently I said to a young boy whose mother was walking with him and pushing his IV, "You can walk, talk, and push your own IV pole." I told him he was spoiled and he said he is and he loves it. But in the long run this isn't going to be good for him. We have a philosophy about giving pain medication because we expect people to be able to do something later—not just to alleviate pain, but to help people do something with pain-free good time.

This type of team philosophy can be called the articulation of norms that are the unwritten rules that govern any group. "When they are understood as such, or just 'felt,' they are powerful determinants of how team members behave. They constitute 'the way we do things around here.' They're most obvious when contravened. The dissenter may be met with quiet uneasiness, irritation, or a joking reminder of the norm" (5, p. 465).

The group of people that consistently reported a philosophy were those who worked in hospices where oftentimes they had spent a great deal of time in attempting to articulate a team philosophy. At one prominent hospice the general philosophy was, "We don't attempt to be the perfect hospice, but we have the notion of being a 'good enough' hospice which allows people to have a 'good enough' death." This philosophy can keep staff members from inappropriately suffering personally when patients do not die in the "ideal way." It allows staff to be open to constant learning without having unrealistic expectations that everything will be perfect. A hospice team in a midwestern Canadian province were interviewed together and said that they found that as a hospice they had to decide who they were and what they were trying to do. Fairly early on they attempted to handle the issue of rivalry so that it wasn't a major problem for them. They spoke of the fact that a good team allowed for overlap and extension of roles.

> When the team is working right you get a sense that you don't have to take everything on your own shoulders, that you're not alone. No one on this team has to do a solo— sometimes it can be a chorus. Our team lets you ask questions, give suggestions, be hurt, or even kick someone. We manage to stick together in part because we don't have strong attachments to our own professional discipline. We allow for considerable role blurring, overlap and sharing of work. We know for example that the pharmacist who's there is a resource to us and we can listen to the pharmacist criticize other members of our discipline without taking it personally. Gradually over time we've built up a sense of trust. We can all work at being a team and we can *now* pull an individual out, and the team can still function. When there's an opportunity to go to a conference, some- times people will say, "I won't go because my staff needs me." We do this because the ward is considered more important, not because the ward can't survive.

Mount and Voyer (5) comment that in a successful hospice, it is necessary for each member of the team caring for patients to know what all the other involved team members are doing and why they are doing it. This is crucial to a philosophy of sharing information rather than hoarding it to oneself and attempting to have individual "special relationships" with patients. Doyle (6) comments that good terminal care demands role overlap and a mutual appreciation and support of one another's role that can be so difficult that some caregivers will find themselves unable to work in this kind of a setting because their own personal insecurity may become evident to them.

A physician who directs a palliative care unit commented on the difference between palliative care and intensive care work. She observed that in an intensive care unit it is often possible for colleagues to disagree about a particular treatment approach but in a palliative care unit such disagreements become major problems.

> I had a colleague with whom I had serious conflict and a personality clash. We had different expectations of the role of physician, a whole different approach to work, and a difference in philosophy. In an intensive care unit, if two physicians had been at variance, it probably wouldn't have mattered that much. By and large the matters discussed in an ICU are more technical. The more philosophical questions just don't get addressed at the same level that we attempt to address them on a hospice unit. On an ICU you may be talking about discontinuing a respirator or not going for a third bypass. These decisions however, are generally taken by physicians and the nurses are told what the decision is. With the role of the team, the practical issues of making decisions become much more difficult. There are similarities between the hospice unit and the intensive care unit, but the way that the team works is often very different. An ICU has a much more structured hierarchy where professional skills matter much more than personal skills. Here on a hospice unit, it's much more democratic. All decisions aren't team decisions, but hopefully all have team input. Here personalities are often more important because people as individuals are seen as more important. We need to have both personality and personal skills combined with good technical

skills, more than one needs in an intensive care unit; therefore serious personality conflicts become more important in this situation than in an ICU.

In a successful team, group norms also allow for people to comment to one another and to provide some kind of positive and hopefully helpful criticism. A nurse on a burn unit commented that they admitted a woman who was over 60 with burns over more than 60% of her body. She had attempted suicide and said on admission that she didn't want to be rescued. Generally if the probability of survival is minimal on this unit, then patients are asked what they want done and their wishes are followed. In this situation however, the family wanted the woman to be rescued. On the third or fourth day on the respirator, the nurse spoke to the physician who was treating a burn patient for the first time. She said, "You look like you're pushing a wheelbarrow full of rocks up a mountain and it's raining and muddy." The physician responded, "And someone is pushing the other way; I think I'll talk to the family about discontinuing treatment." The nurse said, "It's his first patient and we have to help people to understand how far to push." Obviously such sharing allows for a fair amount of role blurring. It is only with time and an understanding of team philosophy that teams are able to believe and trust one another well enough to be able to do this.

Team Building

Team building implies the development of the skills that a team member will need in order to function as a member of this particular team. It is presupposed that an individual team member comes with a reasonable number of skills of their own professional discipline before beginning to work on any multidisciplinary team. It is often only after caregivers have been able to see themselves as functioning adequately and competently in their own professional role that they are ready to become members of a team where there might be considerably more role blurring than is the norm. Then it behooves the team to which they are coming to attempt to help them to build on their own previous professional skills and to develop the skills that will be needed in this particular setting. A family practitioner spoke of how difficult it was for physicians to learn to become team members.

> We're not taught to work on a team. Things don't usually go well even on a medical team, and we're not taught even within the strictly medical team system. There is always a pecking order and you don't share anything, even though we all may be doing the same thing and could benefit from sharing. Even in medical school I could see that there were lots of people who had expertise that I didn't have and I recognized other people's skills. Most physicians don't, but I think that's what enabled me to move into palliative care and to function effectively on a palliative care team.

In speaking of team issues, Florence Slepian (7) commented that each team writes its own history and has its own norms regarding humor, intimacy, confidentiality, and socializing after work. Each may have its own ways of decreasing tension during stressful situations. Each may decide about socialization outside of work and these relationships then may lead to role confusion, role ambiguity, and role overlap. Someone coming into a team needs to have a sense of the norms that govern this particular team. An important concept of team building is that one needs to have some understanding of these unwritten rules. When one is accepted into a well-integrated team, then there's often the sense of feeling very worthwhile because one has become a member of an august group. This then may increase one's sense of self-esteem.

Frequently, however, the new employee finds that the team is trying so strongly to defend its boundaries that no time is taken to help someone new to become integrated into a team membership role, and self-esteem is thereby decreased. Coming into such a team the person may simply feel part of a group, not a team, which negates any sense of identity and sense of consequence. Meyer (8) says that to alleviate this confusion and to avoid "demotivation" people need orientation as individuals and follow-up with the person who initiated the original "psychological contract" about 6 weeks after hiring. Such contact should continue to take place periodically and concentrate on the ways in which the individual's role on the team could be enhanced.

Vaillant (9) comments that in the process of learning, one's adaptation is enhanced by an apprenticeship. We learn to anticipate future pain effectively, only if someone first sits beside us as we learn to bear current anxiety. Applying this concept to team building, one can see that it is helpful if initially a caregiver has the sense of interest and support from colleagues who do not leave one to attend to problems completely alone. A coordinator of a program for survivors of suicide states that in her process of team-building, she helps the volunteers to assess their own vulnerability and their own risk in doing this work periodically.

> I attempted to have a mix so that people are more or less vulnerable at certain points in time. If someone has had a child suicide then I don't have them only work with bereaved parents or people in similar situations. Everyone has a partner and their work with people is time-limited. There is supervision provided after each 2-hour interview and we have monthly support meetings. If one individual is a bereaved parent, then I make sure that their partner is not also a bereaved parent. Partners are there to rescue one if you get too involved. They can also be mutually helpful in identifying sources of stress in supervisory sessions. In our program we mix both volunteers who have survived a suicide themselves as well as those who haven't had such an experience, and we find that such a mix is very helpful.

In an emergency room situation nurses spoke of how they attempted to team build by supporting one another in difficult situations, sharing the kind of work that they liked as individuals but also by enabling others to have learning experiences. One nurse commented: "I can't deal with both the patient and the family if the patient has died. If I've been involved with the arrest, I find it hard to deal with the family. Because my colleagues know this, someone will often volunteer, 'You handle the patient, I'll do the family.' "

Another nurse spoke up and said that she particularly liked dealing both with the patient and the relatives, but she felt that she needed to hold back so that someone else could get the experience. "By my not doing it, I'm doing a favor by exposing my younger colleagues to the situation of needing to deal with bereaved families. Then I'll help them with whatever feelings have evolved."

An oncologist spoke of the fact that in his previous work situation there were no teams. In setting up a new clinic he decided that he wanted to have a well integrated multidisciplinary team that was composed of oncologists, nurses, a psychiatrist, a social worker, psychologist, and home care personnel.

> We initiated large rounds where everybody meets to share their expertise. The way the system works is that the patients call the nurses with the problems that they're having.

Nurses are then able to bring their expertise to benefit the patients. This makes life easier for the doctors and everyone else and leads to enhanced job satisfaction for nurses, and decreased stress. When there are problems that need counselling, the social worker, psychologist and psychiatrist meet together and try to clarify their roles. Meeting together is essential because if you fail to communicate, then you're in trouble. We have regular team development meetings and have an outside consultant who helped us initially and who helps us when we're involved in stressful situations. When we started team building we realized we needed a central philosophy and we set up our philosophy within the team meeting.

Team Support

Social support from one's colleagues and team members is a crucial part of coping with potential job stressors. Social support is a function of a team which seems to evolve over time and which probably is most effective only after the team members have become secure in themselves and are able to reach out and trust one another. While some new teams will start by having a strong philosophy of team support, it takes a considerable amount of time before the philosophy can become a reality and before caregivers are really able to reach out and meet the needs of other people on the team. Support for colleagues implies a level of reciprocity which is sometimes lacking. Some caregivers can only support, other can only take, while still others feel that one should take care of one's own support needs.

Mount and Voyer (5) have noted that while mutual support may be an important aspect of team work, the caregiving team must also be aware of the fact that their primary mandate is to patient and family care. "They are called on to be sensitive to one another, not to endlessly support one another. The aim of the therapeutic intervention should be the patient and family—not the needs of co-workers" (5, p. 468). They suggest that if team members keep this awareness as a primary focus, then they will minimize the risk of lowered team efficiency through inordinate preoccupation with its own mental health.

Team support that caregivers reported was both informal as well as formal. It included being able to get support from one's colleagues on a PRN basis, having organized support systems available, and having supportive contact with one another outside of the work situation. PRN support was sometimes provided by nursing team members to one another during periods like staff report time. At other times PRN support consisted of having someone hug another caregiver, or reach out to listen and share a cup of coffee following a difficult situation. Caregivers spoke of the help that their colleagues provided in listening to them as they needed to talk about their own personal stressors outside of the work situation.

A chaplain spoke of his experience with ministering to his team members in the following anecdote:

One of the times I really ministered to the team was in a situation where they were keeping a young child alive for a transplant. They took the person to the O.R. and in a few minutes a nurse who had worked in the O.R. for 22 years came out screaming. She just freaked out. She realized that the whole team was there to remove the kidney— all but the anesthetist. It really hit her and she fell apart. I sat and talked with all of them about what it all meant.

This ability to share at a time of personal stress and in times of crisis was very much appreciated by caregivers. The sense that one's colleagues could understand

and be supportive to one during times of crises provided immeasurable help in both getting through these situations and in being able and willing to come back the next day and confront new potential stressors. Mount and Voyer say that when caregivers are sensitive to one another, team members will be quick to discern distress in a colleague. At that point, a statement of concern, with honoring of confidentiality, a complete freedom to choose when and with whom confidences will be shared, should be tactfully offered. It is also helpful for caregivers to be able to let their colleagues know when they feel they are in an overload situation and need to back away. A social worker said that she found it helpful that on her team, ". . . anyone can go up and say to another team member, 'I'm tired, I have a headache.' People will move in and you can back off. That goes for anyone on the team. We have a strong sense of team in our hospital and are very supportive of one another. If you're deeply engaged with a patient who then dies, there will be an arm around you and a sense that it's okay to cry. I feel a great sense of family and a great sense of support from my colleagues." This type of team support or team camaraderie has been called a "truly caring community" (10).

Social support can also be provided in a more formal way. A physician who runs a chronic care unit spoke of the way in which her unit handled stress.

> We do a lot of discussing on our unit. Because we have so many patients with problems like multiple sclerosis and subarachnoid hemorrages, we often come to discuss issues like whether we're best to keep people alive or allow them to die. Someone supports the staff so that they don't depersonalize patients who aren't able to talk to them. This support may come from the team leader, the head nurse, or the in-service coordinator. We have programs to maintain staff's awareness that these chronically ill, nonverbal patients still often know what's going on. We have interdisciplinary case conferences every month with everyone attending. If we have problems with particular patients (if, for example they die or die in an unpleasant way) then we call a conference to talk about what's going on. We have family conferences regularly and that's often helpful for everyone. We, as a staff, are able to cry together. We've all been together for a long time, and we're quite open with each other. We've come to realize if we have a clumping of deaths all together, then our anxiety level increases and people get irritable and tired; so we try to be particularly careful with ourselves and meet around those difficult times.

A final way for staff to get support for one another is by having outside activities together. Caregivers often spoke of having opportunities to get together with one another for pot-luck dinners, sports activities, a drink after work, prayer meetings, or a wide variety of other activities that they shared together and which sometimes involved their family members. There are numerous advantages in this kind of social get-together, presuming that caregivers can get beyond simply "talking shop." One other problem that may occur with these get-togethers is the development of sexual liaisons between team members which can then sometimes cause difficulty in team dynamics when back in the work situation.

STAFFING SELECTION AND STAFFING POLICIES (15%)

Appropriate staff selection and staffing policies were the most important environmental coping mechanisms in intensive care units. In addition, caregivers in pediatric intensive care units, pediatric chronic care, emergency rooms, and adult chronic care rated it as being an important environmental coping mechanism.

Perhaps not surprisingly, it was more important to those in the under thirty age category who probably had not yet attained a great deal of control over their personal work environment and who found it very important to have good rotation schedules to allow them to have the freedom and flexibility for a social life or for dealing with the early stages of marriage and family building.

Staff Selection

Of crucial importance in this coping mechanism was the selection of the right candidate for the job in order to maximize person-environment fit. Anyone who has attempted to hire staff members realizes, however, that it is not always possible to have as wide a selection of candidates as one might wish, nor is it always possible to completely assess any candidate before seeing the person perform in the work situation. Nonetheless, a few guidelines have been suggested as being effective in staff selection (5, 11-13).

Insofar as it is possible, caregivers who are to work primarily with the critically ill and dying should have developed and tested their professional skills in other settings before beginning to meet the demands peculiar to these particular settings. If the caregiver is to function on a multidisciplinary team there are distinct advantages to having established one's professional role before entering into an environment in which considerable role blurring will be demanded. This does not mean that caregivers should have a rigid sense of their professional role, but rather, that they should have a good idea of what it is before it blurs to encompass many other roles (12).

Much of the writing that has been done in this area has come from the palliative care field (5, 11-13). Mount and Voyer have noted in their experience with the now renowned Royal Victoria Hospital, that the most significant staff selection problems have occurred when there was an inadequate understanding of the specific requirements of the job in question, an incomplete understanding of what the job really entailed and required, or an inadequate appraisal of the caregiver's character and work profiles. They included in some of their errors, the placing of people who did not have leadership skills in positions of leadership, skilled solo artists in group situations, and those requiring support in solo roles. These authors note that the job incumbent usually receives the lion's share of the resultant distress and the blame of colleagues when the results of person-environment misfit become obvious. Unfortunately, all too often much of this blame for inadequate role performance often comes from those who are responsible for staff selection.

A physician who directs a palliative care service commented that one of the primary selection factors for a caregiver in palliative care is for someone with a high need to serve. She observed that one of the biggest challenges in palliative care was to match the personality and character traits of the individual with the conditions and needs of the job.

> Currently we have a physician who is very capable with exactly the right orientation towards whole person medicine. He's a gangbuster, compassionate, and it simply isn't working. What we need on the unit is a constant clinical presence with a high need to serve. What we got was a person with academic ambitions who functions best as a consultant. He likes popping in and out and having a broad variety of interests in which he can tinker. He doesn't want to develop the depth of knowledge in symptom control which we need.

This same physician suggested, however, that in searching for someone with a high need to serve it was important to avoid hiring people with the high neurotic component that often accompanies this personality characteristic. Vachon (14) has warned that those who are motivated by a sense of religious or humanistic "calling," such as is implied by this need to serve, may run into difficulty. Such caregivers tend to approach their jobs with a missionary zeal and they may become quite involved with their patients, patients' families, and their jobs. "No demand is too great. They are on call 24 hours a day, 7 days a week. Such involvement can lead to depletion, however, unless one has some outside source of replenishment—spiritual, interpersonal, or both" (14, p. 118). Such a sense of calling can lead to overinvolvement and overinvestment in patients which can lead to severe grief each time a patient dies. In addition other caregivers may have difficulty when exposed to the surfeit of virtue these people may exhibit. "They may admire such dedication but it may also make them feel guilty and useless, as well as hostile and resentful. Patients may also feel guilty and be unable to speak of their lack of religious faith or past sins to a person who seems unable to understand certain aspects of people's humanity" (14, p. 118).

LaGrand (13) has listed guidelines that should be considered in hiring caregivers for the helping professions and death education movement. These include: careful analysis of the motivation to serve others; analysis of personality and job characteristics; an ability to relate well and to be sensitive to human needs; past history in meeting high stress problems; realistic goal oriented work habits as well as physical condition and work habits.

Other factors that should be considered include the life-event stressors that the caregiver is currently experiencing as well as reactions to previous deaths and losses. There is some concern that caregivers who have previously unresolved grief reactions might do well to take the time to resolve their grief before being exposed to a setting in which they are going to be constantly exposed to grief. In addition there are many working in this area who feel that any caregiver who has had a major bereavement within the last year should be hired with caution and with help being immediately available if grief should be exhibited in such a way as to cause problems in patient care or personal stress.

Staffing Policies

Staffing policies are an attempt to maximize both patient care and staff survival within a work setting. In many of the work situations studied there were clear-cut policies about the amount of work that caregivers would be expected to do, either on a particular shift or over time. For example, nurses on intensive care units might be expected to deal with only one ventilated patient who was to have their full attention.

In other settings an attempt might be made to simultaneously acknowledge the needs of the patient and the caregiver by considering both in patient assignments. For example, a head nurse in an ICU spoke of the fact that she tried to limit nurses' assignments to particularly difficult patients. "When there are difficult patients like young MVAs (motor vehicle accidents), the nurses care for them only on one set of days on their 12-hour shifts—otherwise it's too difficult for them. The doctors frequently don't visit these patients and their families are usually fairly frantic."

Intensive care nurses were not the only ones to attempt to carefully organize staffing assignments. Nurses in a visiting nurse agency spoke of the way in which they handled their palliative care patients. "If the patient is going to be for palliative care, we feel that one nurse shouldn't handle the patient and family alone. Therefore we'll have two share the patient/family responsibility." Nurses from an emergency room commented on an approach that worked to improve patient care. "At one hospital they had a nurse receptionist. I really hated that job but I came to see it as being very important. That nurse could be free to comfort relatives and spend time with them after a death or during the crucial time that the person was in emergency."

In some settings which potentially can have a high degree of stress, the caregivers in administrative positions had often devised ways in which staff members rotated off of high stress units at least for certain periods of time (15). The director of social work in a university hospital said that he rotated his staff from unit to unit every 2 years—although sometimes they stayed as short a time as 18 months and other times they stayed as long as 3 years. It was his belief that it was helpful to have new challenges. He felt that in this way no one was buried in a particular department, nor were they constantly exposed to trauma. He felt that with too long an exposure to trauma, one was apt to become hardened and not very responsive to traumatized individuals. Staff members had a choice as to the units to which they would be assigned. In addition they had a mutual support system whereby there was a backup social worker to each unit. This was helpful if a particular individual became overloaded, was off sick, or on vacation—there was always someone familiar with the unit who could cover or talk with a colleague about a particularly stressful event.

Volunteers were a group who needed to have some clear-cut limitations on their involvement with clients. A director of volunteers on a palliative care unit said that she began to hear through the grapevine that volunteers were wondering if they would ever be able to get any time off. She told them that of course they could take a leave of absence and then if they wanted to come back after a period of about 2 months, they would be more than welcome. She said that with the exception of volunteers for the summer, she tried to get a 1-year commitment from volunteers because "lots of time and effort goes into helping them and we need something back."

For nurses and caregivers who had to rotate shifts, a staff rotation schedule given well in advance was crucial. There were many preferences given for shift rotation and off-duty time. Many caregivers felt that they preferred to have 12-hour shifts because they got significant time off. Sometimes, however, those in administrative positions expressed concern about 12-hour shifts because of the fact that caregivers were quite exhausted at the end of their shift and wound up losing a fair amount of their off-duty time because of a need to catch up on sleep. Occasionally nurses felt so virtuous because of working so hard that they "rewarded" themselves with trips or expensive clothes or household articles. They got into debt and then had to work overtime to pay off their debts. Discussion of a variety of shift patterns can be found in the literature (16-18).

For caregivers who have to rotate shifts, Mount and Voyer (5) have several suggestions to decrease difficulty with shift rotation. They suggest arranging important activities in their normal peak hours and using food and alcohol sparingly during the first 3 days of the new schedule. Alcohol, tranquilizers, and hypnotics decrease REM sleep and increase psychopathology so should be used very carefully. In addition they suggest arranging one's personal schedule to maximize sleeping; that is to shorten the "day" rather than the "night."

With regard to an on-call system, a neonatologist reflected on the one his group had developed.

> Most ICUs don't have people on call for a week or a month so that you can get called in any time. We have staff sleep-in for certain periods of time. The rest of the evenings (a) you aren't in the hospital and (b) you aren't likely to get called. It's a great help. You have a period of acute stress but then you can say to your wife, "this is when I'm on and off." I can go out without a bellboy and we can go to a party without needing to go in two cars. That's a real stress factor in medicine. I think we've minimized stress as far as we can in the intensive care unit.

One of the major difficulties that came up in several units was the fact that there was inadequate staffing and the need to have outside staff from other agencies rotate through the hospital. The staff members in a chronic care hospital solved that problem in a way that was satisfying to them and avoided having their own staff needing to come in on days off. They made a conscious decision to improve their treatment of agency staff, to encourage them to get to know their patients, to avoid "dumping" difficult situations on them, and to encourage them to return to their hospital—thus they developed a special group of relief staff.

ADMINISTRATIVE POLICIES (13%)

This section includes both formal administrative policies as well as areas that these policies might affect, both directly and indirectly. These include: administrative recognition of achievement; provision of support services and the organizational milieu, which includes patients and the physical setting. Administrative policies were rated as being most important to those in obstetrics and palliative care. Their importance increased somewhat with age and they were more important in community settings.

Formal and Informal Policies

Kahn (19) speaks of strategies of coping that attempt to bring the organization more nearly into congruence with human needs and abilities. These involve the distribution of power, allocation of rewards and division of labor. Harrison (20) notes that organizations need to have programs that allow for individual workers. "The relationship between each worker's needs and values in the work environment must be considered. This relationship can be considered at one point in time, over the time the individual holds the job, and over the career of the individual" (20, p. 197). These issues should be considered during the hiring process. We should come to know how to measure an individual's ability and then to fit this ability into specific job demands. This requires however that we develop dimensions describing what the job can give to the individual in terms of how much appreciation and respect goes with this job and what are the opportunities for achievement. An employer needs to periodically review these with the employee while he is in the job. Those with person-environment misfit can have counseling, training, job transfer, or promotion. It is important to consider person-environment fit with respect to the individual needs and values in addition to fit with the individual's abilities. Degrees of misfit can be tolerated if they are of short duration and leading to a desired goal but they are more pronounced if no opportunity for change is seen. Effective utilization of staff also involves the recognition of what Hertzberg (21) refers to as the motivating factors of: responsibility, recognition, achievement opportunity, and accomplishment opportunity.

A nurse administrator who had recently completed a Master's in Business Administration spoke of how she was going to attempt to integrate many of these concepts into her own work role.

> The nurses feel a lack of support and we have to begin to figure what can be integrated into the nursing administrative role. The first issue is going to be communication and keeping people informed—not 100% but well enough for them to feel that they know what's going on. We need to help them to realize the limitations on what resources are available by clearly spelling out the issues. If we need X machines at X price and we have X dollars to spend we can only purchase X machines. We also need to concentrate on giving positive as well as negative feedback. The head nurses will be reporting directly to the directors who are on the administrative council of the hospital with all the administrators from other disciplines. Nursing managers have not previously been represented on the administrative council so now we will have direct feedback to the top and a link with top administration. This will hopefully improve the communication between the directors of nursing and the head nurses but the real problem will be between head nurses and staff nurses. We are going to have to help people to develop priorities and we as administrators will have to be seen on the units so that the head nurses will know that we know what's going on out there and we'll have to demonstrate that we really can help. If the head nurses feel that they have been heard then they'll accept reality when we present it to them. The important thing is for them to feel that someone is at least listening. The role expectation of the head nurse job is also going to need to be clarified and we're going to have to help head nurses to define that role. This new role will need to be interpreted to the head nurse so that she comes to realize that she can't take all of her administrative work to do at home because she's been feeling guilty and has been out dealing with patients all day. I learned that myself in my last job. These approaches, in addition to giving feedback to the person regarding actions on problems being taken are some of the ways in which we're hoping that we are going to be able to turn around some of the stress in our particular organization.

Other administrators spoke of the need to develop clinical ladders for staff nurses so as to be able to allow them to have a reasonable amount of job enrichment. Malanka recently reported on a number of approaches being used at Memorial Sloan-Kettering to improve job satisfaction (22). These included not only a career ladder but also the autonomy deemed necessary to give good patient care; specializing in one type of cancer nursing; being responsible for patient teaching; and developing a resource book of nurses and their specialties. With this book, for example, a nurse having difficulty with a plugged chest tube can call a colleague in thoracic surgery, rather than having to wait to speak to a physician about the problem.

As is the case at Memorial, the ability to delegate authority appropriately is crucial in maximizing job satisfaction. A funeral director commented, "It takes a long time for some of the homes to change to make the job more rewarding for the funeral service personnel by sharing and allowing them to follow clients through. In one of the homes we used to joke 'if X is here none of us have a brain in our heads, but if he's gone, if the Queen dies any of us can handle it.' "

Administrative policies that allowed for adequate time off were crucial. People talked about being able to take a mental health day; time off in lieu of over-time, or to be able to take a vacation as they felt they needed it. Nutritionists working in a cancer hospital commented that it seemed important to them to be able to have a vacation about every 6 months in this type of setting. Originally it had been the administrative policy that people could have a vacation only after they had worked for a full year but because of staff complaints that policy was changed.

The issue of staff terminating or being terminated is a difficult one. A staff member who watched many of her colleagues leave the organization spoke of the fact that it was becoming important for administration to begin to investigate why caregivers were leaving as well as for caregivers to assume the responsibility of being honest about their reasons for leaving. It is only with openness and honesty that necessary administrative changes can be made.

In other situations it was sometimes necessary to dismiss caregivers for a variety of reasons. A hospital administrator spoke of the need to dismiss incompetent staff members.

> I've had to get rid of two doctors. I go through the Medical Director and let him know it's gotten to the point where these people are no longer safe to practice. I finally said, "Either you do it, or I will and I don't have your experience in dealing with these issues." I said "Imagine it was your wife or mother who was an emergency admission tonight. Would you trust them to treat her?—If not then how can we have them on the staff?" Keep that idea in your head and go to deal with them.

Recognition of Staff

While poor performance needs to be punished, good performance needs to be rewarded. Veninga (23) states that in order to avoid burnout there must be commensurate financial and psychological rewards for responsibility because it grates to know one is working for less than others of commensurate responsibility. In addition it is crucial to have recognition for a job well done and also to have the flexibility to take time away from clients or to spend time with clients if that would be an effective job reward. All of these require that there be administrative policies that in fact acknowledge and appreciate the work that caregivers are doing.

One area that administration often finds difficulty in acknowledging is the grief that caregivers experience when a particular patient dies. Several caregivers spoke of feeling that they had to have at least a little while to grieve for the death of one person before they immediately had to care for someone else in the same bed. Dr. Eric Wilkes the renowned physician of St. Luke's Hospice in Sheffield, England, spoke of the fact that their institution has a 24-hour gap between patients when one dies in the hospice. This type of a gap allows caregivers time to grieve for one person before another one fills the bed and also means that the person who comes into the bed of the individual who just died does not suffer from having caregivers so busy with their own grief that they are unable to move on and deal with the new people to whom their energies must now turn. When it is impossible to keep beds empty because of economic necessity or, more importantly because there are other people who really need the bed, then caregivers might either be assigned to someone other than the new admission or else have time to themselves before taking over the care of the new person.

Provision of Support Services

The work supervisor has a crucial role to play in providing support to caregivers as well as in buffering them against a wide variety of stressors and with regard to a large range of health outcomes (5, 24). House and Wells (24) have suggested that while many supervisory training programs emphasize goals related to social support for reasons other than reducing occupational stress and/or its impact on health, that the supervisors might be taught to provide this social support as a part of their job responsibility and thus might serve to decrease work stress.

It is also important for caregivers to feel that administration recognizes the stress that they experience in that administration is willing to bring in extra resources to help them deal with particularly difficult situations. When caregivers felt that they wanted or needed mental health professionals either for their own support, to run support groups, or to work directly with patients, it was helpful when administration was able to acknowledge this need (26).

Often times employee assistance programs have also been used to deal with employees who were experiencing work-related or personal stress (27). The important issue is not so much how these problems are dealt with but the fact that administration is willing to meet with staff and begin to look at how together they might jointly work to solve some of the recognized and as yet unmet needs within a particular organization.

Organizational Milieu

The milieu of the environment included the appropriate selection of patients or clients, attention to the physical plant, and the more general milieu or environment. In some settings it was very important that only predefined "appropriate" patients be admitted or that numbers of particular types of patients be restricted. A head nurse in a palliative care unit compared the unit in which she worked to that of another unit in the community. She spoke of the other unit as being much more selective:

> Here we have a good screening process but we don't have an age limit. At the other hospital they have an age limit of 75 and prefer that the patient be going to die within 3 months or less. On our unit we'll take even convalescent patients. This is an advantage to staff and patients to see people going home. It helps to keep staff morale up when patients go home. We see them coming in for symptom relief and then going out. Personally, I prefer this type of mix. We're also very careful when we come to admit a patient to keep in mind the staff we have and the kind of patients we already have on the unit. If we have three people with tracheostomies we know that these are long-term patients and we would turn other people with trachs down.

The physical environment was also important with regard to the type of care that could be provided. One caregiver observed that the physical surroundings in which we work give messages that either soothe or offend our eyes, ears, nose, sense of touch, and the need that we have for variety and stimulation. A physician spoke of the palliative care unit which she set up that allowed for maximum natural light, the avoidance of stark colors, and particularly avoidance of the color yellow which might make jaundiced patients look even more jaundiced. They attempted to have good ventilation and the whirlpool bath was a very important aspect of their environment. Unlike some other hospices theirs chose to have some private rooms in recognition that not all patients find it helpful to watch several room-mates in a row die.

Hospices have invested considerable effort in attempting to understand the importance of physical environments on patients and caregivers alike. Caregivers spoke of the pleasure it gave them to work in milieus that were designed so that patients and families' needs were really recognized. They made comments such as "It was a real pleasure to be able to give that kind of care." Stedeford (28) comments that the person who feels secure in the warmth of a therapeutic environment wherein physical symptoms are alleviated is more open to change. Patients may also be more open to their own families and to the care that caregivers are so anxious to provide. When patients and families benefit from the environments in which they are treated, caregivers likewise benefit and job satisfaction increases.

COLLEAGUES AT WORK (12%)

Talking with colleagues at work was the most important environmental coping mechanism for those in emergency rooms where in fact it accounted for one third of the environmental coping strategies. It was also a crucial element in oncology and was more than twice as common in younger colleagues than in those in the group over 30. This category differed from team support in that it involved less of a sense of integration into a team and more sense of seeking out a support system that might go beyond one's own team. It sometimes but not always implied more of a sense of isolation from a team and the need to get help from a single individual as opposed to jointly from one's colleagues and often it was less structured than team support. It sometimes occurred with spontaneous end-of-shift contact or at times of crisis. Caregivers spoke of consciously forming social networks within their work situation that consisted of people to whom they could go when they were having difficulty. They spoke of social networks of other head nurses or other nurse clinicians or more informal social networks such as the group of physicians who passed on to one another the names of nurses with whom they were having difficulties so that the new physicians knew what nurses they could trust coming on to a new unit. A chaplain commented that "I have to be able to talk to others and one of the physicians here is my best sounding board. I don't have a family so I have to go to someone for understanding the hospital situation and I've developed such people."

A gynecologist had a broader support system that was somewhat different than that reported by many other people.

> I was able to talk to the hospital chaplain when I was feeling stressed. In addition, I find it helpful to be in an educational institution. The students buoy you along because they're refreshing and they keep me honest. The antiabortion gang which criticizes me a lot also keeps me honest and on target. The pro-choice group keeps all my feelings at the surface. I am a member of the divison of sexology and my colleagues are a wonderful support system for me. In addition my family is aware of the work I do and they're supportive particularly if the press has been especially difficult with me recently. When I get tacked to the cross for doing abortions it's helpful to know that my family and friends know my true position on the subject and who I am as a person. Support is essential at those times or else I'd really go crazy.

Sometimes the support that caregivers wanted came from members of their own department or their own professional discipline. A social worker commented:

I get my support from the rest of the social work department. We're very close—like a family. We don't usually see each other outside but we do have parties and dinners occasionally and they're very supportive and close. Everyone is supportive and always joking. When you want to talk there's always a willing ear. I found it helpful to sit down with them at lunch and discuss patients and the humorous points of the day. Everyone in the department has a sense of humor and it's really helpful for us.

Shaffer (29) has observed that "When people are happy and enjoy working together, the positive emotional climate generated by their interaction makes work pleasurable and satisfying. On the other hand if there is an air of tension on the job, people sense it and begin to reflect that tension in their work or in their relationships with co-workers" (29: 153).

Shaffer goes on to say that when there is dissatisfaction, discord, or chaos in the workplace then these negative feelings can permeate the atmosphere and create a climate that workers want to avoid because no one wants to be tense or miserable 5 days a week. It is sometimes in these situations that caregivers seek relationships with people outside of their own direct team situation. Some of the situations in which staff members sought this kind of interdisciplinary collaboration came about because of work tension. A nurse in a community hospital working with cancer patients observed:

It's not like in the teaching hospitals where you can get the doctors to make changes and do what you think is best. Here they say "He's my patient and I want this and I'll order this drug." So sometimes we get another doctor to suggest to them that they order aqueous morphine and see if it would work. It's getting better and now the nurses make suggestions and sometimes the physicians listen.

The exact opposite comment was made by a physician who was having difficulty with his medical colleagues. "As a physician I couldn't get doctors to change their orders but if a nurse brought it up at rounds then my colleagues would be willing to change."

Corridor consultations were also helpful in dealing with stressful situations. These consisted of one person stopping another to get advice in a casual and informal way. Some caregivers who function in the mental health role resented these corridor consultations because they felt that they interfered with the group meetings which they had which were not always completely satisfactory. Others came to appreciate corridor consultations both from the point of view of getting others to begin to develop a relationship with them and as an indirect way of beginning to affect patient care. When things get difficult for caregivers it is often helpful to involve people in the mental health field and this provides some indirect support for the caregivers as well. An oncologist commented:

It's the young patients that bother me. I guess maybe because I identify with them. Today I have a young man with cancer of the testes. He responded well to chemotherapy and radiation and then relapsed. Then he responded to surgery, radiation, and chemotherapy and then he relapsed. Now there's nothing left but a few drugs that won't do much. He has a pushy family, he's well connected to the medical establishment, and he got married between his second and third relapses. Now there's nothing left so I referred him to the social worker.

This kind of referral can be seen as a "dumping job" and yet frequently it can serve not only to provide the patient with the help that the social worker can give but also to help the physician with his feeling of impotence.

Other people also spoke of going to their colleagues when they were in a difficult situation. A physician spoke of having a patient commit suicide in front of the hospital.

> It would have been more difficult in front of my office then in front of the hospital because at my office I would have been alone with my guilt. Here there was a bond among the physicians who knew and they talked to me about it. We spoke about the fact that as physicians you're always taking a chance. You make a decision and it may or may not be right. Whether you are deciding on chemotherapy or a treatment of depression, you take risks and the risk of malpractice is always there. I had lots of support from physicians who either had been there or knew that they could be. I was doing his assessment and decided that he was suicidal and was just calling to admit him when he bolted from the emergency room and jumped from the parking garage.

For many the support system within their work setting was crucial to enabling them to defuse sufficiently so that they did not need to use their outside personal support system primarily as a way of supporting them with their work stress.

FORMALIZED WAYS OF HANDLING DECISION–MAKING AND DEATH (12%)

The importance of having formalized ways of handling decision-making and death was mentioned most often by caregivers who worked in acute care settings where decisions often had to be made quickly. These included pediatric and adult intensive care units, emergency rooms and, as well, pediatric chronic care wherein there were often specific approaches to handling decision-making. There were no differences with regard to age or practice setting but physicians were somewhat more apt to endorse this coping mechanism than were other caregivers.

Although few mentioned relying on professional codes of ethics, standards of care, or statements of patient's rights to guide them in their decision-making, these can be quite helpful and should be reviewed by caregivers as individuals or groups (30–34). As well caregivers should be familiar with systematic studies of the ethical, medical, and legal issues involved in decision-making (35–36).

Hospital or Team Procedure

Some hospitals or teams had clearly delineated philosophies about handling difficult decisions. The most widely known of these are the policies of the Massachusetts General Hospital and Beth Israel Hospital which were the first two hospitals to develop and publish official policies in which they defined the circumstances in which it would be acceptable or even desirable to issue "orders not to resuscitate" a dying patient (37).

Dr. Chuck Cartwright spoke of the way in which decisions to initiate life-support systems were made in one large Canadian hospital.

> The decision to intubate and ventilate is not a big one here. We have the facilities so we generally do it. Our major criteria is generally the reversibility of the primary disease process—if there is any chance of reversibility then our belief is that the person should be treated. If a person has widely disseminated cancer and has pulmonary metastasis then our job is to keep the person comfortable. If he is intubated then I'll be very upset.... The stressful part is when it becomes blatantly clear that we've made a mistake. The patient doesn't have a reversible disease. The resources have been used

inappropriately. Then what do you do? . . . My "gut" feeling is that the decision should be made by those who know the patient—the ICU team, and the primary physician who knows and can talk to the family. . . . We get together with the primary physician and ask that person to speak to the family. If anyone disagrees and says "go another week" and try something else, then we do.

Reverend Ruth Nevens reflected that even with formalized ways of handling decision-making, life is not always easy. "Whenever we make the decision to discontinue aggressive treatment whether with a cancer patient, a palliative care patient, or a person involved in a rigorous treatment program, it's done not knowing for sure what decision should be made but that's the world we live in."

An intensivist from Australia said that the best intensive care units in which he had worked had a consistent nurse/physician team to make difficult decisions. Although the composition of the team might vary from week to week, the staff knew which two people were responsible. He also spoke of settings in which "DNR" orders were written on patient charts. Such orders had to be renewed every 2 days by a physician who was not a resident. This avoided the orders becoming "enshrined" and caused the team members to carefully reconsider the appropriateness of the orders every 2 days.

In other settings ethics committees have begun to have an important role in helping individual physicians or hospital teams with difficult ethical decisions. Carol Levine has reviewed the state of such committees (38) and found they may serve an entire hospital or a special unit such as a neonatal intensive care unit or a cardiac intensive care unit. In some settings existing committees are used to deal with ethical issues rather than having ethics committees. Levine reviews the benefits and possible disadvantages of ethics committees and states that not all hospitals necessarily have to consider having such a committee, particularly if existing policies and recommendations work well and there is little staff conflict. She suggests that hospitals that do not see much of a need for such committees because of their client population and referral system might consider banding together with other hospitals to form a committee. In any case, she recommends that hospitals should have policies to govern the types of cases that typically arise such as DNR policies, informed consent, and the like.

Involvement of the Patient in Decision Making

Conscious and competent patients who are in a position where decisions need to be made about their treatment have the right to be told about their diagnosis, prognosis, and the decisions that need to be made. They have the right to refuse treatment or to withdraw from research studies if they should so choose. Patients may also have the right to choose not to know their exact diagnosis and prognosis but caregivers must be careful to ascertain that this is the patient's wish and not the projection of the caregiver or family's preference. If the caregiver feels that the patient is giving verbal or nonverbal messages that he does not want to know this information then there is an ethical obligation to check this out on other occasions to ensure that the person has not had a change of attitude.

An oncologist spoke of the way in which patients needed to be involved in decision-making. "If one is using a treatment modality that's not fully established then one must ask 'Am I justified in subjecting anyone to this treatment?' And then I must speak to the patient. I spend time with patients and like to get to know how aggressive they would like to be at critical points. We arrive at a mutual understanding."

An approach used by Dr. Ernest Rosenbaum of California can be useful in such situations (39). In order to enhance communication with patients and families he tape records family interviews so the patient and family can listen to the tape at their leisure and carefully consider any of the issues involved. While the use of tape recordings might be questioned with seriously ill patients, they could certainly have a value in being used with significant treatment decisions that patients might want and need to ponder.

Involving patients in decision-making can be painful for caregivers who may have to watch them struggle with these decisions. The situations in which patients with severe life-threatening burns are given the choice of aggressive or palliative treatment when they are in the emergency room and before the edema has occurred that will necessitate their being put onto a respirator is just such a painful choice. So too are the decisions of people with chronic obstructive lung disease, cystic fibrosis, or amyotrophic lateral sclerosis who may make informed decisions not to go onto a respirator with the next episode of pneumonia or respiratory failure.

Family Involvement

Frequently it is not possible to involve the patient in decision-making because an unexpected illness or accident has resulted in the patient's being unconscious and therefore unable to make decisions, or the patient is an infant or very young child. In these situations family members must be involved in making decisions. Sudnow (40) has referred to one aspect of this phenomenon as "breaking it to them gently." This refers to the fact that staff may have to prepare family members for the fact that difficult decisions may have to made by them. A neonatologist said that when he has a woman in labor with a 25-week fetus he realizes that she knows the condition is serious. "At 25 weeks no one expects an okay baby but we can give one three quarters of the time. Even before the birth I say 'This baby will need a lot of help. We're prepared to give all the help we can as long as things look reasonably normal. Otherwise we'll all ask ourselves whether we are doing the right thing in carrying on.' "

Sometimes in such situations family members can become involved in their infant's care in a way that gives them a sense of constructive participation with the staff in both the care and the resulting decisions (41).

Caregivers who wish to have clear cut ethical guidelines to which they can turn in difficult situations will find that they do not exist. The issues are too complicated and will require continued communication amongst clinicians, consumers, the legal profession, ethicists, theologians, and others. We must all continue to struggle with the issues but can be helped to cope with the stress we experience through the writings of others who also struggle (42–48).

Caregivers who find their own ethical principles being compromised need to have a well-developed personal value system on which they can rely. A ICU nurse in a community hospital found herself in just such a situation and decided that she had a moral responsibility to make sure the relative acting on behalf of the patient really understood what she was doing. In making her decision she was guided by the value that her primary role was as patient advocate (49) rather than physician assistant. The nurse's belief that the ethical concept of informed consent took precedence over her responsibility to her medical colleagues led to the following result.

> The residents decided to do a kidney arteriogram on Mr. A who was within hours of death. I asked "Why are you going to do it? It's going to take three nurses, an X-Ray tech., anesthetist, and you. Why would you put him through all of this when he's dying? Will you do anything if you find a blockage?" The answer was "no," but we want to do it for scientific curiosity.
>
> I had to witness the phone call to get the family consent—we're big on consent around here. The doctor called the sister and said "Your brother needs this procedure performed immediately. It's very important that we do it." He then told her a little. I got on and said "Do you really understand what the doctor just said?" She said "No, not really." They're going to cut him—or are they? Will he go to the O.R. or not? Is it to put a tube in? No, I don't know, but if the doctor says he needs it done then I'll trust him." I said "I won't accept your consent until you really know what they're going to do. I'm going to put the doctor back on the phone." He glared at me, but there wasn't much that he could do.

Sometimes caregivers make a conscious decision that they should make decisions to terminate life supports, rather than having the family responsible for a decision that may haunt them in years to come. In such situations those involved must be sure that it is the family's welfare and not their own that is being considered, and if family members want the treatment to be continued their wishes have to be seriously considered and may well have ethical priority.

Training of Team Members for Decision Making

An intensivist spoke of the manner in which the residents in his service were trained to make such decisions. The senior medical resident was chosen very carefully, "We want the one who can do it all, who knows the importance of dealing with families. We want the cream of the crop—the good guys who'll be doing ICU in the future." Such a resident is then responsible for the running of the ICU 24 hours a day with no other responsibilities for running clinics or doing surgery. "They need to learn how to make the choices about admitting, discharging, putting in Swans Ganz, doing tracheostomies, knowing when to be conservative or aggressive—making all these decisions that need to be made every day. They need to be comfortable with it all because they are going out in 6 months after they finish with us to be on their own."

An oncologist said that an experience with a friend whose sister died in emergency while the husband waited thinking the problem was minor convinced him of the importance of notifying families of any change in a person's condition. "I feel a social and legal responsibility to let the family know if there is a problem." If a resident phones me in the middle of the night that a patient has unexpected bleeding. I say 'What are you doing? Has anyone phoned the family?' I may not come in but I want to know how they're handling it and if a nurse or the resident has let the family know what's going on. An unexpected death is the worst to handle."

Decisions Regarding Caregiver Involvement with Death

The expectation of the way in which caregivers should be involved at the time of death may be an individual or team decision. Oftentimes those most involved with the patient will choose to be present to care for the person at the time of death. In some settings there are clearly defined policies, however, that if a caregiver is not scheduled to be on duty then he or she should not attempt to be present at the time of death. There are obviously some instances in which caregivers become overinvolved with one or more patients and may tend to want to spend considerable extra time with these people. Occasionally this can be very helpful to the dying person, the family, and the caregiver, while at other times it can be a burden to all concerned.

In some situations, which may pose ethical problems for certain caregivers, for example, dealing with women having abortions or when patients with chronic severe lung problems are on respirators and are being medicated with morphine while the respirator is gradually turned down, then caregivers must have the option to request a different assignment, providing of course that this does not subject the patient to a greater risk—such as being unattended.

It is also helpful for teams to have carefully considered the manner in which families should be handled at and immediately after the time of death. All too often the emphasis is on maintaining a certain amount of decorum within the unit setting and getting family members out as soon as possible. Many approaches to "death-telling" are reflective of the strong dislike that caregivers have for this difficult task and reflect the lack of training they have received and their feelings of inadequacy as they undertake this task (50). Caregivers should remember that as difficult as the task is for them—the news is more difficult still for the family involved. The aim in such situations—whether with an expected or unexpected death should be to provide a supportive, private atmosphere in which family members can naturally express the grief they feel. This may take place in open weeping or wailing; anger towards caregivers who must realize that this is a natural response and try to avoid feeling guilty or angry in response; feelings of guilt and self-recrimination, shock and complete denial; a desire for all of the relevant facts; or an apparent calm acceptance. It is important to realize that whether or not the death has been anticipated and even openly discussed may not appear to have any impact on the way in which the news is accepted. Cultural mourning patterns will also in part determine the way in which mourners will respond. Caregivers should become aware of the variations in normal responses to grief and the manner in which these may be culturally determined. In addition they should realize that the way in which they handle a family at the time of a person's death often becomes imprinted on the minds of the survivors who relive the scene for days or years to come. The goals of dealing with a family at the time of a death should be to allow them to begin their process of grieving in *their* way; to get their questions answered; to begin to say their "goodbyes," which may involve being able to see and spend time with the body of the person—perhaps to get some of their guilt expressed and perhaps assuaged—or at least hopefully not inappropriately exacerbated; to have the practical help they require; and to be able to leave the hospital and return home safely. The latter may involve either calling a friend, relative, taxi, or perhaps having police assistance in returning home. Effective help to grieving families also involves teams making a conscious decision as to their involvement in bereavement follow-up.

Several years ago Dr. Elizabeth Kübler-Ross made the suggestion that when a death occurred in an emergency room then the caregivers involved with the death should contact the bereaved relatives about a month later in order to allow them the opportunity to return to the setting where their loved one died and ask any questions they might now have about what happened at the time of death. Did he die in pain? Did he call out for me? What did you do to save him? Physicians working in neonatal intensive care units sometimes call the parents a few weeks after death in order to give relevant autopsy findings, discuss implications for future pregnancies, and to provide support. Family physicians or obstetricians sometimes assume this role with deaths of other family members or stillborns. Caregivers in other settings where there has been long-term involvement with family members such as may occur in oncology, cystic fibrosis, or kidney dialysis units may either formally or informally make contact with family members. Hospice programs often have formalized bereavement follow-ups (51) that may range from a sympathy card with an offer of follow-up if needed, to one or more phone calls to family members, home visits, or invitations to attend group sessions for bereaved relatives. When bereavement follow-up becomes a formal part of a program it acknowledges that we as caregivers have a responsibility to families, rather than just to patients. Such contact acknowledges that we understand that family members have not only lost their relative to death—they have also lost contact with the caregiving staff that might have become quite important to them. Such a call allows the family members to ask any questions they might have, to speak again of the illness and death, to reminisce with others who cared and were present at important moments. In addition it allows caregivers to assess whether any additional intervention might be needed. If intervention is needed then it might be provided through individual grief counseling or therapy, the principles of which are most clearly articulated in the work of Dr. J. William Worden (52). Some family members will benefit most from self-help groups at which they can have contact with others who have gone through similar experiences (53-56).

Caregiver Bereavement

Family members are not the only ones who must grieve for the death of patients, so must caregivers. While not all caregivers are going to experience each death equally, there must be an opportunity to grieve when the loss is felt. One of the more effective methods caregivers have devised is that practiced at the St. Boniface Terminal Care Unit in Winnipeg, Manitoba. There the nurse who is present when a person dies tape records the circumstances surrounding the death, who was present and how they coped, who might be at particular risk following the death as well as sharing whatever feelings the nurse might wish to discuss. (Other settings have the nurses write in a "Last Moments Book," or hold Psychosocial Autopsies [57]). On Friday mornings death rounds are held and team members listen to each tape. This provides for an opportunity to discuss each person who has died in detail. Such discussion allows team members to discuss what they learned or gained from each person, how the treatment might have been improved, how they feel about the circumstances surrounding the death, and the feeling of grief that they are experiencing. As caregivers discuss the person who died they simultaneously each sign a sympathy card that will go out to the survivors one month after the death.

This type of exchange allows the team to share one of the most important experiences of mourning—the recognition that we have survived this death. We are not to blame for the death and we deserve to continue to live. The presence of food at a wake, shiva, or death rounds is symbolic of our right to survive.

Other specialties have other ways of handling their grief. A physician who works with children with cystic fibrosis observed "The nurses go to the funerals; I go to postmortems." Many caregivers mentioned how helpful it was to go to funerals at least occasionally and some mentioned that in their settings fellow patients might either go to a funeral or attend a hospital memorial service for those who have died. Physicians as a profession have institutionalized mortality rounds as a way of ascertaining whether or not a particular death could have been prevented and to deal at least in part with the issue of responsibility and the phenomenon of survivor guilt.

ORIENTATION AND ONGOING EDUCATIONAL PROGRAMS (7%)

The importance of programs that prepared caregivers to effectively function in their professional roles was mentioned somewhat less than might be expected. In part this might be the result of the caregivers being inclined to be fairly experienced in their roles, to the fact that they took inservice education programs or the ability to attend conferences or meetings for granted, or perhaps they had found the programs they had attended had not been particularly helpful.

In developing an education program for caregivers it is first necessary to consider doing a needs assessment to ascertain what is particularly needed. Several international studies have been done in this area (57–60).

A number of approaches have been used to teach the care of the critically or terminally ill, their families, and their caregivers. Doyle (61) discusses the role of the hospice as a training center for those who will care for the terminally ill in a variety of settings. Their program centers on inculcating three things: awareness, general principles, and technical details. Awareness includes the teaching and demonstrating of the physical, emotional, social, spiritual, and communication problems common to this work. In addition there is a focus on professional potential and limitations and an examination of personal faith, fears, and philosophy. Their approach encourages medical students to work as auxilliary nurses or nurse aides, rather than as junior doctors in the hope that this intimate and intensely demanding contact will lead to improved awareness and the absorption by osmosis of the principles and technical details crucial to this work.

Other work to sensitize caregivers to the needs of people with life-threatening illness has been done with medical students working with cancer patients using didactic and clinical experiences (62); in teaching empathy and communication skills (63); in seminars on loss and mourning for medical students and graduate nurses that focused on both clinical and personal experiences (65); and with all health professionals working with cancer patients (64). Benoliel (66) writes of the educational and personal needs of death counselors who she sees must be familiar with human development across the life span, including the communication problems that exist across differences in age, sex, culture, and cohort experiences. She also sees the need for knowledge about the impact of different death-related experiences on individuals, families, and providers and stresses the need for goals reflecting the integrity of those involved. In addition she notes that the counselor needs access to an ongoing support system that can provide for personal development and an increasing awareness of one's own value system.

Formal structured orientation programs for both nursing staff and housestaff to prepare for the technical and emotional demands of work are essential. In addition ongoing educational experience on the unit led by members of one's own discipline as well as by other disciplines is also essential as is the ability to attend outside conferences (67). Orientation can sometimes be enriched by having a "buddy system," a role model, or a mentor. An experienced ICU nurse observed: "I say to the younger nurses 'You're nursing the machine, not the patient. Look him in the eye. Stand at the foot of the bed and look at him, don't just go by the numbers on the monitor. . . . They get so busy trying to get the numbers on the pump that they don't have time to look at the person and tell him 'You're doing well. You will get better.' "

A family physician commented:

I try to teach the students to be more accepting of uncertainty in diagnoses, to live with uncertainty, to accept your own feelings about patients. I encourage them to see themselves as people and to develop a practice which reflects their personality. We find that with this philosophy the residents stay in their practice longer, are more satisfied, spend more time with patients and are less concerned about making money.

An experienced oncologist at a prestigious hospital spoke of the way in which he served as a role model, "When residents come to me I say to them 'I can teach you very little about medicine (in fact they have a lot to teach me), but I can teach you judgement and how to handle patients through our one-to-one preceptorship.' " An oncologist at another center handled situations in a similar manner. "I can't teach interns formally how to handle patients. They have to see what happens and where I go with each discussion. I may finish a discussion today or have to come back tomorrow. . . But they have to see what I do, where I push, where I draw back. I could never explain it. They have to see it in action."

Other programs have tried to formally teach some of these skills (40, 68-69). There is also a trend at many medical schools to use the study of the humanities to improve physicians' understanding of the issues that patients confront. Considerable work in this area with professionals of many disciplines has been done by Sandra Bertman and her colleagues who work to teach a humanistic framework for dying (70).

Lastly, there has also been considerable emphasis in educational programs on effective stress management techniques for caregivers. McCue (71) suggests honest discussion by physicians on the psychological difficulties of medical practice and the feelings they experience during difficult encounters with patients as a way of identifying maladaptive behavior. He also suggests direct exploration of productive adaptations to stress as a way of avoiding suppression of feelings and/or excessive distancing from patients. Payne (72) reviews the work of Meichenbaum (reference in original) on stress innoculation training which helps people to use cognitive approaches to analyze stress and deal with it by means of internal speech, steady breathing, rehearsing what one will do, and using positive suggestions. Lattanzi (73) shows how stress reducing techniques can be applied in the effective education of hospice staff and volunteers.

JOB FLEXIBILITY (6%)

The ability to have flexibility within one's position and to have at least some possibility of upward mobility if one so chooses was important to some caregivers. It was slightly more important to those under thirty and to social workers than to the others interviewed. For some the ability to alter job descriptions so as to restructure relationships with clients, subordinates, peers, and superiors was helpful as a way of reducing stress (74). A nutritionist commented, for example, that she found it much easier to work with patients with cancer when they were mixed in with patients with ulcers than she did when assigned to work only with cancer patients. Several caregivers said that they appreciate the ability to periodically change their caseload or to switch from a more to a less intensive environment, for example from an inpatient to an outpatient setting.

In addition nurses with expertise in certain areas such as psychiatry or palliative care symptom relief are sometimes used to consult on other units, thus enhancing their sense of job satisfaction. It must be noted, however, that not everyone wants or considers this to be job enrichment. Some caregivers prefer to have a structured job that does not change. Hopefully organizations can have the flexibility to be able to meet the needs of the various employees.

SUPPORT GROUPS (4%)

The final organizational coping strategy is the use of support groups. This has been one of the most commonly prescribed techniques for dealing with work related stress in caregivers in a variety of settings and yet was the least commonly mentioned technique in the present study. In one-third of the instances in which it was mentioned it was to comment that it was not a particularly effective technique.

Most of the literature on support groups is descriptive in nature and is written from the perspective of the group leaders who describe any problems they have with the groups as being due to resistance. These meetings are probably helpful for some groups (75–84) but they should not generally be prescribed as a panacea for all stress reactions. The most helpful way in which support groups seemed to work was if the caregivers involved had asked for the group and had input into the format of the group. Meetings in which patient/family issues or specific management problems could be discussed with the topic of team feelings being addressed as people were ready to do so seemed to be the best model. When unstructured group meetings were used caregivers made comments such as:

> If you have weekly meetings with a psychiatrist then you are making an implicit assumption that there is staff stress. Maybe the meetings were started originally to prevent a problem. Now there is a feeling that if you have a meeting then you must be having problems. It used to be that everyone at the meetings was angry and if I wasn't angry then I'd be given the message that I was repressing my feelings. That then made me feel paranoid about not feeling angry.

Other caregivers spoke of scapegoating which would go on in group meetings that seemed to lead to additional problems in the work setting.

Joint support groups for caregivers and family members have been suggested by some authors (13, 24) as a possible way of dealing with some of the overlap between work stress and job/home interaction.

SUMMARY

In summary, there is no one way of avoiding or coping with work stress. We are exposed to a variety of potential work stressors throughout our work lives. The manner in which we respond will in large measure be determined by the person-environment fit that exists. We can grow from exposure to stressors, respond neutrally to them, or eventually be destroyed by them. Our response to these stressors will depend in large measure on who we are as people, what else is going on in our lives, the nature of our social support systems, our individual appraisal of the stressors over time, and the personal coping mechanisms we have developed. Equally important is the work environment in which we function and the organizational coping strategies that are available to us. Work environments that acknowledge the needs of employees, appreciate their efforts and provide a safe and caring atmosphere for the critically ill, dying, and bereaved people with whom we work then allow for an interaction in which the demands and supplies of caregiver and work environment can be to our mutual advantage. This will allow us to provide the care that those whom we seek to serve so richly deserve without sacrificing ourselves to so many symptoms of stress that we can no longer cope.

REFERENCES

1. Pearlin, L., & Schooler, C. (1978). The Structure of Coping. *Journal of Health and Social Behavior, 19,* 2–21.

2. Scholom, A., & Perlman, B. (1979). The forgotten staff: Who cares for the caregivers? *Administration in Mental Health, 7*(1) 21–31.

3. Beckhard, R. (1974). Organizational implications of team building. In *Making health care teams work.* H. Wise, Beckard, R., Rubin, I., & Kyte, A. L. (Eds.). Cambridge, MA: Ballinger. pp. 69–94.

4. Hayden, W. R. (1982). Support systems for caregivers: The physician. In R. E. Marshall, C. Kasman & L. S. Cape (Eds.), *Caring for sick newborns.* (pp. 66–81). Philadelphia: Saunders.

5. Mount, B. M., & Voyer, J. (1980). Staff stress in palliative/hospice care. In I. Ajemian & B. M. Mount (Eds.), *The R V H manual on palliative/hospice care.* (pp. 457–488). New York: ARNO.

6. Doyle, D. (1982). Nursing education in terminal care. *Nurse Education Today, 2*(4) 4–6).

7. Slepian, F. W. (1981). The team: How to make it work. In *Social work and cancer care proceedings.* Social Work Oncology Group, Boston: Sidney Farber Cancer Institute.

8. Meyer, M. C. (1978, May). Demotivation—Its cause and cure." *Personnel Journal,* pp. 260–266.

9. Vaillant, G. E. (1977). *Adaptation to life.* Boston: Little, Brown.

10. Roach, Sr. M. S. (1978). The experience of an academic care giver: Implications for education. *Death Education, 2*(1–2) 99–111.

11. Vachon, M. L. S. (1979). Staff stress in the care of the terminally ill. *Quality Review Bulletin, 5*(5) 13–17.

12. Vachon, M. L. S. (1985). Staff stress in hospice care. (2nd ed., pp. 111–127). In G. Davidson (Ed.), *Hospice: Development and administration.* Washington: Hemisphere.

13. LaGrand, L. E. (1980). Reducing burnout in the hospice and death education movement. *Death Education, 4*(1) 61–75.

14. Vachon, M. L. S. (1978). Motivation and stress experienced by staff working with the terminally ill. *Death Education, 2,* 113–122.

15. Goodell, A. S. (1980). Responses of nurses to the stresses of caring for pediatric oncology patients. *Issues in Comprehensive Pediatric Nursing, 4*(1) 2–6.

16. Anderson, C. A., & Basteyns, M. (1981). Stress and the critical care nurse reaffirmed. *Journal of Nursing Administration, 11*(1) 31–34.

17. Eaton, P., & Gottselig, S. (1980). Effects of longer hours, shorter week for intensive care nurses. *Dimensions in Health Service, 57*(8) 25–27.

18. Ward, R. T., & Fuhs, P. A. (1981). Change in nursing shift patterns improves emergency department. *Hospitals, 55*(20) 64–68.

19. Kahn, R. L. (1973). Conflict, ambiguity, and overload: Three elements in job stress. *Occupational Mental Health,* 3:1:2–9.

20. Harrison, R. V. (1978). Person-environment fit and job stress. In C. L. Cooper & R. Payne (Eds.), *Stress at work.* (pp. 175–205). Chichester: Wiley.

21. Hertzberg, F. (1972). *Management of organizational behavior.* Englewood Cliffs, NJ: Prentice-Hall.

22. Malanka, P. (1984). Reaching for excellence: A look at what nursing can do. *Nursing Life, 4*(3) 41–46.

23. Veninga, R. (1979). Administrator burnout—Causes and cures. *Hospital Progress, 60*(2) 45–52.

24. House, J. S., & Wells, J. A. (1978). Occupational stress, social support and health. In *Reducing occupational stress: Proceedings of a conference.* A. McLean, G. Black, & M. Colligan (Eds.). U. S. Department of Health, Education and Welfare, H.E.W. (NIOSH) Publication No. 78-140.

25. Jacobson, S. P. (1978). Stressful situations for neonatal intensive care nurses. *The American Journal of Maternal and Child Nursing, 3,* 144–150.

26. Fawzy, F. I., Wellisch, D. K., Pasnau, R. O., & Leibowitz, B. (1983). Preventing nursing burnout: A challenge for liaison psychiatry. *General Hospital Psychiatry, 5*(2) 141–149.

27. Podboy, J. (1980). A counselling service for hospital staff members. *Hospital and Community Psychiatry, 31*(3) 206–207.

28. Stedeford, A. (1983). Psychotherapy of the dying patient. In C. A. & D. M. Corr (Eds.). *Hospice care: Principles and practice.* (pp. 197–208). New York: Springer.

29. Shaffer, M. (1982). *Life after stress.* New York: Plenum.

30. Davis, A., & Aroskar, M. A. (1983). *Ethical dilemmas and nursing practice.* (2nd Ed.) Norwalk, CT: Appleton-Century-Crofts.

31. Annas, G. J., Glantz, L. H., & B. F. Katz ((1981). *The rights of doctors, nurses and allied health professionals.* New York: Avon.

32. International Work Group in Death, Dying and Bereavement (1979). Proposal for standards of care for the terminally ill. *Canadian Medical Association Journal, 120,* 1280–1282.

33. National Hospice Organization. (1979). *Standards of a hospice program of care.* (6th Revision), Unpublished booklet.

34. Joint Commission on Accreditation of Hospitals. (1983). *Hospice Standards Manual.* Michigan.

35. President's Commission for the Study of Ethical Problems in Medicine and Biomedical and Behavioral Research (1983). *Deciding to forego life-sustaining treatment.* New York: Concern for Dying.

36. Law Reform Commission of Canada. (1982). *Protection of life: Euthanasia, aiding suicide and cessation of treatment.* Working Paper 28. Ottawa: Ministry of Supply and Services.

37. Culliton, B. J. (1976). Helping the dying die: Two Harvard hospitals go public with policies. *Science, 193*(4258) 1105–1106.

38. Levine, C. (1984). Questions and (some very tentative) answers about hospital ethics committees. *The Hastings Center Report,* 14(3) 9–12.

39. Rosenbaum, E. (1982, October). Aids toward improving communication with patients. Paper presented at The American Cancer Society Meeting on Human Values and Cancer: Dilemmas in Cancer Care, Portland, Oregon.

40. Sudnow, D. (1967). *Passing on: The social organization of dying.* Englewood Cliffs, NJ: Prentice-Hall.

41. Sahler, O. J. Z., McAnarney, E. R., & Friedman, S. B. (1981). Factors influencing pediatric interns' relationships with dying children and their parents. *Pediatrics, 67*(2) 207–216.

42. Murray, T. H. (1984). On the care of imperiled newborns. *The Hastings Center Report, 14*(2) 24.

43. Arras, J. D. (1984). Toward an ethic of ambiguity. *The Hastings Center Report, 14*(2) 25–33.

44. Kett, J. F. (1984). The search for a science of infancy. *The Hastings Center Report, 14*(2) 34–39.

45. Fiedler, L. A. (1984). The tyranny of the normal. *The Hastings Center Report, 14*(2) 40–42.

46. Gallo, A. (1984). Spina bifida: The state of the art of medical management. *The Hastings Center Report, 14*(1) 10–13.

47. Steinbock, B. (1984). Baby Jane Doe in the courts. *The Hastings Center Report, 14*(1) 13–19.

48. Murray, T. (1984). At last, final rules on Baby Doe. *The Hastings Center, 14*(1) 17.

49. Winslow, G. R. (1984. From loyalty to advocacy: A new metaphor for nursing. *The Hastings Center Report, 14*(3) 32–40.

50. Clark, R. E., & LaBeff, E. E. (1982). Death-telling: Managing the delivery of bad news. *Journal of Health and Social Behavior, 23*(4) 366–380.

51. Lindstrom, B. (1983). Operating a hospice bereavement program. In C. A. & D. M. Corr (Eds.), *Hospice care, principles and practice.* (pp. 266–278). New York: Springer.

52. Worden, J. W. (1982). *Grief counselling and grief therapy: A handbook for the mental health practitioner.* New York: Springer.

53. Rogers, J., Vachon, M. L. S., Lyall, W. A. L., Sheldon, A., & Freeman, S. J. J. (1980). A self-help program for widows as an independent community service. *Hospital and Community Psychiatry, 31*(12) 844–847.

54. Vachon, M. L. S., Lyall, W. A. L., Rogers, J., Freedman-Letofsky, K., & Freeman, S. J. J. (1980). A controlled study of self-help intervention for widows. *The American Journal of Psychiatry, 137*(11) 1380–1384.

55. Vachon, M. L. S. (1983). Bereavement programmes and interventions in palliative care. In E. A. Mirand, W. B. Hutchinson, and E. Mihich (Eds.), *Thirteenth international cancer congress, Part E Cancer Management.* (pp. 451–461). New York: Liss

56. Vachon, M. L. S., & Rogers, J. (1984). Primary prevention programming and widowhood. In D. P. Lumsden (Ed.), *Community mental health in action.* (pp. 143–52). Ottawa: The Canadian Public Health Association.

57. Weisman, A. D., & Kastenbaum, R. (1968). *The psychological autopsy: A study of the terminal phase of life.* New York: Behavioral Publications. *(Community Mental Health Journal* Monograph 4).

58. Garfield, C. A., Larson, D. G., & Schuldberg, D. (1982). Mental health training and the hospice community: A national survey. *Death Education, 6*(3) 189–204.

59. Tehan, C. (1984). Hospice in America: The reality. Paper presented at the Fifth International Seminar on Terminal Care, Montreal, Quebec.

60. Doyle, D., Parry, K. M., & MacFarlane, R. G. (1982). Education in terminal care. *Journal of the Royal College of General Practitioners, 32,* 335–338.

61. Doyle, D. (1982). Hospice–An education center for professionals. *Death Education, 6*(3) 213–225.

62. Glick, J. H., & Cassileth, B. R. (1981). Teaching models for medical students. In *Proceedings of the American Cancer Society Third National Conference on Human Values and Cancer.* (pp. 89–95). Washington, DC: American Cancer Society.

63. Poole, A. D., & Sanson-Fisher, R. W. (1979). Understanding the patient: A neglected aspect of medical education. *Social Science and Medicine, 13A,* 37–43.

64. Rainey, L. C., Wellisch, D. K., Fawzy, F. I., Wolcott, D., & Pasnau, R. O. (1983). Training health professionals in psychosocial aspects of cancer: A continuing education model. *Journal of Psychosocial Oncology, 1*(2) 41–60.

65. Shanfield, S. B.(1981). The mourning of the health care professional: An important element in education about death and loss. *Death Education, 4,* 385–395.

66. Benoliel, J. Q. (1981). Death counselling and human development: Issues and intricacies. *Death Education, 4,* 337–353.

67. Marshall, R. E., Kasman, C., & Cape, L. S. (1982). *Coping with caring for sick newborns.* Philadelphia: Saunders.

68. Miles, M. S. (1980). The effects of a course on death and grief on nurses' attitudes toward dying patients and death. *Death Education, 4*(1) 245–260.

69. Wolraich, M., Albanese, M., Reiter-Thayer, S., & Barratt, W. (1981). Teaching pediatric residents to provide emotion-ladened information. *Journal of Medical Education, 56*(5) 438–440.

70. Bertman, S. L., Greene, H., & Wyatt, C. A. (1982). Humanistic health care education in a hospice/palliative care setting. *Death Education, 5,* 391–407.

71. McCue, J. D. (1982). The effects of stress on physicians and their medical practice. *The New England Journal of Medicine, 306*(8) 458–463.

72. Payne, R. (1980). Organizational stress and social support. In C. L. Cooper & R. Payne (Eds.), *Current concepts in occupational stress.* (pp. 269–298). New York: Wiley.

73. Lattanzi, M. E. (1983). Learning and caring: Education and training concerns. In C. A. & D. M. Corr (Eds.), *Hospice care, principles and practice* (pp. 223–236). New York: Springer.

74. Edelwich, J. (1980). *Burn-out: Stages of disillusionment in the helping professions.* New York: Human Services Press.

75. Vachon, M. L. S., Lyall, W. A. L., & Freeman, S. J. J. (1978). Measurement and management of stress in health professionals working with advanced cancer patients. *Death Education, 1,* 365–375.

76. Baider, L., & Porath, S. (1981). Uncovering fear: Group experience of nurses on a cancer ward. *International Journal of Nursing Studies, 18,* 47–52.

79. Artiss, K. L., & Levine, A. S. (1973). Doctor-patient relationship in severe illness. *The New England Journal of Medicine, 288*(23) 1210–1214.

80. Billig, N. (1981–1982). Liaison psychiatry: A role in the medical intensive care unit. *Psychiatry in Medicine, 11*(4) 379–386.

81. Strain, J. J. (1981). Communication problems between staff members: Methods to improve interaction. In *Proceedings of the American Cancer Society Third National Conference on Human Values and Cancer.* (pp. 69–73). Washington, DC: American Cancer Society.

82. Hale, R., & Levy, L. (1982). Staff nurses coping an NICU. In R. E. Marshall, C. Kasman, & L. S. Cape (Eds.), *Coping with caring for sick newborns.* (pp. 103–130). Philadelphia: Saunders.

83. Gentry, W. D., & Parkes, K. R. (1982). Psychological stress in intensive care unit and non-intensive care unit nursing: A review of the past decade. *Heart and Lung, 11*(1) 43–47.

84. Weiner, M. F., & Caldwell, T. (1981). Stresses and coping in ICU nursing: II nurse support groups on intensive care units. *General Hospital Psychiatry, 3*(2) 129–134.

Appendix

METHOD

The data for this book were gathered from a variety of sources—individual and group interviews, anecdotes told to me by people who attended workshops or lectures I conducted or who knew of my interest, from groups of caregivers at conferences and workshops, and from my own clinical work and observations. I have taken a developmental approach starting prebirth and going through old age. To gather data I have talked with caregivers working in the fields of obstetrics, pediatrics, critical care, oncology, palliative care, chronic care, gerontology, and bereavement.

In approaching caregivers, I told them that I was writing a book dealing with occupational stress in the care of the critically ill, dying, and bereaved. I showed them earlier versions of the model of occupational stress seen in Figure 1 (Chapter 1), and asked them to describe to me what caused them stress in their work, how this was affected by factors in their personal lives, how their stress was manifest, and what they did to cope with the stress they experienced. The model itself seemed sufficiently easy to understand that most caregivers just examined it briefly, put it aside, and began to talk. The interviews were loosely structured so that I could attempt to gather data in each of the areas.

These interviews lasted from 30 minutes to 2½ hours, the average interview being approximately one hour. Most of the data were gathered from individual interviews but other forms of data collection were used as well. Group interviews were used in a number of instances where caregivers had similar experiences. For example, I met with a group of ten nurses who worked in emergency rooms in ten different hospitals in one large city. In one community hospital I met with 12 nurses who worked in a variety of wards within the hospital—they talked both about the stressors particular to their units and to that hospital as a whole. In another community hospital I went to a number of different units and interviewed three to five caregivers on each of the units. In other instances I interviewed all caregivers on two shifts on one particular ward.

Other data were obtained from anecdotes told publicly at workshops or lectures, or recounted to me personally following lectures. The final way of gathering data was to have small groups of participants at workshops brainstorm about their stressors, manifestations, and coping strategies. I explained to caregivers that I was gathering data for a book, and that any anecdote would be anonymous and disguised if appropriate. Those caregivers interviewed individually were asked if I could thank them in the preface to the book. Most agreed, but due to the large number of interviewees and space limitations, I have been unable to include their names. Interviews were conducted in hospitals, offices, in cars on the way to and from airports, at receptions, and in a variety of informal settings.

All data were recorded by the author on file cards that were then coded as to specialty and subcategories of the model. These were then recoded for the computer analysis that will be discussed below.

SAMPLE

The sample was gathered in a variety of ways: (1) by approaching caregivers I knew locally and asking to interview them and to suggest others who might also be willing to talk about occupational stress; (2) by asking for volunteers at conferences and workshops I attended and conducted throughout Canada, the United States, Australia, and Europe; and (3) by contacting administrators or program organizers in cities to which I would be travelling to ask if they would be willing to set up interviews.

The locations ranged from rural communities in Canada, to medium and large cities across Canada and the United States, to meetings in Australia, England, and Sweden. Wherever I went I gathered data and I went wherever to gather data.

Caregivers represented a number of specialty areas as will be noted below, but it should be mentioned that the sample included caregivers new to the profession, experienced direct care providers, administrators, and some of the leading, well-published experts in the field. However, all of the data will be presented anonymously and will be disguised in many instances. Table 1 shows the types of interviews conducted and the number of caregivers in each category.

The sample size will be considered to be 327, representing the total number of interviews. The reader should be aware, however, that group data have been coded as though just one individual responded. In reality, the 43 group interviews

Table 1 Description of interviews

Individual	144
Anecdotal	140
Small group (2–5 caregivers)	22
(approximate number of subjects = 66)	
Medium group (6–10 caregivers)	12
(approximate number of subjects = 96)	
Large group or workshop data (groups of 10 or more)	9
(approximate number of subjects = 135)	
Total	327
(approximate number of interviewees = 581)	

represent approximately 300 caregivers which means that the data to be discussed were actually obtained from 581 caregivers.

The sample gathered has obviously been a convenience sample. It is reflective of caregivers who were willing to talk about the stress they experienced. This implies a willingness to be open to looking at oneself and one's work situation—obviously not all caregivers are willing to do this. I was, however, very impressed with the number of caregivers who were willing to be interviewed. I had only one direct refusal, that from an oncologist who said, "Surely you don't really want me to talk about my bleeding gastric ulcer, trick knees, and manic behavior."

A description of the caregivers who were interviewed can be found in Table 2. The caregivers represent a variety of disciplines and include social workers, clergy, psychologists, physical and occupational therapists, nutritionists, volunteers, funeral directors, police, etc. Most however, are nurses (49%) or physicians (24%) as these two groups represent the majority of those employed in work with the dying. Female caregivers represent 71% of the sample, reflecting the fact that over 80% of health service and hospital workers are women (1). Of the physicians interviewed, 22% were female and I am embarrassed to admit that only one male nurse was interviewed. Males and females were interviewed in the categories of social work, clergy, psychologists, and funeral directors, but the volunteers, nutritionists, and physio and occupational therapists interviewed were all female.

Most of the caregivers interviewed were experienced practitioners. Only 14% were under age 30, half (50%) were 30-45 years of age, while 35% were over 45. This bias in favor of more experienced people is reflective of my attempt to discover how caregivers manage to cope and survive within the system. Other authors (2-6) have studied the problems more particular to entry into the profession. By studying how people manage to continue to work it is then possible to teach some of their survival skills to other practitioners.

Caregivers worked in a variety of clinical specialties with oncology (25%), palliative care (18%), and critical care (17%) being the largest subsamples. More than half of the caregivers worked in teaching hospitals (53%), but community hospitals (28%) and other practice settings are also represented. Caregivers in all specialty areas represented both teaching and community hospitals. Most of the caregivers were Canadian (74%) but it should be noted that the data gathered in the United States coded as 18% of the sample is in fact reflective of a number of group interviews. Data were also gathered from respondents from Australia, England, Sweden, India, South Africa, and the West Indies.

The majority of caregivers were primarily clinicians (54%), although 21% combined clinical work with teaching, research, or administrative activities.

ANALYSIS OF DATA

As I conducted the interviews, I took notes and then transcribed the data onto index cards using exact quotations from caregivers in so far as this was possible. These data were then coded using the constant comparative method of content analysis described by Glaser and Strauss (7) and since used by numerous other authors including Degner, Beaton, and Glass (8). In this method of analysis each incident or anecdote is coded for its content and compared with other incidents to begin to develop repetitive patterns. In this study, initial areas were devised

Table 2 Description of sample

	Number	Percentage of sample*
Profession		
Nurses and nursing assistants	161	49
Physicians	79	24
Social workers	23	7
Clergy	12	4
Psychologists	9	3
Physiotherapists/occupational therapists	5	2
Volunteers	5	2
Nutritionists	5	2
Other (funeral directors, police, radiotherapy technologists, ambulance attendants, respiratory therapists, biomedical engineers, etc.)	28	9
Sex		
Male	95	29
Female	231	71
Age		
20–29 years	45	14
30–45 years	162	50
45+ years	115	35
Unknown	5	2
Clinical specialty**		
Obstetrics	25	8
Pediatrics, critical care	19	6
Pediatrics, chronic care	26	8
Oncology	81	25
Adult, critical care	55	17
Emergency room	12	4
Palliative care	60	18
Chronic care	13	4
Bereavement	6	2
General	25	8
Multiple specialties	5	2
Practice setting		
University teaching hospital	174	53
Community hospital	91	28
Community practice	30	9
Chronic care facility	25	8
Hospice	6	2
Other	1	.01
Country of practice		
Canada	243	74
U.S.A.	60	18
Other–English speaking	22	7
Other	2	1
Major work focus		
Clinical	178	54
Research	2	1
Teaching	3	1
Multiple roles	68	21
Administration	37	11
Other	39	12

*Numbers will not always equal 100% because of rounding.
**The reader is reminded that many of these were joint interviews representing more people that the number shown. In particular, group interviews were common in obstetrics, pediatrics, critical care, emergency, palliative care, and chronic care.

Table 3 Major anecdotal categories

	Number of anecdotes	Percentage of total
Environmental stressors	3101	36
Personal variables	561	7
Manifestations of stress	1553	17
Coping strategies	3297	37
Total	8912	100

based on earlier models of occupational stress that were developed from the literature and from my own previous experiences and research.

As the data were collected they were compared with the original model, which gradually evolved to its present state. The current model seen in Figure 1 (Chapter 1) is a representation of occupational stress as it evolved from the analysis of the data gathered.

Initially, my intention was to use a grounded theory approach (7) to present the data. Early attempts to use this qualitative approach proved cumbersome because of the extent of the data gathered. I therefore recoded the data using the constant comparative method of content analysis and used a computer analysis to enable me to more appropriately focus my comments.

A total of 8,912 anecdotes were coded; these fell into the following major categories: Environmental Stressors (36%); Personal or Mediating Variables (7%); Manifestations of Stress (17%); and Coping Strategies (32%). An exact break-down of these variables can be found in Table 3.

Because the method of data gathering allowed subjects to expand upon whatever areas they found stressful, some caregivers may have given a few responses in certain areas. For example, Ms. Adams may have named three instances where she strongly identified with particular dying patients and experienced severe grief when they died. This would then be coded as three instances of "Patient/Family-Identification" and three instances of Manifestation-Psychological-Depression." Because of this method of data analysis I will be referring to percentage of anecdotes reflecting certain variables as opposed to percentage of subjects.

Table 4 Rank ordering of environmental stressors

	Number of anecdotes	Percentage of total
1. Team communication problems	193	6
2. Patient/family personality or coping problems	192	6
3. Nature of the unit	161	5
4. Role ambiguity	161	5
5. Role conflict	157	5
6. Identification with patient/family	155	5
7. Patient/family communication problems	153	5
8. Inadequate resources/staffing	151	5
9. Communication problems with others in the institution	143	5
10. Unexpected/tragic illness or accidents	104	3
Total (50% of total environmental stressors mentioned)	1,570	

Table 5   Rank ordering of occupational stressors and professional role

Total group	Nurses (N = 161)	Physicians (N = 79)	Counselors* (N = 44)
1. Team communication problems	1	6	3
2. Patient/family, personality, or coping problems	2	8	2
3. Nature of the unit	3	7	–
4. Role ambiguity	6	10	1
5. Role conflict	5	10	9
6. Identification with patient/family	7	5	7
7. Patient/family communication problems	8	4	6
8. Inadequate resources/staffing	3	9	–
9. Communication problems with others in institution	8	1	10
10. Unexpected/tragic illness or accidents	10	–	8
11. Role overload	–	2	–
12. Difficulty in decision-making (role strain)	–	3	–
13. Communication problems with administration	–	–	3
14. Unrealistic expectations of organization	–	–	5

*Includes social workers, psychologists, and clergy.

The remaining tables include a rank ordering of environmental stressors (Table 4); a rank ordering of occupational stressors by profession (Table 5); the coping mechanisms identified by caregivers (Table 6); and the top ten coping mechanisms (Table 7).

Table 6   Coping mechanisms identified by caregivers

Personal*	Percentage of total
1. Sense of competence, control, or pleasure in one's work	19
2. Control over aspects of practice	19
3. Life-style management	13
4. Personal philosophy of illness, death, or one's professional role	12
5. Leave the work situation	11
6. Avoid or distance from patient/family	7
7. Increased education	11
8. Outside support system	5
9. Sense of humor	3

Environmental**	
1. Team philosophy/support building	31
2. Staffing policies	15
3. Administrative policies	14
4. Colleagues at work	12
5. Formalized ways of handling decisions	11
6. Good orientation and ongoing educational programs	7
7. Job flexibility	6
8. Support groups	4

*Average response per subject/interview = 6.66; number of responses = 2,179.
**Average response per subject/interview = 3.4; number of responses = 1,118.

Table 7 Top ten coping mechanisms identified*

	Number of anecdotes	Percentage of total
1. Sense of competence, control, or pleasure in one's work	423	13
2. Team philosophy, building, support	348	11
3. Control over aspects of practice	314	10
4. Life-style management	295	9
5. Personal philosophy of illness, death, and one's role in life	271	8
6. Avoiding or distancing from patients/families	229	7
7. Leave the work situation	213	6
8. Staffing policies	172	5
9. Increased education	164	5
10. Administrative policies	151	5
Total (78% of total responses)	2,580	

*Total number of coping responses = 3,297; Total number of interviews = 327; Average responses per subject/interview = 10.08.

REFERENCES

1. Marieskind, H. I. (1980). *Women in the health system.* St. Louis: Mosby.

2. Kramer, M. (1974). *Reality shock.* St. Louis: Mosby.

3. Coombs, R. H. (1978). *Mastering medicine.* New York: The Free Press.

4. Bosk, C. L. (1979). *Forgive and remember: Managing medical failure.* Chicago: University of Chicago Press.

5. Schmalenberg, C., & Kramer, M. (1979). *Coping with reality shock.* Wakefield, MA: Nursing Resources.

6. Cherniss, C. (1980). *Staff burnout: Job stress in the human services.* Beverly Hills: Sage.

7. Glaser, B., & Strauss, A. (1967). *The discovery of grounded theory: Strategies for qualitative research.* Chicago: Aldine-Atherton.

8. Degner, L., Beaton, J. I., & Glass, H. P. (1981). *Life-death decision making in health care: A descriptive theory.* Winnipeg: University of Manitoba (Mimeo).

Index

Abortion, 1
   administrative response, 58
   ambivalence, caregiver, 58, 81–82, 83–
      84, 86–87
   caregiver motivation, 23, 86
   coping mechanisms, caregiver, 86–87,
      127–128, 190, 226, 232
   demographic variables, caregiver, 87
   manifestations of stress, 86–87, 128,
      139, 157, 164
   patient/family as stressor, 87, 98–99,
      106–107, 113, 115, 117
   religious beliefs of caregivers, 19
   societal values, 58, 81–82
   technique, 87, 127–128
   work environment stressors, 58
   value conflicts, caregiver, 86–87, 98
Absenteeism, 131, 138–139
Abuse, child/wife, 117–118, 126–127
Acquired Immune Deficiency Syndrome
     (AIDS), 130, 145, 155–156
Adams, D., 132
Aderman, D., 29
Administration:
   abortion, response to, 58
   anger, response to, 163
   authority, 52, 66, 71, 78–79, 85, 88
   avoidance of, caregiver, 34
   caregiver illness, response to, 44
   communication problems with, 62,
     68–71, 82, 88, 206

Administration (*Cont.*):
   expectations of, 69
   fiscal restraints (*see* Fiscal restraints)
   leadership difficulties, 57–58, 66
   terminating staff (*see* Administrative
     decisions/policies)
   (*See also* Work environment stressors)
Administrative decisions/policies, 86–87,
     180, 181, 222–226
   formal and informal, 222–224
   organizational milieu, 225–226
   recognition of staff, 224
   supervisor's role, 225
   support services, provision of, 225
   (*See also* Coping mechanisms; Staffing
     policies; Staffing selection)
Affiliation, need for, 24
Age of caregiver, 11–15, 243
   coping mechanisms, 13–15, 137, 180,
     189, 192, 194, 195, 197, 199–
     202, 204, 206, 207, 212, 219,
     226, 228
   fear of death, 195, 196
   life event stressors, 13, 17–18, 40, 42
   manifestations of stress, 13, 92, 137,
     153, 165
   occupational role stressors, 13, 87
   patient/family stressors, 12
     (*See also* Family of patient; Patients
      as stressor)
   response to death and dying, 12